welfare:
needs
rights
and
risks

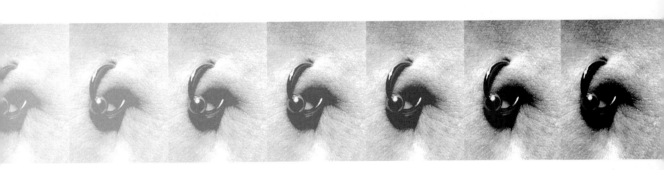

London and New York

in association with

The Open
University

edited
by
**mary
langan**

First published 1998 by Routledge
11 New Fetter Lane, London EC4P 4EE

Simultaneously published in the USA and Canada
by Routledge
29 West 35th Street, New York, NY 10001

© The Open University 1998

The opinions expressed are not necessarily those of the Course Team or of The Open University

Edited, designed and typeset by The Open University
Printed and bound by Scotprint Ltd, Musselburgh, Scotland

British Library Cataloguing in Publication Data
A catalogue record for this book is available from The British Library

Library of Congress Cataloguing in Publication Data
A catalogue record for this book has been requested

ISBN 0-415-18127-5 (hbk)
ISBN 0-415-18128-3 (pbk)

1.1

NORTHBROOK

welfare:
needs
rights
and
risks

social policy: welfare, power and diversity

series editor: john clarke

This book is part of a series produced in association with The Open University. The complete list of books in the series is as follows:

Embodying the Social: Constructions of Difference, edited by Esther Saraga

Forming Nation, Framing Welfare, edited by Gail Lewis

Welfare: Needs, Rights and Risks, edited by Mary Langan

Unsettling Welfare: The Reconstruction of Social Policy, edited by Gordon Hughes and Gail Lewis

Imagining Welfare Futures, edited by Gordon Hughes

The books form part of the Open University course D218 *Social Policy: Welfare, Power and Diversity*. Details of this and other Open University courses can be obtained from the Course Reservations Centre, PO Box 724, The Open University, Milton Keynes MK7 6ZS, United Kingdom: tel. (00 44) (0)1908 653231.

For availability of other course components, contact Open University Worldwide Ltd, The Berrill Building, Walton Hall, Milton Keynes MK7 6AA, United Kingdom: tel. (00 44) (0)1908 858585, fax (00 44) (0)1908 858787, e-mail ouwenq@open.ac.uk.

Alternatively, much useful course information can be obtained from the Open University's website http://www.open.ac.uk.

Contents

Preface

Welfare: Needs, Rights and Risks is the third of five books in a new series of introductory social policy texts published by Routledge in association with The Open University. The series, called *Social Policy: Welfare, Power and Diversity*, examines central issues in the study of how social welfare is organized in the UK today. The series is designed to provide a social scientific understanding of the complex and fascinating issues of social welfare in contemporary society. It specifically examines the key issues arising from questions concerning the changing nature of the welfare state and social policy in the UK, giving particular emphasis to the processes of social differentiation and their implications for social welfare. The series also emphasizes the ways in which social problems and solutions to them have been socially constructed and are subject to historical change. More generally, the books use social scientific theories and research studies together with, and in contrast to, other forms of 'knowing' about social welfare and social issues (such as common sense). This is done in order to raise key questions about how society 'works', how social change occurs, and how social order is maintained.

The five books form the core components of an Open University course which shares the title of this series. The first book, *Embodying the Social*, examines the central issue of how patterns of social difference are socially constructed. It traces the implications of such constructions for social policy – for example, the effects of shifting conceptions of disability – and examines their contested character. In exploring these concerns, the book begins to establish the central focus of the course and series on *diversity*, the formations of *social difference*, and *power*, in particular the power to define our understanding of such differences.

The second book, *Forming Nation, Framing Welfare*, addresses the relationships between nation, state and social welfare by tracing the historical conflicts and constructions that have shaped our modern conceptions of national belonging and welfare rights and duties. The book explores the making of the nation – the inclusions and exclusions of different social groups – and the role of social policy in that process.

This third book, *Welfare: Needs, Rights and Risks*, focuses on a rather different issue, namely the questions of who gets welfare and under what conditions. The book examines how categories of need, desert, risk and rights play a central role in constructing access to welfare, particularly in circumstances where arguments over rationing, priority setting and limited resources are central to the forming of social policies.

The fourth book, *Unsettling Welfare*, deals with the rise and fall of the welfare state in the UK, and traces the ways in which the relationship between social welfare and the state has been reconstructed at the turn of the twentieth century. In particular, it focuses on the consequences of the break-up of the political, economic and social settlements that had sustained the 'old' welfare state in the thirty years after the Second World War.

The fifth and final book, *Imagining Welfare Futures*, looks at the prospects for the further remaking of social welfare around the focal points of citizenship, community and consumerism.

Because these books are integral elements of an Open University course, they are designed in distinctive ways in order to contribute to the process of student learning. Each book is constructed as an interactive teaching text, and this has implications for how the book can be read. The chapters form a planned sequence, so that each chapter builds on its predecessors and each concludes with a set of suggestions for further reading in relation to its core topics. The books are also organized around a series of learning processes:

- *Activities*: highlighted in colour, these are exercises which invite you to take an active part in working on the text and are intended to test your understanding and develop reflective analysis.

- *Comments*: these provide feedback from the chapter's author(s) on the activities and enable you to compare your responses with the thoughts of the author(s).

- *Shorter questions*: again highlighted in colour, these are designed to encourage you to pause and reflect on what you have just read.

- *Key words*: these are concepts or terms that play a central role in each chapter and in the course's approach to studying social policy; they are highlighted in colour in the text and in the margins.

While each book in the series is self-contained, there are also references backwards and forwards to the other books. Readers who wish to use the series as the basis for a systematic introduction to studying social policy should note that the references to chapters in other books of the series appear in bold type. The objective of this approach to presenting the material is to enable readers to grasp and reflect on the central themes, issues and arguments not only of each chapter, but also of each book and the series as a whole.

The production of this book and the others that make up the series draws on the expertise of a whole range of people beyond its editors and authors. Each book reflects the combined efforts of an Open University course team: the 'collective teacher' at the heart of the Open University's educational system. Each chapter in these books has been through a process of drafts and comments to refine both its content and its approach to teaching. This process of development leaves us indebted to our consultant authors, our panel of tutor advisers and our course assessor. It also brings together and benefits from a range of other skills – of our secretarial staff, editors, designers, librarians – to translate the ideas into the finished product. All of these activities are held together by the course manager, who ensures that all these component parts and people fit together successfully. Our thanks to them all.

John Clarke

Introduction

by John Clarke and Mary Langan

This book explores some of the conditions by which people come to receive welfare. As a consequence, it also examines the conditions by which people are excluded from welfare. Although questions of social inclusion and exclusion have become topical areas at the turn of the twentieth century, the ideas of needs, rights and risks have a much longer history in the politics and policies of social welfare. These three terms – needs, rights and risks – identify the sorts of legitimate demands to which social welfare has traditionally been addressed. Social intervention, whether through the agency of the state or through other means, has been designed to meet rights-based entitlements, assuage recognized needs, and manage or control potential risks. Each of these terms, then, identifies a possible route to receiving welfare.

Nevertheless, people do not intrinsically have either rights or needs. Nor are people intrinsically risky or dangerous. Each of these conditions represents the result of social processes: constructions, conflicts, negotiations and evaluations. Let us take the issue of needs. Individuals or groups use the term 'needs' in order to make a claim on social attention or resources. Groups talk about 'having needs' or 'being in need' because the word 'need' itself is part of political discourse: it is a legitimate term through which claims may be articulated. Such claims are subject to processes of acceptance, negotiation or rejection before they can appear as legitimate needs to which collective resources will be devoted. What emerges at the end of these processes is not necessarily the 'need' first presented. The original construction may have been rejected as inappropriate, unreasonable or even utopian (imagine a claim which asserted that everyone needed paid employment or a permanent place of shelter). The original construction of need may have been negotiated – reconstructed – so that its final, publicly legitimate form is different. Such mutations through political or policy processes have been common in social welfare. Take, for example, the introduction of unemployment insurance in Britain in 1911. The provision of such benefits was identified as meeting a need for income security in the context of labour market uncertainties. This was somewhat different from the original claim, made by working-class organizations, to a 'right to work' as being the defence needed against both labour markets and the power of employers (see Langan, 1985).

'Rights' and 'risks' are equally the products of processes of social construction, and equally shaped by contested and conflicting perspectives. However, they may have social and political implications that are different from those associated with 'need'. As several chapters in this book indicate, many groups seeking to improve their well-being have found that a rights-based approach to social welfare is preferable to one based on need. 'Need' tends to be variable and negotiable, often involving the power of experts to assess and evaluate the 'special needs' of groups and individuals. In the process, groups have often come to be defined and treated in terms of their 'special needs'. This sort of experience has been very influential in shaping the demands of disabled people's organizations for an approach based on rights.

'Risk' arises from different processes and concerns. It has tended to be a political, managerial and professional category rather than one through which lay claims to welfare are made. It has been embodied in a range of welfare services where the evaluation of who is 'at risk' of harm, injury or abuse, or who poses 'a risk' to themselves or the public, has become an increasingly significant issue. The evaluation of risk has been closely connected to the trends towards rationing, prioritization and targeting within welfare services, subject to resource limitations. Again, this theme is taken up in several of the following chapters.

The idea of risk also provides an important reminder that 'receiving welfare' is not simply a good – or desired – condition. Most of the discussions about welfare provision in the 1990s have tended to assume that people want welfare and that the issue is how to ration its supply. As a consequence, the terminology used to describe those who receive welfare benefits or services has tended towards positive images. We have learnt to talk of them as consumers or customers exercising choice, or as service users. Nevertheless, there remain people who are less than enthusiastic recipients of welfare services. Some are simply obliged by law to 'receive' services; others find themselves receiving forms of services that feel inappropriate, demeaning or even oppressive.

This book explores a range of issues about the interrelationship of 'needs, rights and risks' and the provision of social welfare. In particular, it emphasizes the socially constructed character of those relationships, giving attention to the shifting social and political conflicts that have shaped the constructions of needs, rights and risks. Some of the chapters begin from a focus on particular services (health care in Chapter 2 and social care in Chapter 3, for example), while others begin from specific groups to examine how their 'welfare needs' have been constructed (children in Chapter 4, adolescents in Chapter 5). Chapters 1 and 6 have a rather wider focus: they address the changing politics of need and the question of who gets to be included in the 'welfare community'. The contested construction of needs, rights and risks links these political conflicts to the policy processes explored in Chapters 2–5. Finally, Chapter 7 reviews and concludes the book by looking at different levels of contestation and construction of need in relation to social welfare.

Reference

Langan, M. (1985) 'Reorganising the labour market: unemployment, the state and the labour movement, 1880–1914', in Langan, M. and Schwarz, B. (eds) *Crises in the British State 1880–1930*, London, Hutchinson.

CHAPTER I

The Contested Concept of Need

by Mary Langan

Contents

1   Introduction

All humans have certain basic requirements to ensure survival – food, clothing, shelter. As we are social beings, our continued existence is only conceivable in relationships with others. Hence the basic requirements of human survival include the means to sustain participation in society, at whatever level of development it has reached.

need

It is immediately apparent therefore that the concept of need includes an element that arises from nature (whatever is required to guarantee physical survival in a hostile environment) and an element that arises from society (which varies according to the development of that society). It is also clear that, in the course of human history, the balance between the contribution of the individual and that of the wider society to the satisfaction of needs has varied considerably.

In neolithic hunter-gatherer communities, for example, where social organization was minimal, most needs were met by individuals themselves working within a simple division of labour. By contrast, under the welfare state in the post-war UK, many needs formerly regarded as the responsibility of the individual – for housing and health care, for example – were for many people met by social institutions. In the same period in the USA, the state played a much smaller role in welfare, and a greater burden of meeting needs fell on individuals and families. The ways in which any particular society defines and meets the needs of its individual members reveal much about the nature of that society and about the relations between the individual and wider social structure that prevail within it.

The concept of need has often been regarded as self-evident: everybody has certain basic needs and the welfare system exists to make sure that they are met. From this perspective the problems of welfare policy are about how best to deliver services to meet these needs. The underlying needs themselves are largely taken for granted.

Yet, as long-running controversies in welfare policy confirm, the concept of need cannot be considered to be so straightforward. A glance at the framework of welfare services that exists today reveals two complicating factors. The first is that there is a spectrum which stretches from services provided in response to individual demand, on the one hand, to welfare interventions that are imposed on individuals, whether they ask for them or not, on the other. The second is that the structure of welfare services in the UK today is different from that which existed 50 or 100 years ago, and is also different from welfare systems in other countries around the world today.

The central theme of this chapter is that the concept of need that underlies any particular system of welfare is a product of a particular society at a particular time: it is, in short, a social construction.

■ In section 2 we begin by exploring the tension between the individual and society in defining and meeting needs and draw attention to the historical fluidity of needs which are commonly taken for granted today.

■ We then examine how needs were defined and met in a familiar and still influential historical context – that of the post-war welfare state in the UK.

■ In section 4 we look at the way in which the concept of need became the focus of conflict as part of the wider polarization of social and political forces in the UK in the 1970s and 1980s.

4

- Section 5 explores the debate about rationing in the 1990s that provided the context for the strategy of dampening welfare demand and curtailing public spending.

- Finally, section 6 examines the discourse of needs-led welfare associated with the reforms of welfare services in the 1990s and the resulting major shift in the responsibility for meeting need from the state back to the individual.

This chapter, and indeed this book, is concerned with demonstrating and analysing the changing social construction of need. In order to do this, we will interrogate key issues and moments in the development of the post-war welfare system. We focus attention on the shifting relationship between the individual and the state reflected in different ideas and discourses of need and the way in which these discourses have a role in the resolution of wider social tensions and conflicts. (These issues are taken up in **Hughes and Lewis, eds, 1998**.)

ACTIVITY I.I

1   Think of some examples of needs which are met by the state in the UK today, but which would not have been 100 years ago.

2   Think of some examples of needs no longer met by the state in the UK today that would have been met twenty years ago.

3   Taking one example in each category, think about what you know about the changing definition of need. What was happening at the time? Was it the focus of popular/public demand? Were professionals or politicians keen to promote certain issues?

COMMENT

You have probably identified a number of issues. Here are some of my examples.

In the 1890s the state provided only the most meagre and stigmatized welfare benefits, minimal health care, only primary school education and no housing. The dramatic expansion of the state's role in all these areas in the first half of the twentieth century was the outcome of a complex combination of popular demand and state initiative.

The retreat of the state in the 1980s and 1990s from the provision of earnings-related unemployment benefits and pensions, cosmetic surgery and free university education was clearly not the result of popular demand, but a redefinition of need imposed on individuals in response to what were considered unsustainable pressures on public spending. We will explore some of these issues in the rest of the chapter.

■ ■ ■

2   Defining needs

The statement 'I need' followed by a particular benefit or service may be taken as a clear indication of an individual's demand for welfare provision. However, it is important to recognize that such a statement is based on a number of presuppositions. An individual can only identify a need for something when the provision exists: thus, though somebody might in the past have complained of pain and stiffness in the leg, it is unlikely that they would have limped into their doctor's surgery and declared 'I need a hip replacement'. Furthermore, an individual's expression of need is likely to be qualified by their judgement of whether or not their demand to have this need met would be considered legitimate by the appropriate welfare professionals or authorities. Thus somebody might say to themselves, 'I need a new car', but they would be unlikely to present this demand to their local benefits agency.

A more difficult situation arises where somebody presents what they consider a legitimate demand for a service to meet a real need – for example, 'test-tube baby' treatment for infertility – but the health authorities declare that they are ineligible for such treatment. The difficulty here is compounded by the recognition that this provision might have been available in the recent past, before the tightening of eligibility criteria in response to pressures to rationalize health service spending, and that it continues to be available in the private sector, but at a cost prohibitive to a substantial section of the population. In all these ways, then, *supply*, or provision, conditions *demand*, or the expression of individual need.

individual need

Turning to the other end of the spectrum, the statement 'what you need is' followed by some intervention by an agency of the welfare state can be understood in different ways, which may be communicated by subtle changes in the tone of the statement. Thus it may be delivered in a benign or neutral tone in relation to a service which is provided by the state and for which the need is generally acknowledged – for example, primary and secondary schooling or child health and ante-natal clinics. At the same time, anybody who refuses to have their needs met in the officially prescribed manner is likely to experience at least disapproval, and perhaps the further attentions of welfare professionals such as health visitors, midwives or educational welfare officers. In cases where parents refuse to send their children to school, they may even face prosecution.

The statement 'what you need is' may be delivered in a more authoritative tone, in circumstances in which the need in question is not recognized or acknowledged by the person concerned. Decisions to place a child or family on the 'at risk' register under the child protection regulations of the Children Act 1989 or to arrange a compulsory admission to hospital under the provisionss of the mental health legislation or to place a young offender in an intermediate

needs of society

treatment programme are typical examples. Here the needs of society as a whole, as interpreted by the state, codified in legislation and enforced by welfare professionals, take priority over the rights of individuals who are judged to be a danger to themselves or others. (These issues in relation to children and young offenders are explored further in Chapters 4 and 5 respectively.)

Where the need is identified as what society needs rather than the individual, there is clearly scope for problems. This is particularly the case in societies where there is a high level of social inequality, differentiation and antagonism.

social inequality

Such societies are likely to experience difficulty in reconciling individual demands and social provisions and the needs identified by the state may conflict with the perception of needs by individuals.

The second factor which complicates the question of need is the fact that, despite the commonsensical notion that basic human needs are universal, societies reveal dramatic differences in the way that need is conceptualized and met. For example, in nineteenth-century Britain, many needs which are now met through the more or less comprehensive services of the welfare state were managed, if at all, through private arrangements between wealthy individuals and their personal professional attendants, and piecemeal public provisions for the poor. For example, Victorian Britain offered relief from poverty only on the most stringent and punitive terms, effectively excluding 'paupers' from citizenship (**Mooney, 1998**).

The post-war welfare state reduced both the stigma and the harshness of the Poor Law system (see Chapter 6), offering benefits to those considered in need as a means of including the whole of society in a wider conception of 'social' citizenship. However, traces of the distinction between the old notions of 'deserving' and 'undeserving' persisted in the social security benefits system, the former receiving universal benefits based on insurance, the latter selective, means-tested payments. A moral component of the concept of need remains influential today: though people may have similar needs, some are considered more deserving of welfare provision than others.

If we look at different Western countries, say the USA, the UK or Germany, we see marked differences in the way in which needs are defined and met under different welfare systems. In the USA there is a greater emphasis on private provision through the market than in Europe, where the state takes responsibility for a wide range of publicly provided welfare services. If we look further afield, at some of the countries of sub-Saharan Africa (where the basic needs of a substantial section of the population are scarcely met at all) or at the more economically successful societies of East Asia (where the patriarchal family continues to play a major role in meeting basic welfare needs), or at countries in the Middle East or Latin America (where both family and religious institutions as well as the state and the private sector play important welfare functions), we see even wider differences, influenced by cultural and religious factors as well as by economic and social considerations.

Needs, in short, are socially constructed, historically specific and contested. To understand how needs are defined and met, we need to examine the wider social and historical context and the influences of ideological and political conflicts as well as questions of resources and policy.

Can you identify some of the social factors that affect the construction of need? How have these changed?

3 The concept of need in the post-war welfare state

The striking feature of the period in the 1940s in which the welfare state was established in its modern form, and indeed of the immediate post-war decades, was the absence of much controversy around the question of need. There were heated debates about matters such as the form of the new health service, the pace of the house-building programme and the level of spending in different areas of welfare, but the nature and extent of the needs which the welfare services were designed to meet were largely taken for granted. However, if we look at the broad framework of services provided through the welfare state, we can clarify some of the underlying assumptions about need.

3.1   Social solidarity

The Beveridge Report of 1942, which is generally accepted as the 'mission statement' of the post-war welfare state, famously identified the 'five giants' of Want, Disease, Ignorance, Squalor and Idleness which were to be vanquished under the new welfare regime. It is worth recalling that Beveridge's main concern was not the oppressive burden of these tyrants on individual members of war-torn British society, but that they were 'five giants on the road to reconstruction' (Timmins, 1995, p.7). In other words, the motivating force of the post-war welfare state was not a concern with meeting the needs of British citizens for a higher quality of life, but rather a preoccupation with overcoming the barriers to the reconstruction of a new social order. For Beveridge and the other architects of the welfare state, the project began from the needs of society rather than from the needs of the individual.

For example, in the sphere of social security, the immediate concern of the Beveridge Report itself, the over-riding preoccupation was not with raising the living standards of those experiencing 'Want' most acutely – the unemployed, the sick and disabled and the elderly – and still less with reducing inequality in society. The central emphasis was on guaranteeing a basic minimum income below which nobody would be allowed to fall, which would thus enhance a sense of collective belonging within society, a spirit of what Marshall later termed

social
citizenship

'social citizenship' (Harris, 1977; **Hughes, 1998a**; Marshall, 1950).

In setting the level of the proposed 'national minimum', Beveridge used survey data on working-class patterns of consumption, nutritionists' assessments of the quantities of carbohydrates, fats and proteins required to sustain life and statistical information on rents and other prices, to calculate the benefits required. These were set at a level adequate to provide 'basic nutritional needs' plus an element taking into account what was considered a 'customary' and 'acceptable' standard of living (Harris, 1977, Ch. 6). Thus, assessments of need made by official experts based on quasi-scientific techniques, rather than the judgements expressed in popular demands, formed the basis of welfare provision.

paternalism

Though the needs of society took priority over the demands of the individual, the ethos of the post-war welfare state was paternalistic rather than authoritarian. The state acted as a benevolent father-figure, administering services according to its own judgement of what the needs were of the national family. Given the considerable level of public acceptance of the political and social order, there was no need for the state to impose its welfare regime on a hostile or resentful population. Thus in the sphere of education, the state developed the framework of secondary schools (establishing the tripartite 'grammar', 'technical' and 'modern' division, later superseded by the 'comprehensive' model) and inaugurated a steady expansion of further and higher education, according to the educational and training needs of the post-war labour market. In housing, central and local government encouraged grand programmes of slum clearance, and the creation of new towns, new suburbs, garden cities and new estates. Though discontent with state provision in both spheres became widespread in the 1970s, in the preceding decades the trends towards expansion and innovation ensured that education and housing reforms were generally popular.

3.2 Power to the professionals

The ascendancy of the determination of need by experts over popular demands for services in the post-war welfare state was linked to another key feature: the consolidation of professional power (Johnson, 1972). The model of occupationally-derived status and autonomy, towards which other groupings aspired, was provided primarily by the medical profession.

professional power

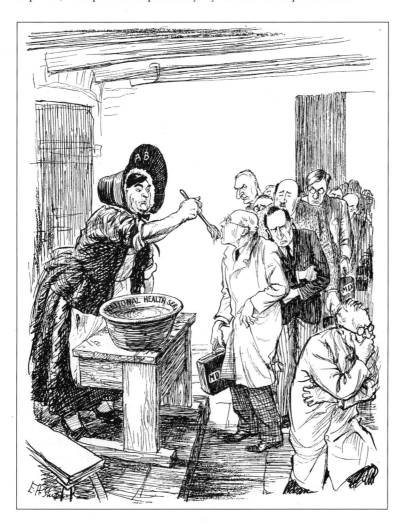

Dotheboys Hall
"It still tastes awful"
Such cartoon images of Labour's health minister, Aneurin Bevan, forcing the NHS on a reluctant medical profession, disguised the concessions he made to medical power (Source: Punch, *21 January 1948)*

As a profession whose power was already fairly well entrenched before the Second World War, doctors were in a relatively strong bargaining position when negotiations opened over the structure of the proposed National Health Service. The outcome of this prolonged and well-documented process was a series of major concessions by the politicians to the doctors. These gave substantial financial rewards to senior consultants, allowing them to continue to run the hospitals through an administrative system with a high degree of autonomy from local or national government and, indeed, from popular accountability, and allowed general practitioners to retain their status as sub-contracting 'small businesses' within the state system.

gatekeepers

Though highly autonomous, doctors enjoyed great powers of discretion in the allocation of resources within the health service, acting as gatekeepers regulating access of individual patients to both primary (GP) and secondary (hospital) care and influencing the distribution of spending at national and regional level. However, at a time when medical prestige was running high – and, from the development of antibiotics in the 1940s to the advent of transplant surgery in the 1960s, it appeared to rise and rise – few challenged the power of doctors to define both the need for health care and the manner in which it was met.

Other professional groupings working within the framework of the welfare state – such as teachers, nurses and physiotherapists – attempted to emulate the medical model. However, lacking the doctors' distinctive combination of a highly-regarded body of expertise and skills with a high degree of cohesion and a tradition of forceful political organization, they were unable to achieve the same status. Yet, as the late emergence of the professional social worker following the reform of the personal social services in the early 1970s indicates, the framework of state welfare could be helpful to a fragile professional grouping **(Pinkney, 1998)**. Once given powers to assess need – whether for community care provision, compulsory psychiatric admission, or for child protection intervention – social workers acquired new status as professionals.

3.3   The ambivalent legacy of universalism

universalism

The boldest claim of the post-war welfare state was that its services were universal. They were available to everybody in society according to need. Most significantly they were provided without the historic restriction of the market system on access to goods and services – the capacity to pay. Thus everybody was entitled to basic social security benefits, to education, health care, housing and, at a later stage, to the services provided by the local social services department. Furthermore these provisions were either – like health and education – 'free at the point of use', or, like council housing or the early charges for prescriptions and dentures, so highly subsidized that cost should not deter anybody from taking up the service. Though some selective benefits continued – 'national assistance' provided for those not eligible for benefits based on prior national insurance contributions was still based on means testing – Beveridge and the other ministers in the post-war Labour government anticipated that such benefits would become of marginal importance in a full-employment labour market (Harris, 1977, pp.392–3).

For Beveridge, universality was the key to transcending the stigma of selectivity associated with the earlier system of means-tested benefits, and crucial to the higher sense of social inclusion considered vital to the progress of post-war reconstruction. However, the continuation of the distinction between those eligible for 'universal' national insurance benefits ('deserving') and those receiving 'selective' national assistance benefits ('undeserving') reflected the persistence of the moral outlook of the Poor Law into the post-war period. The fact that the numbers claiming national assistance benefits steadily increased, rather than dwindling as anticipated, only underlined this flaw at the heart of universalism.

As a system of services provided by the state to everybody in society, the post-war welfare system had a bureaucratic style. Services were provided in a standardized way, based on decisions by government officials, professionals and other experts. Distribution was to every citizen. For example, every child was given one-third of a pint of milk every day at school. No-one questioned that they all needed it. The welfare state also had a patriarchal character. Thus the framework of benefits assumed the model of a working man, earning a family wage to enable him to support his non-working wife as well as any other dependants. According to Harris (1977, p.392), 'to Beveridge the archetypal insurance contributor was … the adult male worker whose income was derived solely from earnings and who needed protection when such earnings were interrupted by unemployment, accident or disease.' The welfare state was thus founded on the projection of the particular interests of the male worker as the universal interests of society. In the 1950s and 1960s the welfare state thus ratified the established sexual division of labour in society: the effective exclusion of women from the world of work and their confinement to the domestic sphere. However, as women's participation in the labour market steadily increased in subsequent decades – together with male unemployment – the assumptions of the post-war welfare state came into growing conflict with the realities of late twentieth-century society (this is taken up in Chapter 6).

exclusion

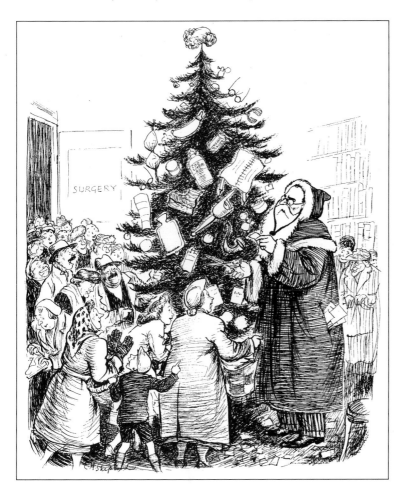

Dear Doctor Christmas
The Universal Provider
(Source: Punch, *22 December 1948)*

ACTIVITY 1.2

The following table illustrates some contrasts between British society in the early years of the welfare state and forty years later.

1945–55	1985–95
Full male employment	Prolonged high male unemployment
Low female participation in labour market	High female participation in labour market
Working father/homemaking mother	Working father/working mother
Stable families	High divorce rate, family breakdown
Rising living standards	Growing inequality in living standards
Consensus	Fragmentation, pluralism, multiculturalism

In what ways did the welfare system – including social security, education, health and housing – designed to meet the needs of society in 1945, appear inappropriate for society in 1995?

COMMENT

The post-war welfare state assumed a society composed of nuclear families, headed by a wage-earning, breadwinning father (with a job for life in manufacturing industry), a homemaking mother ('housewife') and a small number of well-behaved children. The experiences of depression in the 1930s and the Second World War, followed by the post-war boom and Cold War, all contributed to an unprecedented level of social harmony and political quiescence. Popular respect for British institutions – the monarchy, parliament, the Church, the NHS, the BBC – reflected some sort of common allegiance to the values of democracy, equality and social justice.

The demise of the framework of post-war British society also brought its welfare arrangements into question. The decline of manufacturing and the rise of services, the return of long-term (particularly male) unemployment and the expansion of part-time (and full-time) female employment – together with the dramatic rise in divorce and illegitimacy – rendered obsolete the assumption of male breadwinner/ female homemaker on which the social security system was built. The struggles and demands of migrants from Ireland, the Caribbean and the Asian subcontinent for the right to recognition of their cultural forms established the UK as a multi-cultural and multi-faith society. Economic decline and political disillusionment led to a loss of respect for traditional institutions, including those in the sphere of welfare.

■ ■ ■

The assumptions of the welfare state concerning needs and the ways in which it organized to meet the needs defined by these assumptions remained fairly uncontroversial for the first two post-war decades. The demonstrable achievements of the welfare system in at least substantially reducing the stature of all five of Beveridge's giants undoubtedly contributed to the success of the wider project of reconstruction. Steady economic expansion ensured, if not quite 'full employment', persistently low levels of male unemployment and a decline in class conflict contributed to an unprecedented period of social and political consensus. However, the breakdown of these conditions, which began with the recession of the early 1970s, also pushed the question of need into the realm of controversy (see **Hughes, 1998a**; **Lewis, 1998a**).

social and political consensus

4 The politicization of need

The 1973 recession marked the beginning of the end of the post-war welfare state. Though more than two decades later the basic framework of welfare services was still recognizable, it was also apparent that major changes had taken place. The years of steady expansion and low unemployment were followed by a series of recessionary downturns each succeeded by a more sluggish recovery and persistent mass unemployment (see **Gazeley and Thane, 1998**). Economic decline and slump contributed to the collapse of the social consensus on which the welfare state was founded.

From the perspective of both the individual and society, need came to the fore. In terms of individual need, the emergence of permanent mass unemployment generated a demand for unemployment and other welfare benefits on a steadily expanding scale. The sense of growing insecurity and social malaise also provoked both an increased demand for welfare services (notably for health services, but also in education and other areas) and a growing sense of dissatisfaction with the poor quality and bureaucratic character of the services provided.

From the perspective of the state, welfare spending began to be experienced as an increasingly unsupportable burden from the mid 1970s onwards (Bacon and Eltis, 1976). The result was a growing pressure to curb public expenditure on welfare, first manifested in 'spending cuts' provoking extensive national and local protests, and subsequently taking the form of measures to shift the responsibility for welfare away from the state onto other agencies, or simply into the marketplace, and onto individuals and their families. The drive to curtail welfare spending at a time of growing need for welfare services inevitably heightened political conflicts within the welfare sphere.

The politicization of the concept of need emerged out of a series of critiques of the inadequacies of the post-war welfare state in the new circumstances of the 1970s and 1980s. These controversies have in turn shaped the reconstruction of the framework of welfare in the 1990s. Let us look briefly at some of the criticisms coming from widely different political and academic directions.

4.1 The persistence of inequality

From the late 1950s onwards the welfare state came under criticism from academic commentators influenced by a broadly social democratic outlooks whose studies revealed that social inequalities – considered a useful indicator of need – had not significantly altered in the two decades following the Second World War (Titmuss, 1958). Though, as we have seen, reducing inequality was not regarded by Beveridge as a legitimate objective of social policy, many more radical advocates of the welfare state certainly believed that it could achieve a significant redistribution of resources in society in favour of the poor. Now, however, several studies showed the persistence of significant levels of deprivation despite twenty years of policy aimed at relieving 'Want' – a trend dubbed the 'rediscovery of poverty' (Abel-Smith and Townsend, 1965).

redistribution

rediscovery of poverty

Furthermore, others claimed that, far from benefiting the underprivileged, the post-war proliferation of welfare benefits and services (from employers and other private sources as well as in the public sector) had provided further

13

advantages to the better-off. This effect was particularly striking in health and education, where, as Titmuss (1965, p.360) put it, 'the major beneficiaries of the high cost sectors of social welfare are the middle and upper classes'. The radical GP Julian Tudor Hart (1975) expressed the distribution of resources in health in

inverse care law

the inverse care law: the greater the level of need, the lower the level of resources allocated, and vice versa. In 1982 another social policy academic Julian Le Grand (1982, p.151) concluded from a detailed survey of the impact of different welfare services over the post-war period, that 'the strategy of equality through public provision has failed'. Whereas the 1960s generation concluded from their surveys that there should be some reorientation of social policy in order to effect a more equitable distribution of welfare resources, by the early 1980s Le Grand (1982, p.137) was pessimistic about the prospects of achieving any reduction in social inequalities in this way. Noting that 'public expenditure on the social services has not achieved equality in any of its interpretations', he could not see much chance of overcoming the problem 'through only piecemeal reform'. He concluded that 'the forces which create inequalities in the first place and which perpetuate them, seem to be too strong to be resisted through indirect methods such as public expenditure on the social services.' Ironically, Le Grand turned to the market to effect the redistribution that the state had failed to achieve. A decade later he pronounced 'a broadly positive view of the market reforms introduced into the NHS by the Conservative Government' (Robinson and Le Grand, eds, 1994, p.250).

4.2   The radical critique

In the 1970s the welfare state came under a wide-ranging radical critique focusing on its inadequacies in meeting the growing needs of an increasingly diverse and conflictual society. Such criticisms came from the traditional left, from radical

new social movements

the radical critique

academics and from feminists and representatives of other 'new social movements' (Gough, 1979; Ginsburg, 1979, Doyal, 1979; Illich, 1977). The radical critique contained a number of distinct themes.

One element was a critical evaluation of the role of professional power in the world of welfare, concentrating in particular, but by no means exclusively, on the medical profession (Illich, 1975, 1977). The attack on medical authority was bolstered by a growing scepticism about the efficacy of what became known as 'Western biomedicine' in dealing with the 'diseases of civilization' – heart disease, cancer, chronic degenerative conditions. Challenging the medical profession's own account of its heroic conquest of infectious disease, radical epidemiologists insisted that the demise of the old epidemics was more the result of improvements in diet and living conditions than of the impact of immunization and antibiotics.

As the deferential spirit of post-war welfare gave way to a more questioning approach to professional authority, medical claims to scientific objectivity were subjected to rigorous scrutiny: 'Contrary to the popular image of a scientifically-based medical profession, the reality is that few of the techniques used by doctors have been evaluated in a scientific manner' (Radical Statistics Health Group, 1977, p.25). If doctors' judgements were not based in science, then how could they claim objectivity in defining need and allocating resources?

The radical challenge to the medical profession as a self-serving elite opened the way for the definition of need in different ways by different people. It also encouraged a wider questioning of professional power in the public services, extending rapidly to teachers and social workers, whose professional prestige was rather less secure.

Another element in the radical critique of welfare was the assertion of the needs of particular groups through the mobilization of pressure groups and self-help organizations. These organizations were concerned with both formulating specific demands to be met by some arm of the welfare state and with expressing dissatisfaction with the existing services. Thus claimants unions advanced the demands of the unemployed and other welfare dependants for higher and more accessible benefits and condemned the bureaucratic and stigmatizing character of social security procedures; tenant groups, community activists and squatters organizations articulated their particular requirements to the housing and other local government authorities.

self-help

While numerous local campaigns against hospital closures challenged the consequences of 'the cuts', attempts to co-ordinate their efforts at a national level and to advance a wider agenda of health service reform made little headway. However, the take-over of Tadworth Hospital from the NHS in 1983 by a private trust headed by the Spastics Society (now Scope) after a prolonged campaign against closure, signalled a new role for voluntary organizations and pressure groups in the new world of welfare. Self-help groups such as Alcoholics Anonymous and Weight Watchers offered a model that was rapidly taken up in relation to hundreds of different medical and social conditions.

The most coherent and comprehensive challenge to the definition of need and the provision of services under the welfare-state umbrella came from the women's movement, which gathered momentum from the early 1970s. Feminists challenged the assumption of the family wage by the social security system and the intrusive and discriminatory operation of regulations, such as the practice of reducing benefits to women 'cohabiting' with men. They challenged the patriarchal way in which the medical profession asserted control over issues of women's health, particularly in the spheres of contraception, abortion and childbirth (Doyal, 1979). They exposed discriminatory practices and sexist assumptions in other areas of welfare, notably education and social services.

women's movement

While the women's movement demanded extensive reforms to make welfare services more responsive to women's needs, other social movements also campaigned for change. Organizations of black and others defined as minority ethnic communities began to press their particular needs and to expose the patterns of discrimination that developed under the surface of the 'colour-blind' welfare state. Organizations of people with disabilities of different kinds have pursued a similar approach. These forces challenged the welfare state as reproducing the forms of inequality and oppression of the wider society (see **Hughes, 1998b**; **Lewis, 1998b**). They exposed the universalist propositions of welfare provision as incapable of meeting the needs of *different* social groups. From a position that recognized inequalities among groups, activists from these movements identified the welfare provision as having a key role in replicating disadvantage and discrimination.

Perhaps the most radical element of the radical critique was its perception of the increasingly coercive character of state intervention in society in the form of welfare services. This was most forcefully articulated by the radical social work movement, which identified the expansion of personal social services in the 1970s as part of a wider drive to strengthen the controlling influence of the state over an increasingly fragmentary society (Bailey and Brake, eds, 1975). The 'anti-psychiatry' movement, which enjoyed only marginal influence in the medical world, had wider appeal among social workers, particularly among those involved in the growing use of powers of compulsory detention in hospital of those considered to be suffering from mental illness. An anti-pedagogical tendency in education challenged what it identified as a parallel trend of using the schools to turn out passive and acquiescent workers (Bowles and Gintis, 1976). For adherents to these views, nothing less than a fundamental transformation of society would suffice; mere reforms could only reinforce the oppressive structures of the welfare state.

4.3   Welfare dependency: the New Right critique

Though some conservative proponents of the virtues of the free market and the evils of state intervention, such as Hayek, had never been reconciled to the welfare state, they remained a marginal force for much of the post-war period (Hayek, 1944, 1949; Friedman, 1962). However, in the 1970s, as the various dimensions of the 'crisis of the welfare state' became generally acknowledged, they gained growing influence, particularly within the Conservative Party in its years in opposition after 1974 (Brittan, 1973; Bacon and Eltis, 1976). When the Conservatives returned to power in 1979, their ideology and policies were shaped by what had become known as the 'New Right'. Organized in a number of think-tanks and pressure groups, the New Right advanced a wide-ranging critique of the welfare state and a radical agenda for reducing its role in UK society (Levitas, ed., 1986).

From a traditional free market perspective, the New Right objected to the burgeoning of state expenditure in the post-war period, which it identified as a key factor in the stagnation of the wider economy. It particularly condemned state provision of welfare services as inherently wasteful and bureaucratic. In principle the New Right favoured any measure to shift the delivery of services from the public sector to the private sector, where the price mechanism would both increase freedom and choice for the consumer and ration scarce resources, that is **market-led welfare provision**. It opposed the provision of universal benefits and services as paternalistic and inefficient, though it accepted the need for selective welfare provision, so long as it was 'targeted' at those in 'real need'.

The New Right disputed the assumptions about need which underlay established welfare services. It argued that, apart from some exceptional circumstances, the giants identified by Beveridge had been effectively vanquished in the years of post-war prosperity. From this perspective the radical 'rediscovery of poverty' was depicted as the 'reinvention of poverty' based on a tendentious definition of 'relative poverty' (see Extract 1.1 below). Neo-liberal economists condemned radical social policy academics for inflating need – a practice contemptuously termed 'needology' (Dennis, 1997). They also condemned mainstream politicians for acceding to popular pressures to raise benefits to levels they considered a disincentive to participation in the labour market (Foster, 1983, pp.34–5). As long-term mass unemployment returned and became linked to wider social problems of family breakdown, crime and delinquency in the 1980s, the New Right critique of welfare was expanded to embrace the concept of the underclass. (This is explored more fully in Chapter

market-led
welfare
provision

needology

underclass

6.) The underclass was a section of society that was largely defined in terms of its dependence on welfare benefits and held to demonstrate the demoralizing consequences of the culture of dependency supposedly fostered by the welfare state (Murray, 1990).

culture of dependency

The New Right critique led to a series of proposals for reform, often advocated tentatively at first in recognition of the challenge they represented to post-war welfare traditions. In the course of the 1980s proposals to roll back the state in the provision of welfare, to shift some services into the private sector and to extend the role of the market in the public sector became increasingly bold (No Turning Back Group, 1988, 1990). In practice the structure of welfare proved remarkably durable through the first two Conservative terms of government, reflecting the strength of the post-war consensus and the vested interests with a stake in the existing framework. Even by the end of the decade many commentators were struck more by the degree of continuity than by the extent of change (Hills, ed., 1990).

In the Conservatives' third term, after their 1987 election victory, the pace of change in welfare accelerated. These dramatic developments were the result of a number of factors. The first was the collapse of the late 1980s' boom which disappointed the high hopes it had raised of long-term recovery as recession turned to slump in the early 1990s. The second was the series of events beginning with the demolition of the Berlin Wall in December 1989 which rapidly culminated in the disintegration of the Eastern bloc and the Soviet Union itself and the end of forty years of East–West 'Cold War'. The consequences of these historic events were often paradoxical. The collapse of socialism and the left internationally combined with the long-term decline of the domestic labour movement to remove not only the main force of opposition to conservatism in the UK but also the major force behind the establishment and expansion of the post-war welfare state (Mishra, 1995).

If the initial challenge to the concept of need in the post-war welfare state came from left-wing demands for measures to reduce persistent inequalities in society, the emerging reconceptualization of need in the late 1970s owed more to right-wing arguments about the burden on a financially constrained state of meeting existing welfare demands. Ironically, as the wider balance of forces swung to the right, the concept of need was reconstructed in such a way as to legitimize the growth of inequality in society.

reconceptual-ization of need

One of the great controversies surrounding the social construction of need centred around the definition of poverty. As living standards in general rose through the 1950s and 1960s, the general conviction grew that 'absolute' poverty, meaning a standard of living below that required to guarantee survival, had been abolished. In response, a number of radical social policy commentators and activists (dubbed the 'poverty lobby') insisted on a 'relative' definition of poverty. In their view, poverty should be measured not merely in terms of the survival of the individual, but in relation to the living standards of the rest of society. According to these criteria, poverty not only persisted under the welfare state, but was actually increasing. They argued that those incapable of earning an income (by reason of unemployment, sickness, disability, age) should receive an income determined, not by the minimum necessary to ensure subsistence, but by what was required to guarantee a decent standard of living according to the prevailing norms of society.

'absolute' poverty

'relative' poverty

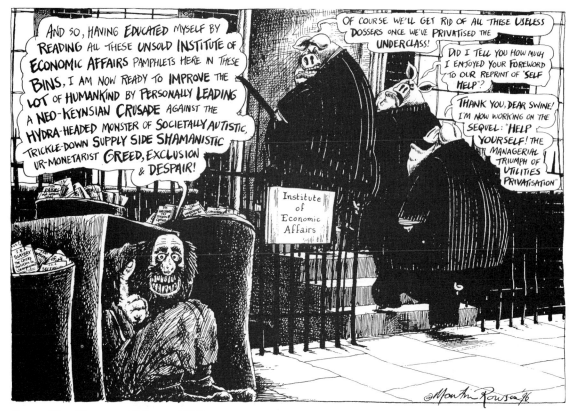

(Source: The Observer, 25 August 1996)

The concept of 'relative poverty' was fiercely condemned by conservative commentators as a device for inflating need and undermining individual responsibility. Norman Dennis was a sociologist who characterized himself as an 'ethical socialist'. However, by the 1980s he had, by his own account, become so alarmed at the consequences of the unrestrained individualism of left and right alike for families and communities, that he became an outspoken advocate of a return to traditional values. In Extract 1.1 he offers a polemical account of the influence of 'relative poverty' and an illustration of the intensity of the conservative backlash against it.

ACTIVITY 1.3

As you read Extract 1.1, try to identify Dennis's main arguments against definitions of 'relative poverty'. How does he think poverty should be defined?

Extract 1.1 Dennis: 'The poverty debate'

Relative poverty

A new, much more durable idea of poverty began to form [in the 1960s]. The benefit rate was quite quickly redefined, not as the sum of money that kept a person *out* of poverty, but the proof that he was *in* poverty. Another refinement was stumbled upon. In order not to disadvantage the prudent, a person was entitled to National Assistance even if he had a few savings or a small income from some other source. As the *average* 'disregard', as it was called, added on average 25 per cent to the National Insurance scale rate, and was therefore the average income of the poorest, … 'it would not be unreasonable' to take resources of not more than 25 per cent above National Assistance scale rates (after rent was paid) as being resources at the poverty line.

On that basis it was estimated that two-and-a-half million British old people were living at or around the poverty line [Cole and Utting, 1962; Wedderburn, 1962, pp.264–5]. Once that idea entered the fund of ideas of the poverty lobby, it proved a powerful yet simple way to increase the number in poverty. For why stop at 25 per cent above social security benefits? Why not 40 per cent above? Why not 50 per cent? From 1953 a random sample of over 3,000 households supplied records of income and expenditure for two consecutive weeks each year.[1] Its unpublished tabulations were soon recognized as a magnificent source for the study of the effect of deriving different proportions of the population in poverty by applying different definitions of poverty to them. 'The higher the poverty line the more we draw in a sizeable pocket of wage earners' [Wedderburn, 1962, p.276]. This allowed much more scope for righteous indignation by inflating the figures more or less at will, rather than following the tedious procedures of the poverty surveys up to the 1950s, of trying to arrive at some empirical measure of what was actually happening over time.

What also began to emerge in the early 1960s was a conceptualization of poverty that was to prove even more fruitful (at least so long as the general standard of living rose). 'If we remember that real disposable income has increased by twice as much as the real increase in National Assistance since 1948, it cannot be thought unreasonable to say that National Assistance rates are a reflection of pre-war thinking about subsistence' [Wedderburn, 1962, p.257]. That was not yet 'relative poverty' in the modern sense. But it was coming close.

It is an anomaly that its really effective take-over dates from Runciman's *Relative Deprivation* of 1966, for (as we have seen) Runciman himself still used the concept principally in the sense, damaging and retrograde to the poverty lobby, of working people comparing themselves with their parents and grandparents, or their present conditions with their own previous, lower standard of living. Runciman had been impressed by the *failure* of the poor in Britain to be resentful of the rich. The results of his own survey research had led him to the conclusion, indeed, that at the standard of living they enjoyed in the post-war 'affluent society' and under the other cultural and structural conditions of British life, 'there was, in fact, no occasion for manual workers to make the sort of cross-class comparisons likely to suggest themselves to academic investigators examining the statistical evidence' [Runciman, 1966, p.90]. To make the poorer members of society aware of their relative deprivation in the here-and-now in the cross-class sense, and to abandon their feelings of relative well-being in the historical and cross-cultural sense, became, therefore, the objective of the emerging poverty lobbies and their academic supporters. Relative poverty in its modern form means *only* the income and possessions of the poorest in the here-and-now relative to the rich in the here-and-now. One of the main uses of the modern concept is to *obliterate* any comparisons with the past not, as in Runciman's usage, to point them out.

In 1992 the Rowntree Foundation published the results of the work of the Family Budget Unit of York University [Bradshaw, 1992]. The standards set up were purely relative and quite immune to any improvements in the absolute standard of living. One, what half the population had, was a 'modest but far from luxurious' lifestyle. The other, lower standard, was what three-quarters of the population possessed. Launching the report, Professor Jonathan Bradshaw, who led the research, said the low cost budget would buy an 'extremely mean' standard of living [Laurance, 1992]. Clothing was budgeted at £29.27 a week, based on the cheapest items available at C&A. Food was budgeted at £58.67, based on 300 basic items priced at Sainsbury's. There could be no car, the budget covered public transport only. Nothing was allowed for either drinking or smoking. Nothing was allowed for an annual holiday; only for a day trip to Blackpool.

In order to reach this 'low' and 'extremely mean' standard of living, a household of two adults and two children (whose weekly state cash benefits amounted at that time to £105 a week) would need another £36 a week.

By the time the 1995 Report was published, insufficiency of income could be defined in these relative terms so effectively and naturally that *The Times* – not to speak of the *Guardian* or *The Independent* – could headline the 'fact' that the average family needed £21,000 a year for 'basics'. Keeping a family provided with what most people regarded as the 'necessities of life', Jeremy Laurance's report said, cost £300 a week. Benefits provided by the state amounted to only £100 a week [Laurance, 1992]. As £21,000 a year was £5,000 above average *earnings* in 1992, the scope for further employment in the poverty lobby was assured.

...

Relative poverty breaks away altogether from the idea, not just of a satisfactory minimum standard of living that the community through the state, or private benevolence, or a combination of both must afford each of its members, but from any idea of a 'satisfactory' minimum standard of living at all.

The concept of relative poverty is a weapon of agitation that the Left wields. But as it has been used so far, it is more effective in securing benefits for the well-to-do in society than for the less well-to-do. For the idea of the ever-rising cash standard of living, the limitless pursuit of commodities, provides a great and continuous stimulus to the economy, providing the well-to-do with the goods, and leaving the poor with the discontent. As an ideological concept, therefore, relative deprivation is far better adapted to modern industry and commerce than any of the old Christian or ethical-socialist notions of what is 'sufficient', either for one specific purpose or another, or for 'a good life'.

Note

1   For details of the earliest surveys, see *Family Expenditure Survey 1957–1959*, HMSO, 1960, and 'The Family Expenditure Survey: some results of the 1960 Survey', *Ministry of Labour Gazette*, December 1961.

References

Bradshaw, J. (1992) *Household Budgets and Living Standards*, York, Joseph Rowntree Foundation.

Cole, D. and Utting, J.E.G. (1962) *The Economic Circumstances of Old People*, Welwyn, Codicote.

Laurance, J. (1992) 'Average family now needs £21,000 a year for basics', *The Times*, 11 November.

Runciman, W.G. (1966) *Relative Deprivation and Social Justice: A Study of Attitudes to Social Equality in the Twentieth Century*, London, Routledge and Kegan Paul.

Wedderburn, D.C. (1962) 'Poverty in Britain today: the evidence', *The Sociological Review*, vol.10, no.3.

(Dennis, 1997, pp.143–6)

In place of the relativizing definitions of the poverty lobby, Dennis upholds his own standard of a 'satisfactory minimum' that each member of the community should be afforded. But how is this minimum to be set? When he tackled precisely this problem, Beveridge concluded that it was necessary to add to the amount calculated to ensure basic nutritional needs, an additional amount required to ensure an acceptable 'customary' standard of living. The 'poverty lobby' would claim that they were merely extending Beveridge's approach into the post-war period. As overall 'customary' living standards rise, then the acceptable minimum must also rise: if the vast majority of families have a television, a fridge and a washing-machine, then these consumer goods, the preserve of the wealthy in the 1940s, become requirements for everybody.

Though Dennis does not specify either the level of his 'satisfactory minimum' or how it should be decided, the implication is that it should approximate to the amount required to guarantee physical subsistence. While there is clearly a danger of shifting the definition of poverty to such a degree that it includes a substantial proportion of a population that is living at a historically unprecedented level of prosperity, there is equally a danger of insisting on a 'satisfactory minimum' which might keep body and soul together, but would not enable its recipients to participate in any real sense in the life of society.

■ ■ ■

One of the most striking consequences of the resolution of more than a century of political conflict in terms of 'left' against 'right' was the way in which elements of the radical critique of welfare were assimilated to the welfare reforms in the early 1990s. If we turn to examine the emergence of an explicitly rationed welfare system, we can see the results of this convergence.

What are some of the main political factors influencing the social construction of need in the post-war period?

5   Rationing welfare in the 1990s

The dramatic changes that affected virtually every area of welfare in the early 1990s had a number of characteristic features. First, the reforms encouraged a much greater role for market forces, both within the public sector (as in the internal market introduced in health care, with trust hospitals competing to sell their services to fundholding GPs, and through the local management of schools) and through privatization (that was most advanced in housing). The community care reforms pushed local councils away from directly providing different forms of care towards acting as purchasers from a mix of public, voluntary and private agencies, as well as encouraging families to shoulder a greater burden of care.

internal
market

purchaser–
provider split

It was striking that many of the radical critics of the inadequacies of the traditional welfare state in reducing social inequalities now adopted a more benign assessment of the potential impact of the market reforms (Le Grand and Winter, 1987; Glennerster, 1992; Hills, ed., 1990). The emergence of a 'market left' in academic social policy paralleled and influenced the rise of 'New Labour' under the leadership of Tony Blair after 1994. According to one social policy expert, Labour's 'reorientation' amounted to 'an inversion of the party's previous emphasis on social rights so that social responsibility is now seen as the lodestone of social policy'; he concluded that 'the major opposition party now seems to have opted for shadowing many erstwhile Conservative social policy approaches' (Sullivan, 1996, p.259).

consumerism

Second, the government took up the cause of the consumer, promoting a series of charters, performance league tables and complaints procedures in every area of welfare (**Clarke, 1998**). These measures capitalized upon the growing distrust of professional power in the definition and dispensation of welfare, whether this was in the hands of doctors, social workers or teachers. The rhetoric of choice, quality and standards echoed around the schools and hospitals. However, whether, given the continuing strictures on public spending, there was any real improvement in the position of the consumer was debatable.

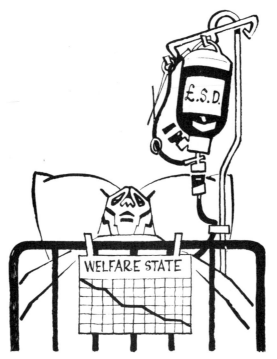

(*Source:* Daily Mail, 13 February 1967)

A third trend was a shift in the emphasis of welfare from care and support towards discipline and surveillance. This is a recurrent theme in surveys of the operation of the Children Act 1989 in the context of the recurrent child-abuse media panics. Nigel Parton (1991) has drawn attention to the shift from the traditional 'medico-social' model of child abuse to the 'socio-legal' approach of current child protection practice, in which the courts and the police have a much higher profile. The launch of the Child Support Agency in 1993, with the purpose of pursuing errant fathers for maintenance for their children – a response to growing concern about the growing number of single parents (mainly mothers) receiving long-term welfare benefits – was another coercive measure.

authoritarian-ism

The authoritarian trend was also striking at the level of terminology and metaphor. For example, the renaming of benefit for the young unemployed as

22

'job-seeker's allowance' was explicitly linked to the exclusion from benefit of those considered to be 'not genuinely seeking work'. Together with the removal of rights to benefit from young people between the ages of 16 and 18, this was part of a wider shift from welfare to 'workfare', where benefits are provided only on condition that the unemployed agree to undergo some form of training (often of dubious value) or 'work experience' programme. The price of this redefinition of need was the effective exclusion from social citizenship of those who refuse to conform. Those who would not participate in the work of society on terms decided by a welfare agency were deemed to have no legitimate claim on society's support.

workfare

The rhetoric of New Labour heralded the emergence of a new – and apparently more austere – welfare consensus. In its major review of the welfare state on behalf of New Labour, the Commission for Social Justice proclaimed that its objective was to 'transform the welfare state from safety net in times of trouble to springboard for economic opportunity' (Commission on Social Justice, 1994, p.1). In its proposals on social security, the Commission emphasized that the welfare state 'must enable people to achieve self-improvement and self-support' (p.8). To that end, 'it must offer a hand-up, not just a hand-out'. The implication was clear that the springboard might recoil on a diver reluctant to take the plunge into the labour market, or that the open hand might deliver a firm clout to anybody who failed to display the required enthusiasm for self-help.

The emergence of a new pattern of welfare provision was accompanied by a more explicit recognition of the concept of need, which followed the controversies of the 1970s and 1980s. On the one hand, there was a new emphasis on identifying and quantifying need at both individual and population level, so that welfare resources could be distributed to maximize efficiency and efficacy. On the other hand, there was a general recognition that, given the overall stagnation of economic development, the resources available for welfare would inevitably be inadequate. Indeed some variation on the formulation 'infinite demand, finite resources' was the prelude to a debate about rationing in every area of welfare. Let us look at this more closely.

5.1 Disparaging need

The notion that need is infinite effectively disparages the concept of need and the demands for resources that follow from it. In the UK in the 1980s a climate of public opinion developed that regarded the growth of needs as an alarming manifestation of the impact of uncontrollable forces (an ageing population, technological imperatives, popular expectations, selfish wants) on a society with limited resources. This gloomy mood was also encouraged by arguments which depicted the expression of need as irrational or irresponsible. Let us take the latter point first.

Denunciations of 'dole scroungers', 'irresponsible single parents', 'bogus asylum-seekers' and others who were said to abuse the welfare system became a recurrent feature of speeches by Conservative politicians. Though such condemnations were not new – Labour's Aneurin Bevan, founding father of the NHS, notoriously justified prescription charges in the early 1950s by denouncing poor people for pouring free cough linctuses down their throats – they became

welfare abuse

more systematic, more wide-ranging and more draconian as the squeeze on welfare gathered momentum. Amplified by the media, these ideas undoubtedly had considerable impact in society. Once it was established that welfare services were being abused, the government could move ahead with measures to make services more selective and restrictive.

Though the assertion that welfare services are facing a crisis of rising expectations appears more neutral than the attacks on scroungers, the consequences are similar. Such statements recurred in discussions about health and community care in particular, where expectations were to some extent raised by the rhetoric of the market and consumer sovereignty. But from the perspective of the free market, rising expectations should be celebrated as a stimulus to enterprise: should not demand stir the hidden hand to supply? In the quasi-markets of UK welfare, however, more demand seemed to induce only despondency. Hence rising expectations were often discussed as a mysterious and irrational development, or as an expression of individual irresponsibility – as in responses to the increased demand for out-of-hours visits by GPs. While making piecemeal attempts to meet such demands, doctors also attempted to reduce them through a 'patient education campaign' launched jointly by the Department of Health and the British Medical Association in March 1996.

The continuing offensive against 'the poverty lobby' and its alleged inflation of need was another component of the conservative anti-welfare campaign (see Extract 1.1 above). In May 1989 social security minister John Moore attacked Townsend's use of the threshold for benefit under the income support scheme as the 'poverty line', arguing that 'the poverty lobby would, on their definition, find poverty in paradise' (quoted in Sullivan, 1996, p.237). Again, in April 1996, another social security minister, Peter Lilley, rejected appeals to introduce a 'poverty eradication plan' as proposed by the United Nations, denying the existence of poverty in the UK (*The Guardian*, 17 April 1996). Though recognizing a problem of 'low income', Lilley pointed out that poverty could not be considered to exist in a society in which everybody had access to clean water and adequate supplies of food, most have central heating, almost half have a car, three-quarters are on the phone and more than half own a video-recorder. By insisting on an absolute definition of need, ministers were moving away from the relative conception, including an element determined by social convention and custom beyond mere physical subsistence, that had been a founding assumption of the post-war welfare state.

technological push

Another argument that effectively devalued need was the emphasis on the way that technological development creates new needs which then remorselessly deplete the resources of a limited national economy (not to mention a limited planetary ecosystem). This argument tends to exaggerate the recent pace of scientific and technological advance – unfortunately rather less impressive than earlier in the twentieth century – and to underestimate the potential savings resulting from such advances (for example, a kidney transplant provides not only a higher quality of life, but is in fact a cheaper option than long-term dialysis). According to one ministerial estimate, in the 1980s technological advances added 0.5 per cent annually to NHS costs (Hills, 1993, p.59).

demographic timebomb

Perhaps the most powerful support for the notion of need as an uncontrollable, even malevolent and threatening force, was the concept of the 'demographic timebomb'. The argument here was that society was sinking under the burden of an increasingly ageing population, whose growing welfare needs had to be supplied by a shrinking economically active population. This concern about the ageing of Western society was often linked to fears about an influx of young 'economic refugees' from the rest of the world where a different sort of 'population explosion' is taking place (Vincent, 1996, pp.3–4). In the world of 'apocalyptic demography' it seems that metaphors are weighed in tons of TNT.

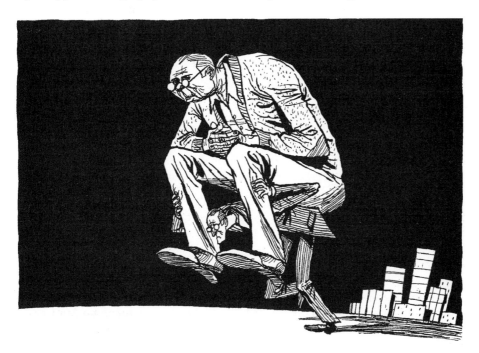

According to Hills, the impact of ageing in the UK was grossly exaggerated: he estimated that the needs of older people could be accommodated by an increase in welfare spending of 0.32 per cent per year over the next half century. Furthermore, he noted that the ratio of people of working age to that over 65 was likely to improve in the UK relative to other Western countries: 'What tends to be forgotten is that the UK went through the ageing process relatively early, by comparison with other countries' (Hills, 1993, pp.12–13). Vincent (1996, p.23) also dismissed the 'demographic timebomb' as a 'pseudo-scientific argument' which allowed the government to redefine the issue of pensions as 'not a moral issue, but a technical one, in which the experts reveal that the state pension system is not sustainable' and 'pensions can be privatized', leaving the elderly 'vulnerable to the whims of the financial markets.'

ACTIVITY 1.4

Health policy analyst Peter Draper argued that the notion of infinite demand was a myth which had 'no mathematical nor other theoretical basis':

> The idea behind this myth is that we all have nothing better to do than to consume health care … If everybody suffers from the proclivity to feign or invent symptoms to secure medical treatment, then genuine need has ceased to exist. But need does still exist, arguably on a growing scale: what has changed is the capacity – and the will – of society to meet it.

(Draper, 1996, p.48)

Draper is clearly motivated by a desire to defend people who may need health care against a campaign to justify curbing spending on health care on the grounds that people's demands are unreasonable. Think about this in the light of what we have discussed and in the light of your experience. Do you think Draper's argument is justified?

COMMENT

Draper implies that the demand for health care arises from the experience of illness: people will only express the need for treatment if they are ill. But what about the demand for treatment resulting from screening and other preventive interventions? What about the demand for new investigations, new drugs and new operations encouraged by features in newspapers and on television? Is it not also the case that much of the demand for specific medical interventions comes, not from patients themselves, but from their doctors – and that such demands vary enormously among doctors practising in different countries, even in different areas of the same country? Is it possible for the state, given wider economic constraints, to cater for all these demands?

■ ■ ■

5.2   The rise of rationing

rationing

All the arguments disparaging need point in one direction – towards the rationing of welfare provision. The move to curtail the resources allocated to meet welfare needs, at a population or individual level, has been further legitimized by a number of arguments. The most important, clearly, is the bottom line: the notion that the overall level of resources is 'finite'. Acceptance of this ultimate limit on the scope for meeting need is contingent upon accepting a number of underlying assumptions. These include the assumption that contemporary capitalist society does in fact mark the highest attainable level of human civilization and that we have therefore reached the 'end of history' (Fukuyama, 1992). Another assumption is that, even given the limits of the British economy, it is impossible to spend a higher proportion of GDP on welfare than at present. All these arguments raged with a particular intensity around the issue of health care, which is examined further in Chapter 2.

One of the most familiar refrains in the rationing debate was the claim that though there has always been rationing, it is better that is done openly. It was ironic that the authorities discovered a new willingness to open up decisions about the allocation of welfare resources to particular services or treatments to public debate and consultation only in the context of an overall drive to curtail welfare-spending. Critics of the government argued that the purpose of making rationing explicit and opening up public debate was to spread the responsibility for unpopular decisions and to legitimize reductions in resources. As Ann Oakley commented in the debate about rationing health care, the point of the more open process of needs assessment and the allocation of resources was not 'to ensure that the people have the health service they want, but rather to persuade them that the health service they are given is the one they have chosen' (in Oakley and Williams, 1994, p.12).

Peter Draper insisted that the key issue is not whether or not rationing is explicit or implicit, but whether it is acceptable or unacceptable. Rationing is acceptable where, for example, a GP refers a patient for specialist treatment on an urgent or routine basis, according to clinical need. It is unacceptable if people are arbitrarily excluded from treatment (on the basis of age or postal code) or subjected to inordinate delays for urgent treatment because the hospital casualty system is overloaded (Draper, 1996).

Rationing was further legitimized by the promotion of quasi-scientific 'need indicators' (a subject we consider in more detail in Chapter 2). The first major exercise in the use of such indicators was the programme implemented under the auspices of the 'Resource Allocation Working Party' (RAWP) in 1976. The proclaimed objective of RAWP was 'to reduce progressively, and as far as feasible, the disparities between the different parts of the country in terms of the opportunity for access to healthcare of people at equal risk' (DHSS, 1976). The working party used a 'weighted population index' which took account of geographical variations in age, sex, morbidity, fertility and marital status. In a comprehensive critique, Sheldon and Carr-Hill (1991, p.23) warned that statistics could 'become a scientific "fig leaf" providing a legitimation of what are essentially political judgements.' The immediate consequence of RAWP in the context of the overall squeeze in public spending in the late 1970s (nobody ever suggested such a redistribution when public spending was increasing) was to produce what Mohan (1995) described as a 'greater equality of misery'.

How has rationing become an issue in the social construction of need?

6   'Needs-led' welfare?

By the late 1990s the broad outline of a new welfare framework in the UK replacing the post-war 'welfare state' could be discerned. The rhetoric of 'needs-led' welfare provision appeared to be supported by a convergence of the major political parties – and academic commentators – around the acceptance of a shift in the centre of gravity of welfare away from the state and towards the individual and the community. The central notion of this was that the provision of welfare services began from the needs of the individual citizen, mediated through the market, rather than from the propositions of state bureaucrats and public sector professionals. But had 'needs-led' welfare become a reality? Could one speak of a new welfare consensus having been formed?

'needs-led' welfare provision

The ideology of needs-led welfare certainly transformed the shape of welfare provision. In community care, 'needs assessment' emphasized the primacy of the needs of the individual service-user and the responsibility of professionals and managers to fit services to those needs. In health, the notion that 'the money follows the patient' through the internal marketplace from GP surgery to hospital and back into the community fundamentally changed doctor–patient and GP–consultant relationships. In education, parental choice, guided by league tables of results, and carried through into local management of schools, became a major force.

The welfare policy of the Labour Party, transformed into New Labour under the leadership of Tony Blair after 1994, was the clearest indication of a new welfare consensus. The elevation of responsibility over rights, of individualism over collectivism, and of community over class, arguably revealed the abandonment of the traditions embodied in the post-war welfare state. The emphasis on the more authoritarian policies associated with 'workfare' rather than the supportive, if paternalistic, traditions of welfarism reflected the degree of Labour's change.

Following the approach pioneered by the Labour government in New Zealand, New Labour in the UK shifted away from the traditional labour movement's concern with economic inequality and collective security to identify with the new social movements' hostility towards discrimination on grounds of gender, 'race', disability or sexual orientation. Procedural rights took priority over substantive rights. As Mishra (1995) observes, from this perspective, what matters is equality of treatment (in the form of equal opportunities/anti-discriminatory polices, which are compatible with the market system) rather than equality of outcome (which implies a challenge to the market system). Mishra further notes that while poverty was increasingly accepted as natural and inevitable, and those in its grip were either ignored or blamed, concern with issues of discrimination was 'stronger than ever'.

In many respects the transformation of welfare appeared as a victory for the New Right. The conversion of New Labour and the academics of the 'market left' to the virtues of the market and a new sense of the responsibilities of the individual was certainly an intellectual triumph for the New Right. The shift in the pattern of welfare provision towards a 'new mixed economy of welfare' in which the private and voluntary sectors played a much greater role and state welfare was increasingly residualized (most successfully in housing) also marked a considerable achievement. On the other hand, the burden of welfare-spending on the public purse was, if anything, even greater. It proved easier for the right to roll over the left than to roll back state spending.

Yet had the individual been set free? A closer look at 'needs-led' welfare suggests that it was led more by the demands of a chronically declining economy than by the real needs of the individual casualties of that decline. The process of 'needs assessment' for community care provision illustrates the character of needs-led welfare (this subject is discussed further in Chapter 3). How was need assessed? The official manager's guide acknowledged that need was 'a complex concept' and helpfully offered clarification:

> In this guidance the term is used as a shorthand for the requirements of individuals to enable them to achieve, maintain or restore, an acceptable level of social independence or quality of life, as defined by the particular care agency or authority.
> (Department of Health, 1991)

The last clause revealed that need was not defined by the individual, but by the authorities. The guidelines further clarified that need was a 'dynamic concept', whose definition varied according to changes in national legislation, changes in local policy, the availability of resources, the patterns of local demand – but not, evidently, in response to changes in the needs or demands of the dynamic individual whose needs were supposed to be 'leading' the whole process. It was not surprising that numerous disputes about 'needs-led' community care ended up in the courts as individuals asserted their rights to resources in face of the authorities' definition of their needs.

The contrast between rhetoric and reality was also evident in the health service. Non-fundholding GPs, who thought that the money would follow the patient if they referred a patient to a particular hospital, discovered that this was only the case if their local health authority had a contract with the hospital –

and if the referral was sent in before their budget ran out. Even fundholding GPs found that the money tended to follow the patient along routes determined more by history and geography than by the invigorating atmosphere of market forces (Audit Commission, 1996). In education, parental choice was also gravely limited by catchment areas, but even more by the evident deterioration in the quality of educational provision at every level of the system, from crumbling infant and junior schools to overcrowded, under-resourced universities.

The deficiencies of 'needs-led' welfare were perhaps most evident in the sphere of social security. Here the long-running debate about the respective merits of selective and universal benefits tended to obscure the overall deterioration in the real value of benefits, with the resulting impoverishment of a growing number of welfare dependants, and the tendency towards the exclusion of people from benefit – and in a sense from society. These trends were most apparent among young people and lone parents – the targets of the workfare drive – and among old people – casualties of the dramatic decline in the value of state pensions as well as of the expansion of private pension schemes of dubious value. It was striking that these groups also suffer public denigration, most explicitly in attacks on young beggars or mothers on welfare, but more insidiously in the 'demographic timebomb' depiction of old people as a threat to the rest of society.

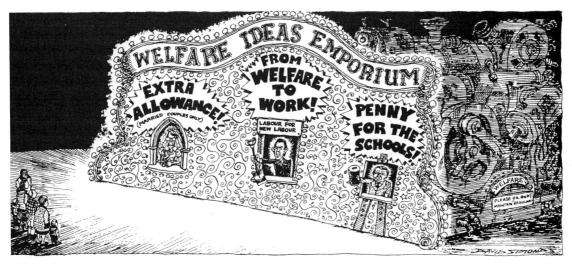

(*Source:* The Guardian, 7 April 1997)

7   Conclusion

We began the chapter with a remark that the concept of need is often regarded as self-evident; we take it for granted. The transformation of the framework of welfare services in the UK is a striking illustration of the process of the *social construction* of need. It illustrates, moreover, in a conspicuous way that 'need' is a contested concept. As we have seen, both the deconstruction of the concept of need embodied in the post-war welfare state and the reconstruction of a new conception in the 1990s were the outcome of a prolonged period of conflict and contestation among the diverse social and institutional forces concerned with the world of welfare. The struggles over definitions of need were struggles involving power – the power to define *legitimate* need. We have been concerned in the chapter to investigate political power, as well as popular resistance. This has led us to examine the way in which definitions of need determine sets of relationships between those who administer services and those who receive them.

In the post-war period 'need' was little questioned and the welfare state provided services of a fairly basic and uniform character to a society already collectivized by the experience of war and austerity. The broad structure of welfare was devised by Liberals (Beveridge and Keynes), introduced by Labour (Attlee and Bevan) and endorsed by the Conservatives (Butler and Macmillan). The big battalions of labour and capital – through the TUC and the CBI – accepted the welfare state, with varying degrees of approval and apprehension, and the civil servants and professionals accepted the prestige of administering the various services. Public enthusiasm for welfare was certainly uneven, and in retrospect exaggerated but, in general, resistances were not fundamental.

Thirty years later, virtually all the assumptions of the welfare pioneers have come into question. Conservatives challenged state intervention in the economy and welfare, while the left defended public provision – and demanded more and better. Political consensus disintegrated as the old power blocs (at home and abroad) collapsed and new social movements emerged demanding rights and recognition of the particular needs of sections of society which had been ignored in the 1940s – women, black people, disabled people, lesbian and gay groups. Bureaucratic and professional elites found themselves under attack from above (from governments determined to curb their control over research) and from below (from citizens empowered by the demise of deference and invigorating influence of market forces).

Whether needs-led welfare could provide for the needs of all members of an increasingly unequal society remains uncertain. But there could be no doubt that the state-led welfare services of the post-war years had gone forever.

Further reading

In studying the concept of need in relation to the development of welfare, there is much to be said for going back to basics: to the Beveridge Report or, perhaps even better, José Harris's acclaimed biography of William Beveridge. Doyal and Gough's *A Theory of Human Need* is a brave attempt to advance a universal concept of need from a radical perspective in face of the adverse tide of events of the 1980s. The pamphlet *Choice and Responsibility*, published by the Tory No Turning Back Group in 1990, is a good brief statement of the New Right position. John Hills' edited collection, *The State of Welfare*, includes many of the LSE commentators and indicates their coming to terms with the market reforms of the Thatcher era and anticipates the direction of New Labour social policy. Ramesh Mishra's article, 'Social policy after socialism', is a prescient assessment from the left of the impact of the demise of state socialism on social policy. **Hughes and Lewis (eds, 1998)** provide an overview of changes to specific areas of social policy change.

References

Abel-Smith, B. and Townsend, P. (1965) *The Poor and the Poorest*, London, Longman Green.

Audit Commission (1996) *What the Doctor Ordered: A Study of GP Fundholders in England and Wales*, London, HMSO.

Bacon, R. and Eltis, W. (1976) *Britain's Economic Problem: Too Few Producers*, London, Macmillan.

Bailey, R. and Brake, M. (eds) (1975) *Radical Social Work*, London, Edward Arnold.

Bowles, S. and Gintis, H. (1976) *Schooling in Capitalist America: Educational Reform and the Contradictions of Economic Life*, London, Routledge and Kegan Paul.

Brittan, S. (1973) *Capitalism and the Permissive Society*, London, Macmillan.

Clarke, J. (1998) 'Consumerism' in Hughes, G. (ed.) *Imagining Welfare Futures*, London, Routledge in association with The Open University.

Commission on Social Justice (1994) *Social Justice: Strategies for National Renewal*, London, Vintage.

Dennis, N. (1997) *The Invention of Permanent Poverty*, Choice in Welfare no.34, London, IEA Health and Welfare Unit.

Department of Health (1991) *Care Management and Assessment: Manager's Guide*, London, HMSO.

Department of Health and Social Security (1976) *Sharing Resources for Health in England: Report of the Resource Allocation Working Party*, London, HMSO.

Doyal, L. (1979) *The Political Economy of Health*, London, Pluto.

Doyal, L. and Gough, I. (1991) *A Theory of Human Need*, London, Macmillan.

Draper, P. (ed.) (1996) *Myths about the NHS and Rationing Health Care*, Banbury, NHS Consultants Association.

Foster, P. (1983) *Access to Welfare: An Introduction to Welfare Rationing*, London, Macmillan.

Friedman, M. (1962) *Capitalism and Freedom*, Chicago, Chicago University Press.

Fukuyama, F. (1992) *The End of History and the Last Man*, London, Hamish Hamilton.

Gazeley I. and Thane, P. (1998) 'Patterns of visibility: unemployment in Britain during the nineteenth and twentieth centuries' in Lewis, G. (ed.).

Ginsburg, N. (1979) *Class, Capital and Social Policy*, London, Macmillan.

Glennerster, H. (1992) *Paying for Welfare in the 1990s*, Hemel Hempstead, Harvester Wheatsheaf.

Gough, I. (1979) *The Political Economy of the Welfare State*, London, Macmillan.

Harris, J. (1977) *William Beveridge: A Biography*, Oxford, Oxford University Press.

Hart, J.T. (1975) 'The inverse care law' in Cox, A. and Mead, M. (eds) *A Sociology of Medical Practice*, London, Collier-Macmillan.

Hayek, F.A. (1944) *The Road to Serfdom*, London, Routledge and Kegan Paul.

Hayek, F.A. (1949) *Individualism and the Economic Order*, London, Routledge and Kegan Paul.

Hills, J. (ed.) (1990) *The State of Welfare: The Welfare State in Britain since 1975*, Oxford, Oxford University Press.

Hills, J. (1993) *The Future of Welfare: A Guide to the Debate*, York, Joseph Rowntree Trust/LSE Welfare State Programme.

Hughes, G. (1998a) '"Picking over the remains": the welfare state settlements of the post-Second World War UK' in Hughes, G. and Lewis, G. (eds).

Hughes, G. (1998b) 'A suitable case for treatment: constructions of disability' in Saraga, E. (ed.).

Hughes, G. and Lewis, G. (eds) (1998) *Unsettling Welfare: The Reconstruction of Social Policy*, London, Routledge in association with The Open University.

Illich, I. (1975) *Medical Nemesis: The Expropriation of Health*, London, Calder and Boyars.

Illich, I. (1977) *Disabling Professions*, London, Calder and Boyars.

Johnson, T.J. (1972) *Professions and Power*, London, Macmillan.

Le Grand, J. (1982) *The Strategy for Equality*, London, Allen and Unwin.

Le Grand, J. and Winter, J. (1987) *Not Only the Poor*, London, Allen and Unwin.

Levitas, R. (ed.) (1986) *The Ideology of the New Right*, Cambridge, Polity Press.

Lewis, G. (1998a) 'Coming apart at the seams: the crises of the welfare state' in Hughes, G. and Lewis, G. (eds).

Lewis, G. (1998b) 'Welfare and the social construction of "race"' in Saraga, E. (ed.)

Lewis, G. (ed.) (1998) *Forming Nation, Framing Wefare*, London, Routledge in association with The Open University.

Marshall, T. H. (1950) *Citizenship and Social Class*, Cambridge, Cambridge University Press.

Mishra, R. (1995) 'Social policy after socialism', *Social Policy Review 7*, Canterbury, Social Policy Association.

Mohan, J. (1995) *A National Health Service? The Restructuring of Health Care in Britain since 1979*, London, Macmillan.

Mooney, G. (1998) '"Remoralizing" the poor?: gender, class and philanthropy in Victorian Britain' in Lewis, G. (ed.).

Murray, C. (1990) *The Emerging British Underclass*, London, Institute of Economic Affairs.

No Turning Back Group (1988) *The NHS: A Suitable Case for Treatment*, London, Conservative Political Centre.

No Turning Back Group (1990) *Choice and Responsibility: The Enabling State*, London, Conservative Political Centre.

Oakley, A. and Williams, S. (eds) (1994) *The Politics of the Welfare State*, London, UCL Press.

Parton, N. (1991) *Governing the Family: Child Care, Child Protection and the State*, Macmillan, London.

Pinkney, S. (1998) 'The reshaping of social work and social care' in Hughes, G. and Lewis, G. (eds).

Radical Statistics Health Group (1977) *In Defence of the NHS*, Radical Statistics Health Group.

Robinson, R. and Le Grand, J. (eds) (1994) *Evaluating the NHS Reforms*, King's Fund Institute.

Saraga, E. (ed.) (1998) *Embodying the Social: Constructions of Difference*, London, Routledge in association with The Open University.

Sheldon, T. and Carr-Hill, R. (1991) 'Measure for measure', *The Health Service Journal*, 1 August.

Sullivan, M. (1996) *The Development of the British Welfare State*, Hemel Hempstead, Prentice Hall/Harvester Wheatsheaf.

Timmins, N. (1995) *The Five Giants: A Biography of the Welfare State*, London, Fontana Press.

Titmuss, R. (1958) *Essays on the Welfare State*, London, Allen and Unwin.

Titmuss, R. (1965) 'Goals of today's welfare state' in Anderson, P. and Blackburn, R. (eds) *Towards Socialism*, London, Fontana.

Vincent, J. (1996) 'Who's afraid of an ageing population?', *Critical Social Policy*, vol.16, May, pp.3–26.

CHAPTER 2

Rationing Health Care

by Mary Langan

Contents

1   Introduction

The conviction that the demand for health care exceeds the resources available for its supply, which must therefore be *rationed*, became one of the central themes in health policy debates in the United Kingdom in the 1990s. Any attempt to allocate health care resources rationally requires some process of assessing health care needs and of deciding health care priorities. The rationing debate therefore brought the question of the social construction of need out of the world of academic discourse and into the day-to-day provision of health services.

social
construction
of need

This chapter focuses on the controversy about rationing health care in order to illustrate the process by which welfare needs in a particular area are defined and redefined in a process of contestation that operates both inside and outside the particular welfare service.

- We begin in section 2 with the rationing debate itself, looking at some of the cases that brought it into the public domain and at the arguments of some of the key protagonists.

- In section 3 we then ask, if it is true – as many supporters of rationing argue – that rationing has always been with us, then what forms has it taken and how has it been implemented?

- Next, we look at the pressures that brought the issue of rationing out into the open, in the 1970s and 1980s, looking at both the 'supply' and 'demand' sides of the health divide.

- We then proceed, in section 5, to consider different attempts to introduce 'rational' rationing, in particular by methods of quantifying the effectiveness of different medical treatments. It includes a rationing initiative from overseas – in Oregon in the USA – that has had considerable influence on the rationing debate in the UK.

- In section 6 we examine different proposals to make the process of rationing and health professionals more open and accountable.

- Finally, we consider rationing as an example of the social (re)construction of need.

2   The rationing debate

In the course of the 1990s a number of highly publicized cases, in which decisions to curtail health service expenditure were contested, opened up the whole issue of health care rationing to wider public discussion.

- In 1993 Harry Elphick, a heavy smoker, was refused surgical treatment for a heart condition because of his inability to quit smoking. There followed a heated debate in the pages of the *British Medical Journal* and further discussion on the BBC television programme, *The Heart of the Matter*, as well as in other news media, before he died.

- In 1995 Jaymee Bowen, a ten-year-old girl with recurrent leukaemia, was refused a second bone-marrow transplant by her local health authority, on the grounds that the chance of success was slight and that the treatment would itself cause considerable distress. Though the High Court at first approved her father's challenge to this decision, on appeal the health authority's stand was upheld. In the event a private donor financed further treatment in the private sector, despite which Jaymee died in May 1996.

■ In 1995 Berkshire Health Authority disclosed plans to refuse financial support for a range of surgical procedures which it deemed not to be cost-effective. In the same year there were reports that elderly people were being deemed ineligible for physiotherapy in one hospital and for palliative treatment for lung cancer in another.

These examples of rationing according to diverse criteria – including a patient's capacity to benefit, the clinical efficacy of a particular intervention and the moral worthiness of the patient – provoked intense public controversy. After a decade of low-key professional and academic discussion, the issue of rationing was placed firmly on the public agenda.

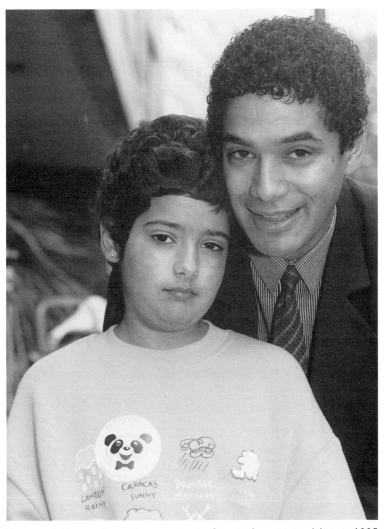

Ten-year-old Jaymee Bowen became a major focus in the rationing debate in 1995 when her father challenged a health authority's refusal to finance further treatment for her leukaemia

2.1   The case for rationing

The leading voices in the call for rationing came from within the medical profession – notably from the Royal College of Physicians and the British Medical Association – and from influential think-tanks concerned with health policy – such as the King's Fund and the Institute of Public Policy and Research. They argued that there had always been a gap between the demand for health care and the available resources, making some form of rationing inevitable. They insisted that, whereas rationing in the past had been a largely implicit and haphazard process, generally conducted behind closed doors, the scale of the gulf now opening up between popular expectations and health care provision dictated the need for much more systematic and explicit mechanisms of resource allocation and decision-making.

Richard Smith, editor of the *British Medical Journal* and a prominent campaigner for a more open and accountable process of rationing, summed up the state of the debate in response to some of the controversies raging in early 1995; his analysis is given in Extract 2.1.

Extract 2.1 Smith: 'Rationing: the debate we have to have'

Britain needs a nationwide, prolonged, systematic debate on rationing

Britain was transfixed last week by two stories that were primarily about the rationing of health care. In one case a court ruled that Cambridge Health Authority did not have to offer a second bone marrow transplant to a 10 year old child dying of leukaemia. In the other case a man with a severe head injury was flown 320 km by helicopter to a neurosurgical unit because none of the many nearer units could take him. The media were filled with these stories, and the debate over rationing exploded into life once again. Unfortunately – because the government is unwilling to be candid on rationing – the debate is likely to die down until we have yet another dreadful case. We need a much better debate.

The medical press has been debating rationing in health care for more than a decade, and two years ago the BMA, the *BMJ*, the King's Fund, and the Patients Association organized a conference on rationing. The secretary of state for health, Virginia Bottomley, opened the conference and was careful to avoid the word rationing. Government, she said, had a role in broad strategic shifts of resources but not in 'priority setting': that had to be done locally. This failure of leadership has meant that Britain has not had the broad, deep, informed, and prolonged debate on rationing that is needed.

What Britain has had is a series of brief, heated, and often uninformed debates about particular episodes. Debates have arisen in response to stories of surgeons refusing coronary artery bypass operations to smokers, people being denied various treatments on grounds of age, older women being treated for infertility, and a woman being given a breast enlargement while other patients were denied apparently more 'worthy' procedures. Each of these cases has illustrated different aspects of rationing, but most people have not had an opportunity to understand the scale of the problem and to give their opinion on issues such as trading off quality against quantity of life. And when it comes to such questions there are no experts: everybody's opinion is as good as everybody else's.

Perhaps these latest cases will prompt the debate we need. Those who know about the fascinating experiments in Oregon may remember that they started after patients on Medicaid were denied transplant operations. Economic pressures forced this step, but medical ethicists and others said that it was foolish to deny transplantation when it might often be much more cost effective than many other – perhaps less spectacular – treatments. So, with the state's encouragement, began a process of consulting the public and merging its opinions with technical measures of the cost effectiveness of all treatments. The outcome was a radically new system for rationing care.

Britain must find its own way of engaging the public in the debate on rationing, but this debate will lead to constructive outcomes only if the government takes the lead. One outcome may of course be an irresistible pressure to increase public expenditure on health care.

(Smith, 1995, p.686)

How did a small number of high-profile cases help to raise public awareness about issues of health care rationing?

2.2 The case against

While individual patients, their families and various voluntary organizations and pressure groups responded angrily when they or those they represented found themselves at the sharp end of rationing decisions, few were prepared to argue a more systematic case against rationing. However, some doctors and other commentators challenged different aspects of the campaign for rationing.

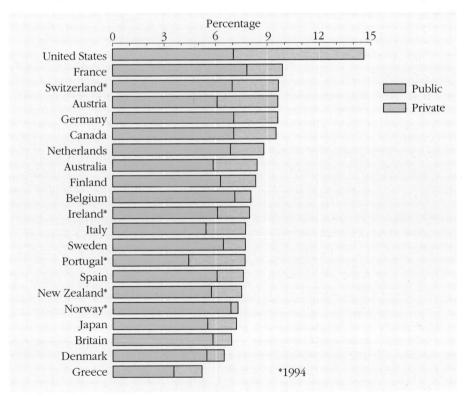

Figure 2.1 Total health spending as percentage of GDP, 1995 (Source of data: OECD; Source: The Economist Election Briefing, 1997, p.14)

The common theme of most critics of rationing was that it evaded the key issue of health policy in the UK – the underfunding of the health service as a whole. This case was particularly supported by international comparisons, which showed the relatively low proportion of GDP spent on health care in Britain: see Figure 2.1. Opponents of rationing argued that if the UK raised its health spending to the OECD average, this would mean an injection of £6 billion into the service and obviate all discussion of rationing. According to Professor Raymond Hoffenberg (BMJ, 1993, p.199), former president of the Royal College of Physicians, if this were done, 'we could probably meet all reasonable clinical demands now and for some time to come at a level inferior to none – that is, serious rationing could be deferred almost indefinitely.' As we have seen in Chapter 1, some critics of rationing also challenged the notion of 'infinite demand' which was a key justification for curtailing expenditure.

infinite
demand

Peter Draper, a leading public health academic based at Guy's Hospital in London before becoming an independent health policy advisor, published the most comprehensive challenge to rationing, reproduced here as Extract 2.2.

Extract 2.2 Draper: 'Myths about the NHS and rationing health care'

There are three main reasons why discussion in the NHS is predominantly about restrictive rationing (or in the government's preferred terms, *priority setting*), rather than about getting a bigger slice of a bigger cake.

First, the creation of the NHS market, as critics allege was intended, has concentrated discussion about resources on local purchasing decisions of the new purchasing agents (the district health authorities and the GP fundholders) rather than about the size of the allocated budget.

To make things worse and actually *create* shortages through misusing the NHS budget, the hefty costs of running the NHS market have had to be found from general resources – for all the extra office staff such as accountants, financial managers, contract officers, public relations personnel, computing staff and extra administrative and clerical staff rather than for more nurses, doctors, or back-up staff.

...

Along with the closure of hospital beds faster than the build up of primary health care and other community services, we have witnessed a new phase of shortages and delays affecting emergencies and inpatient treatment in many areas, particularly in inner cities. This is no way to pursue the laudable policy of providing more and quality services in the community rather than in hospitals.

What is new about recent shortages and delays is that services are *frequently* inadequate and are widely seen by patients, relatives and clinical staff to be inadequate – patients waiting to be admitted for hours on trolleys in A & E departments; patients admitted for operations having to be sent home before surgery in order to vacate beds needed for emergencies and so on. And senior management, right up to the Secretary of State, typically regret but accept frequent inadequacies.

What is different about this phase is that NHS staff are *regularly* having to subject patients to what they know is second or third rate care *and instead of management fighting to improve care, they are concentrating on balancing inadequate budgets*
...

The **second** reason why the public agenda has focused on rationing rather than on seeking a bigger slice of cake is the variety of organizations that have promoted this approach. For instance, the all-party, Conservative-chaired House of Commons select committee on health is engaged on a series of reviews of *Priority setting in the NHS* … Similarly, the Royal College of Physicians recently published *Setting priorities in the NHS.* […]

The **third** factor in directing public discussion to restrictive rationing rather than promoting investment in a cost-effective health sector has been the dissemination of the *myth of the bottomless pit* – the notion that the potential demand for health care is infinite and therefore that any extra funds will make no difference to the overstretched NHS. This illogical and frankly dangerous notion suggests that people have an unquenchable thirst and uncontrollable appetite to spend their lives consuming health services – as if most people are hypochondriacs and as if the NHS had no gatekeepers!

(Draper, 1995, pp.3–6)

2.3 Setting priorities

As Richard Smith indicated in Extract 2.1, the reluctance of government ministers – and even opposition politicians – to take up the cause was a source of some irritation to those in the rationing camp. Given the continuing popularity of the NHS at a time when politicians of all parties had been sliding lower and lower in public esteem, politicians were reluctant to endorse a policy which was likely to be perceived by the public as leading to further cuts in services. Even Margaret Thatcher was forced to confirm that 'the NHS is safe with us' and her Chancellor, Nigel Lawson, once wryly commented that 'the NHS is the only religion the English have'. It was thus not surprising that when she was health minister Virginia Bottomley studiously avoided the word 'rationing', preferring the anodyne 'priority-setting'. It was also not surprising that, in its concern not to upset any potential voters in the long run-up to the 1997 election, New Labour also steered clear of talking about rationing.

priority-setting

Yet, despite the caution of the politicians, the idea of rationing was in the public domain and the medical campaigners were determined to push the debate forward. It was immediately apparent that the issue of rationing opened up a much wider discussion of medical practice and health policy. Thus the question of how resources should be rationed inevitably raised questions about how resources were allocated in the first place. This in turn led to questions about how the effectiveness of any particular medical treatment could be measured and about how health spending and professional performance were monitored, especially, for example, given evidence of dramatic regional variations in different areas of medical practice, such as the use of particular surgical procedures and the success rates of cancer treatments.

Making the process of rationing explicit also raised important questions about who made the decisions at every level from the Ministry of Health to the GP's surgery, about who was consulted and about what sort of democratic accountability existed, if any. The issue of rationing thus opened up a wide-ranging debate about the question of health care needs, about how they could be measured and quantified, and about who should decide how – or indeed, whether – the particular needs of particular people should be met.

In a consultation exercise conducted in 1992, City and Hackney health authority drew up a list of 16 health care services and asked people how they would place them in order of merit in terms of the allocation of resources (highest priority: 1; lowest priority: 16). Complete Table 2.1 according to *your own* judgement of priorities.

Table 2.1 Categories used in the Public Priorities Survey for City and Hackney health authority, 1992

Services or treatments	Priority rank order
Treatments for children with life-threatening illness	
Hospice care	
Medical research for new treatments	
High tech surgery for life-threatening conditions (e.g.transplants)	
Preventive services	
Surgery for people with a disability to carry out everyday lives (e.g. hip replacement)	
Physiotherapy/occupational therapy/speech therapy to carry out everyday lives	
Services for people with mental illness	
Intensive care units for premature infants weighing less than 1.5 pounds (i.e. unlikely to survive)	
Long-stay (hospitals and nursing-homes for elderly)	
Community services or care at home (district nurses)	
Health education services	
Family planning services	
Treatments for infertility (test-tube babies)	
Complementary/alternative medicine	
Cosmetic surgery	

Now look at Table 2.2, which shows how the survey was completed by members of the public, GPs, hospital consultants and public health doctors in East London. How does your list differ from these? To which group does your list come closest?

Table 2.2 Main results of Public Priorities Survey for City and Hackney health authority, 1992 (Values are mean priority ranks: 1 = highest priority, 16 = lowest)

Services or Treatments	Public	GPs	Consultants	Public health doctors*
Treatments for children with life-threatening illness	1	5	2	9
Hospice care	2	4	4	8
Medical research for new treatments	3	11	8	11
High tech surgery for life-threatening conditions (e.g.transplants)	4	12	12	12
Preventive services	5	6	7	4
Surgery for people with a disability to carry out everyday lives (e.g. hip replacement)	6	8	5	5=
Physiotherapy/occupational therapy/speech therapy to carry out everyday lives	7	7	10	5=
Services for people with mental illness	8	2	1	1=
Intensive care units for premature infants weighing less than 1.5 pounds (i.e. unlikely to survive)	9	13	13	15=
Long-stay (hospitals and nursing-homes for elderly)	10	3	6	10
Community services or care at home (district nurses)	11	1	3	1=
Health education services	12	10	11	5=
Family planning services	13	9	9	1=
Treatments for infertility (test-tube babies)	14	14	14	15=
Complementary/alternative medicine	15	15	16	13=
Cosmetic surgery	16	16	15	13=

Note: *Small sample.

Source: Ham, 1993, p. 436

COMMENT

The dramatic differences in the lists drawn up by people with different stakes in the provision of health services indicate the difficulty both of making such choices and of reconciling different perceptions of health care need.

■ ■ ■

3   Perpetual rationing

Rationing is unavoidable today and has in fact been practised within the NHS since its infancy.

(Harrison and Hunter, 1994, p.1)

3.1   The Beveridge fallacy

Beveridge fallacy

Numerous commentators have drawn attention to the 'Beveridge fallacy' – the assumption by the founder of the post-war welfare state that, once the backlog of need was catered for and public welfare improved, the demand for health care would decline. In reality, of course, demand continued to rise, with the result that 'no sooner had the NHS been launched in 1948 than it was overtaken by a series of expenditure crises' (Klein *et al.*, 1996, p.37).

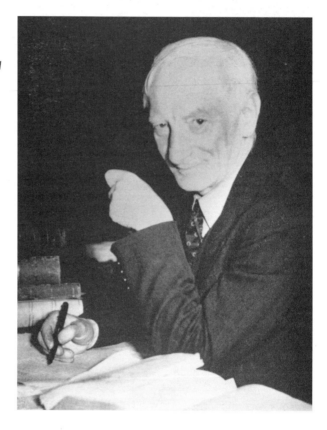

William Beveridge: 'father' of the welfare state – and author of the fallacy that demand for health care would decline once the backlog of need was cleared

The immediate response of the post-war Labour government was to complain about public abuse of the new service and to impose charges on prescriptions. Piloting this measure through parliament in December 1949, health minister Aneurin Bevan, himself a subscriber to the Beveridge fallacy, grumbled about 'cascades of medicine pouring down British throats – and they're not even bringing the bottles back' (quoted in Williams, 1979, p.211). Some sixteen months later, when the cabinet imposed additional charges on false teeth and spectacles, Bevan resigned from the government.

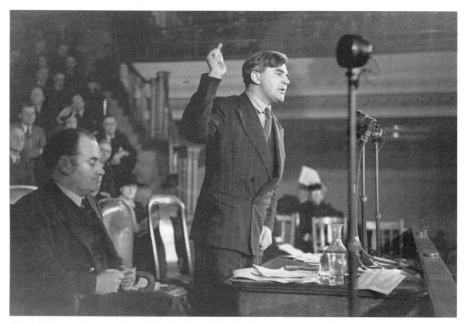

Aneurin Bevan: the founder of the National Health Service was also the first health minister to attempt to ration services by introducing charges

Complaints about the burden of the health service on the Exchequer intensified when the Conservative Party returned to power in the early 1950s, leading to the establishment of the Guillebaud inquiry into the financing of the NHS (Ministry of Health, 1956). The committee's report, published in 1956, vindicated the NHS, describing it as 'the best possible service within the limitations of the available resources'. As Timmins observed in his account of the post-war welfare state, Guillebaud set the terms of the subsequent discussion of the NHS:

> His report saw off the first of the bouts of panic about the service that governments and the public have enjoyed repeatedly over the past fifty years – the belief that NHS spending is out of control, and that the service is a bottomless pit into which any amount of money can be thrown. It also, however, destroyed a then common belief that the cost of the NHS would fall as the nation was made healthier. 'It is still sometimes assumed that the health service can and should be self-limiting, in the sense that its own contribution to national health will limit the demands upon it to a volume which can be fully met. This, at least for the present, is an illusion' [Cmd. 9663, para.98].
>
> (Timmins, 1995, pp.206–7)

3.2 Forms of rationing

Though rationing may not have been publicly discussed at the time, there can be no doubt that rationing did in fact take place in the post-war NHS and indeed continues to take place in a wide range of traditional forms. The following are some of the mechanisms through which resources are preferentially allocated to particular sectors of the population, to particular individuals or to particular forms of treatment.

1 *Deterrence*

Charges for prescriptions and other forms of treatment deter people from seeking health care as well as providing some revenue for the system. First introduced, as we have seen, in 1949, they were temporarily abolished by a Labour government in the 1970s, only to increase at a pace well above the rate of inflation through the 1980s and 1990s.

2 *Delay*

The queue and the waiting-list are the most familiar forms of rationing in the NHS. Both act as a deterrent and as a crude method of ensuring that those whose need is greatest (if, that is, need corresponds to duration of symptoms) are treated first.

3 *Deflection*

Transferring people from the hospital into 'the community' has proved to be a highly effective way of curbing hospital spending over recent decades. The diversification of GPs into family planning, ante-natal care, baby clinics, minor surgery, diabetic, anti-coagulation, travel vaccination and other specialist clinics indicates the growing scope of devolution from the hospital into primary care.

4 *Dilution*

Providing a lower standard of treatment or care, as for example in the old-style residential hospitals for patients with psychiatric illness or people with learning disabilities, or through the declining quality of hotel services in modern hospitals, is a way of cutting costs by spreading services more thinly.

5 *Denial*

Some people are simply refused certain treatments. For years people over a certain age have been refused kidney dialysis in many parts of the country. There has been a growing trend for health authorities not to provide procedures such as cosmetic plastic surgery, infertility treatment and tattoo removal. Regulations governing the eligibility for treatment of immigrants and visitors have also been tightened up.

In some areas of the NHS the insidious effect of these discreet forms of rationing has been quietly but effectively to end public access to particular services. Thus for most adults, dentistry has become a largely private provision; a similar trend advanced rapidly in the services of opticians and chiropodists. The boundary between medical and social care became increasingly hotly disputed as health authorities attempted to pass responsibility for long-term institutional care of older people, and people with mental illness or severe learning difficulties, onto local councils. The combination of rising prescription charges, the growing 'black list' of drugs not made available on prescription, pressures on GPs to curtail prescribing costs, and the increasing availability of former prescription drugs 'over the counter' from pharmacists, all boosted the private pharmaceutical market while significantly reducing the scope of health service prescribing.

3.3 The rationing process

> In short, from the inception of the NHS in the 1940s, the rationing of scarce resources at all levels within the NHS has been largely controlled by the medical profession and has been implicit in nature, making no reference to agreed systems or criteria.
> (New and Le Grand, 1996, p.7)

The established process of allocating resources in the post-war NHS had a number of distinctive features. It had an incremental character, where the dominant influence on both the level and distribution of resources was the pattern established in the past, to which was added an annual increase to account for inflation, population growth and technological advances. The success of the medical lobby in negotiations with the post-war Labour government at the time the NHS was set up, enabled doctors to consolidate their power in the administrative structures of the new service. The persistence of these arrangements ensured continued medical influence at every level of the health service.

A crucial feature of medical authority in the health service was its discreet character. At national and regional level, harsh decisions – such as decisions to refuse kidney dialysis, which resulted in premature deaths for many people with chronic renal failure – were made in a highly informal way by committees of senior doctors and administrators sitting in private offices. The public, the patients themselves and their relatives, voluntary groups, even organizations of other health workers, had no access either to the meetings or to the criteria by which decisions were made. Decisions made by medical gatekeepers at the point of service delivery in the hospital or surgery were cloaked in the mystique of confidentiality and clinical freedom but was in effect the implicit rationing of health service resources. The whole system operated in such a way as to ensure that objections were muted. The rising prestige of doctors in the post-war world of new wonder drugs and dramatic surgical advances, together with the low expectations of a population that had only recently emerged from three decades of depression, war and austerity, guaranteed the popularity of the health service, rationing and all.

implicit rationing

Pause for a moment here and remind yourself about the discreet nature of rationing during this period. What factors account for this?

Though Enoch Powell later became notorious for his anti-immigration views, in the early 1960s he was a highly regarded Minister of Health. In 1966 he wrote a short book drawing on his experience in office and outlining an approach to the financing of health care that anticipated the debates of the 1990s; an excerpt is reproduced as Extract 2.3.

Extract 2.3 Powell: 'Supply and demand'

Medical care under the National Health Service is rendered free to the consumer at the point of consumption – apart, that is, from spectacles and certain dental treatment and appliances. Consequently supply and demand are not kept in balance by price. Since, therefore, resources are limited, both theoretically and in practice at any given time, while demand is unlimited, supply has to be rationed by means other than price. The forms of rationing adopted deliberately or by default, and usually unrecognized – certainly unproclaimed – as such, are among the major irritant ingredients in Medicine and Politics.

Common thought and parlance tend to conceal or deny the fact that demand for all practical purposes *is* unlimited. The vulgar assumption is that there is a definable amount of medical care 'needed', and that if that 'need' was met, no more would be demanded. This is absurd. Every advance in medical science creates new needs that did not exist until the means of meeting them came into existence, or at least into the realm of the possible. For every heart-lung machine or artificial kidney in operation there must be many times that number of cases to which the treatment would be applicable. Every time a discovery is made in, for example, the techniques of grafting, the horizon of 'need' for medical care is suddenly enlarged.

...

The National Health Service, then, must and does apply covert rationing devices in order to limit demand to the actual amount of the supply.

...

Thus, outside as well as inside the hospitals the figure on the supply side of the equation is fixed at any particular time by those complex forces that determine the state's decisions on expenditure. With this figure demand has to be brought into balance. Virtually unlimited as it is by nature, and unrationed by price, it has nevertheless to be squeezed down somehow so as to equal the supply. In brutal simplicity, it has to be rationed; and to understand the methods of rationing is also essential for understanding Medicine and Politics. The task is not made easier by the political convention that the existence of any rationing at all must be strenuously denied. The public are encouraged to believe that rationing in medical care was banished by the National Health Service, and that the very idea of rationing being applied to medical care is immoral and repugnant. Consequently when they, and the medical profession too, come face to face in practice with the various forms of rationing to which the National Health Service must resort, the usual result is bewilderment, frustration and irritation.

The worst kind of rationing is that which is unacknowledged; for it is the essence of a good rationing system to be intelligible and consciously accepted. This is not possible where its very existence has to be repudiated.

(Powell, 1976, pp.26, 29, 37–38)

ACTIVITY 2.2

The striking feature of Powell's argument is how similar it is to that of supporters of rationing some thirty years later. Why do you think his appeal for an explicit mode of rationing attracted little interest in the 1960s? And why do you think an appeal in similar terms in the 1990s should provoke a major debate?

COMMENT

The lack of response to the call for rationing in the 1960s reveals the robustness of the post-war welfare settlement in a period of continuing economic expansion and political stability. The erosion of these foundations of the settlement over the next two decades was the key factor in putting rationing on the agenda.

■ ■ ■

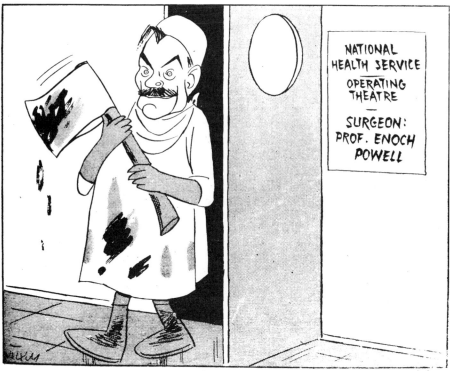

Parliament debates National Health Service costs today.

Surgeon or butcher? Minister of Health, Enoch Powell, was savaged by the press over his proposals for curbing spending in the early 1960s

4   Rationing out in the open

Economists have been peddling these basic premises of scarcity and choice for many years, and so has the NHS – it is just that no one seemed to notice until recently.

(Donaldson, 1993, p.75)

scarcity and choice

The recession of the mid 1970s signalled the end of the post-war boom and the beginning of the process of bringing the issue of rationing in the health service out into the open. The national economic difficulties of this period – stagflation, the return of mass unemployment, the crisis of public expenditure – also led to a growing recognition of a conflict between demands for health care and the finite resources available to the health service. This in turn encouraged the quest for a more systematic mechanism for reconciling supply and demand in the health service, at first among economists and politicians, but gradually also among administrators and doctors. In this section we will trace the evolution of the rationing debate in the 1970s and 1980s. First, we look at the 'supply' side, the squeeze on public spending on health and the various mechanisms promoted by successive governments to reduce the cost and to increase the efficiency of the health service. Then we turn to the 'demand' side and the sources of what has been called the 'crisis of rising expectations' that so preoccupies doctors and other workers in the health service today.

finite resources

4.1 From 'the cuts' to the 'internal market'

'The party's over', Labour minister Anthony Crosland told a gathering of local government officers in July 1975, in a declaration widely recognized as marking the beginning of the end of the welfare state founded thirty years earlier (Timmins, 1995, p.313). Cleaving to fiscal orthodoxy, Labour's Chancellor, Denis Healey, responded to the recession by cutting back government spending and imposing an unprecedented regime of austerity on public services, including health. The main impact of Labour's spending squeeze fell on ancillary workers, whose wages were held down, and on capital expenditure, notably on hospital buildings, which became even more decrepit (many dated back to before the foundation of the health service, and some were still in old workhouses). Protests against 'the cuts' and hospital closures and strikes for higher wages were a prominent feature of the health service in the late 1970s – and contributed to Labour's electoral defeat in 1979.

Labour's policy for the health service was not, however, merely one of spending-cuts and pay-curbs. A number of issues had a significant influence on policy. One was a series of exposures of ill-treatment and poor standards in NHS residential institutions for people with psychiatric illness, those with learning difficulties and the elderly. Another was the revelation of marked imbalances in the distribution of resources around the country, notably the concentration of hospital services in central London, which reflected historical and political factors rather than current population patterns and levels of need. The government's response was what became known by its acronym 'RAWP' – the Resource Allocation Working Party – which set about redistributing resources according to a number of objective indicators of need (see Chapter 1). In place of the traditional formula, aptly summed up as 'what you got last year, plus an allowance for growth, plus an allowance for scandals', RAWP attempted to achieve a more rational distribution, based on demographic trends and on a calculation of levels of ill health from local death rates (Maynard and Ludbrook, 1980).

Though RAWP achieved a more equitable distribution of resources, the fact that it did so in the context of an overall squeeze on health service spending meant that it was experienced as a 'levelling-down' operation rather than as a progressive initiative. It was inevitably fiercely resented in London, which bore the brunt of the cuts, leaving a legacy of problems which remained unresolved until the early 1990s, when a major inquiry under Sir Bernard Tomlinson was set up to deal with the problems of health care in the capital.

Critics noted two further limitations of the RAWP formula: 'First, it only purported to measure *relative* need. It was designed to achieve distributional fairness only and had nothing to say about the adequacy of the allocations that resulted. Second, it only covered expenditure on hospital community services, not primary care' (Klein *et al.*, 1996, p.45). Much subsequent debate centred on the details of the formula and there were various attempts to refine and improve it (Sheldon and Carr-Hill, 1991). Though, as Klein observes, this became 'an increasingly arcane dialogue among statisticians and other methodological experts', it nevertheless marked a significant shift towards a rational and explicit mechanism for distributing – and rationing – health service spending.

Perhaps surprisingly, there was little further discussion of rationing during Mrs Thatcher's first two terms as prime minister from 1979 to 1987. Despite all the 'New Right' rhetoric about rolling back the welfare state, unleashing market

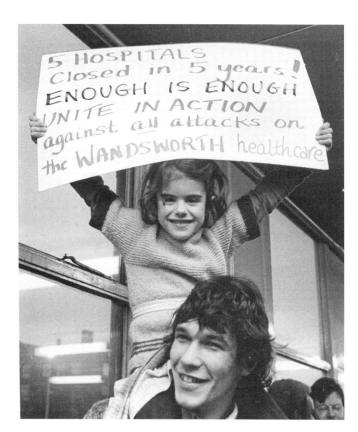

5 HOSPITALS
Closed in 5 years!
ENOUGH IS ENOUGH
UNITE IN ACTION
against all attacks on
the WANDSWORTH healthcare

Campaigning against hospital closures: protests against the consequences of health spending cuts became commonplace in the late 1970s, especially in London

forces and overturning bureaucracy, the NHS at the end of the 1980s appeared remarkably similar to the structure that the Conservatives had inherited a decade earlier (Le Grand, 1990). The Thatcher governments certainly maintained Labour's policy of tight budgetary control, particularly concentrating on squeezing the pay and conditions of ancillary workers through opening up their jobs to 'compulsory competitive tendering' and curtailing the role of the unions. But Mrs Thatcher's most dramatic gesture – the importation of Roy Griffiths from J.Sainsbury with the task of effecting a managerial revolution in the health service – was widely considered to be ineffective (Hunter, 1994; Mohan, 1995, Ch. 6). Griffiths did provoke antagonism, but failed to breach the structure of autonomous medical power.

It was not until her third term of office (which was ended prematurely by the Conservative Party revolt which brought John Major to power in November 1990) that Mrs Thatcher made a real impact on the health service. The 1989 White Paper, *Working for Patients*, recommended the creation of an 'internal market' in the health service by separating the purchasing function of health authorities from the provision of services by hospitals and GPs. It proposed that hospitals should become self-governing trusts, from which health authorities and GPs could purchase services. And it proposed that GPs should be allocated their own budgets, with which they could purchase services from hospital trusts on behalf of their patients. Despite fierce resistance from the British Medical Association and others, these proposals were implemented in full in April 1991.

One consequence of the reforms was to 'lift the veils from rationing', even if ministers still preferred to talk about 'priority-setting' (Klein *et al.*, 1996, p.66).

internal market

The key development was that resources were now allocated by health authorities ('purchasers') according to their assessment of the health care needs of the local population, rather than by hospitals ('providers'), according to the dictates of the doctors. For the first time – in the jargon of the reform process – health care purchasing was 'population-driven' rather than 'provider-driven' (Klein *et al.*, 1996, p.50). Again for the first time, the process through which resources were allocated was explicit and transparent as health authorities were obliged to publish their spending plans each year.

The introduction of the internal market in health care carried one major advantage for the government. Ever since the public expenditure crisis of the 1970s and the various ensuing initiatives by central government to curb spending on health care, central government had inevitably got the blame for the defects of the health service, while local hospitals – and the medical profession – could continue to take the credit for the achievements of the health service and enjoy public approval.

The effect of the internal market, however, was to 'centralize credit and diffuse blame'. Now the government could declare its broad reforming vision for the health service and stand aloof from the day-to-day failures of the service. When people now complained that, after waiting for several hours to see a doctor in casualty, they were then forced to spend several more hours languishing on a trolley before being admitted, the health minister could happily shrug and refer them to the complaints procedure of their local trust hospital. If hospitals were now forced to close or merge, as in London, the blame fell on the local management rather than on the government. Now that everybody accepted that the market offered the most effective mechanism for administering the health service, nobody could complain – at least not to the government – if they objected to particular consequences of its operation.

4.2 The crisis of rising expectations

While economic constraints on public spending dictated a squeeze on the supply of resources for the NHS, a number of factors contributed to a rising demand for health care. These included the growing proportion of old people in the UK, the increasing availability of high-cost new technologies and the replacement of traditional deference by a consumer consciousness fostered by the market reforms.

4.2.1 The 'demographic timebomb'

Discussion of the 'greying' of society as a potential problem, leading to a growing burden on welfare services, gathered momentum throughout the West in the 1980s (see Chapter 1). From the 1960s onwards there was a significant decline in death rates at all ages in the UK, but especially in older age groups. The combination of declining mortality in those aged over 60 and a low and declining birth rate meant a steadily ageing society – and the expectation of a steadily increasing demand for health care (Moon and Gillespie, eds, 1995, pp.36–7). In 1983 the Health Advisory Service raised the spectre of a 'rising tide' of dementia which could 'overwhelm the entire health care system' (Health Advisory Service, 1983).

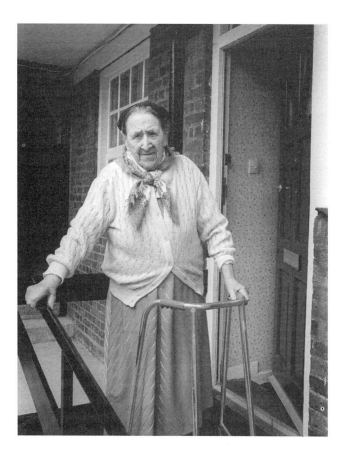

No longer simply an old person in need of help, now a member of a generation increasingly regarded as an unsustainable burden on welfare services

The identification of older people as a growing problem for the health service was reinforced by surveys confirming the increased prevalence of both chronic ill-health and acute illness among older age groups (Moon and Gillespie, 1995, pp.37–8). Furthermore, inquiries into consultation rates in general practice revealed that those over 65 visited their doctors on average six times a year, compared with four times for people aged between 16 and 44 and three for those between 5 and 15. The depiction of the UK as a nation whose future was threatened by an explosive increase of frail, elderly citizens was complete.

The notion of the 'demographic timebomb' did not go unchallenged (see Chapter 1). According to Wilson (1991), most old people remain healthy and independent before succumbing to a brief terminal illness. Hills (1993, pp.12–13) calculated that, even accepting long-term population projections as accurate, an increase in welfare spending at the rate of 0.32 per cent a year for the next half century would be adequate. Furthermore, he showed that in terms of projected shifts in the support ratio, the UK is in a favourable position compared with other European countries, notably Germany. Other international comparisons illustrated a lack of correlation between ageing and health care costs (Wordsworth *et al.*, 1996, pp.8–9).

4.2.2 The technological imperative

A survey of technological advances leading to 'cost-push' in the NHS in 1996 considered four areas of innovation (Wordsworth *et al.*, 1996, pp.11–13):

- *Telemedicine* allowed specialists to use advanced diagnostic techniques and to advise on treatment – even to supervise surgical procedures – from a distant location.

- The *miniaturization* of surgical and diagnostic instruments allowed 'minimally invasive' operations ('keyhole surgery') for hernias and gall bladder removal, and investigations such as twenty-four-hour ECG or blood pressure monitoring, to be conducted routinely.

- *New drugs* promised significant benefits in previously intractable conditions: interferon for multiple sclerosis and chronic hepatitis C, streptokinase for heart attacks, combination chemotherapy for people with HIV/Aids. However, these drugs were invariably expensive and the benefits controversial.

- *Genetic screening*, based on applying some of the breakthroughs of the human genome project, promised major advances in the prevention and treatment of inherited diseases – but these also raised difficult ethical as well as economic issues.

Acknowledging the complexity of calculating the impact of new technology on health service costs, Wordsworth and her colleagues made no attempt to quantify the financial consequences of the advances in these four areas. Indeed, their discussion of day-case and minimal-access surgery revealed how difficult it was to balance the costs against the savings, and how the balance may look different from different vantage points:

> It is not clear that, as a substitute for in-patient care, day surgery actually leads to costs savings as such. It can be argued that day surgery leads to patients being in hospital during the more intensive period of care, when the operation or the procedure takes place … If length of stay is shortened because of day surgery, only some treatment costs (such as drugs) and 'hotel' costs are saved, and, overall, costs may rise as more patients are treated in a given time period. Purchasers may perceive day case care as cost increasing whilst providers may see it as an opportunity to treat more patients.
>
> (Wordsworth *et al.*, 1996, p.15)

The matter may look different again from the perspective of the patient. Somebody who is quite fit, with a comfortable home, few domestic pressures and high levels of support will welcome day surgery. On the other hand, somebody who enjoys none of these advantages may well prefer to stay a few days in hospital.

Some commentators took a gloomy view of the financial impact of new technology on the NHS (Healthcare 2000, 1995). One frequently quoted illustration of the scale of the threat was the estimate that the cost of treating all suitable cases of multiple sclerosis with interferon – at £10,000 per head per year – would add some 10 per cent to the national drug bill (Walley and Barton, 1995). Others were more sanguine, pointing out that not all innovations are costly and that many save resources. Mayston (1996) pointed to the widening role of 'the humble aspirin' in the prevention of heart attacks and strokes, to the savings on expensive anti-ulcer drugs resulting from the (relatively cheap) treatment of Helicobacter pylori stomach infections and to the prevention or premature labour which otherwise results in very costly premature babies.

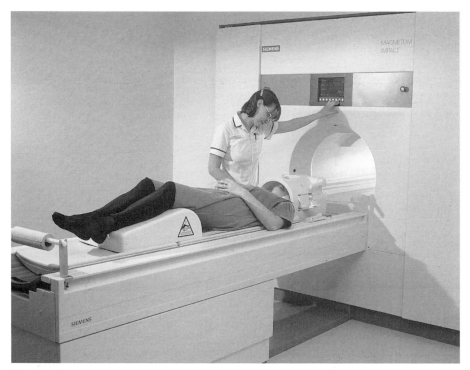

Magnetic Resonance Imaging (MRI): new techniques of visualizing internal organs improve diagnostic accuracy – but at escalating costs

4.2.3 'Customers first'

In retrospect, it is perhaps surprising that the National Health Service enjoyed such high prestige in the immediate post-war decades. As late as 1979 surveys carried out for the Royal Commission on the health service confirmed high levels of satisfaction, though there were criticisms of delays in hospital out-patient appointments and about the early hour at which in-patients were woken up. Yet by any objective standard many aspects of the service were deficient. Hospital buildings were often ramshackle conglomerations of Victorian brickwork and post-war prefabrication, ruled by an elite of consultants experienced by many patients as autocratic and paternalistic. Health centres – promised to GPs as the main incentive to join the NHS in 1948 – failed to appear until the 1970s, leaving many GPs to practise in poor premises, without adequate training, support staff or facilities. The continuing popularity of the NHS was widely regarded as a tribute to the dedication of its staff and the quality of care provided to its patients. It could also be interpreted as evidence of public deference to the medical profession and of low expectations of the health care system.

One of the major sources of the growing pressure on the NHS from the mid 1970s onwards was the breakdown of traditional deference to professional status. Doctors and other health service workers had to deal with 'a better educated, better informed and less acquiescent citizenry' (New and Le Grand, 1996, p.9). The growth in popular demands and expectations was encouraged by the challenge to state paternalism initiated by the Conservative government's promotion of the values of commercialism and consumerism in the NHS in the 1980s and 1990s.

While the Griffiths initiative of 1983 may have made little headway in imposing managerial authority over the doctors, the language of mission statements, 'total quality management', customer relations and satisfaction surveys rapidly permeated the health service. This process was accelerated by the internal market reforms of the early 1990s and by the closely linked Patients' Charter of 1991 which codified existing rights and added more, such as the right to information about local services, the right to hospital admission within two years and the right to complain.

The result was that 'patients' were replaced by 'customers', 'increasingly assertive about what they expect from the NHS and anxious to know why they are not getting it' (New and Le Grand, 1996, p.9). Whereas patients were passive recipients of the expertise and beneficence of state professionals, customers were active agents of their own self-interest, demanding information, choice and quality. Furthermore, they were ready to criticize and complain, even to sue, if they did not get the treatment to which they believed they were entitled.

consumer consciousness Though it is impossible to quantify the effects of rising consumer consciousness in relation to the NHS, there were a number of indicators of a resulting increase in demand for health care services in the early 1990s. Across the country there was a sharp increase in attendances at hospital accident and emergency departments and of resulting hospital admissions; the number of requests for 'out-of-hours' home visits by GPs rocketed, precipitating a crisis in the system. In 1996 the government introduced measures to subsidize local co-operatives and late-night 'primary care centres' as devices for managing the increased workload. Despite an NHS executive to devolve the handling of complaints against GPs to surgery level, both local health authorities and the General Medical Council reported a steady increase in complaints. The growing threat of litigation was reflected in the rapid rise in doctors' subscriptions to medical defence organizations (*British Medical Journal*, 1 February 1997, p.326).

What brought rationing out into the open?

5   Rational rationing

By the mid 1990s the conflict between the rising demand for health care from below and the pressure from above to curtail public spending on health had reached such a pitch that it pushed the debate about rationing onto the public agenda. We can now turn to examine some of the methods proposed to reconcile the conflict over health care priorities.

5.1   Rationing by exclusion

The simplest method of rationing any resource is to appoint a strict doorkeeper instructed to turn away certain people from any form of NHS treatment and others from specific treatments. People in the following categories have, in different ways, been denied access to health care resources:

1   *Foreign nationals and migrant workers (by immigration legislation)*
     New legislation on immigration and nationality in the 1980s restricted
     eligibility to NHS treatment to visitors and migrant workers. As a result many

people who might previously have gained access to NHS resources were obliged to go without or go into the private sector.

2   *Old people (by local treatment guidelines)*
The exclusion of old people – in the past from eligibility for renal dialysis, and more recently from physiotherapy services and from emergency services – has been more controversial. Yet there is a widespread feeling that such discrimination is widely implemented, but in such a discreet and informal way that it attracts little attention.

3   *Poor people (by charges)*
The effect of charges – for prescriptions, dental and ophthalmological treatment – has long been recognized to have a deterrent effect. In areas where charges amounted to substantial sums of money – as, for example, in treatments for infertility – they have effectively denied access to treatments for a substantial section of the population.

4   *The undeserving (smokers, people with alcohol or drugs problems)*
The intrusion of issues of moral worthiness into the rationing debate has inevitably proved highly controversial. The eligibility of smokers for coronary artery by-pass grafts, for surgical treatment of peripheral vascular disease or, indeed, for other forms of treatment for their 'self-inflicted' diseases was hotly debated in the medical and lay press over the cases of Harry Elphick (see section 2 above) and others. The discussion rapidly widened to include matters such as liver transplants for alcoholics – or for those whose liver failure followed deliberate ingestion of drugs, for either recreational purposes or suicide.

ACTIVITY 2.3

Tiny Tim versus Scrooge. The unrepentant, militant smoker versus the ex-smoker who succeeded in giving up after an immense personal struggle. The Nobel-prize winner versus the serial killer. Those who have been waiting a long time for treatment versus those who have only recently acquired the need.

(New and Le Grand, 1996, p.61)

According to New and Le Grand, who set out the above choices, 'in each case it is not difficult to think of more or less convincing arguments that could be put forward favouring one over the other in the allocation of medical care, quite independently of cost-effectiveness.'

Write down your arguments for each of the above choices. Which do you find convincing? Do you think this is a legitimate way to ration health care resources?

COMMENT

Most commentators would endorse the conclusion of New and Le Grand (1996, p.63) that 'in general, we are unsympathetic to the view that patient characteristics unrelated to need should be incorporated into rationing decisions whoever is making the relevant decision.' They reject both measures which discriminate against the already disadvantaged and those which seek to discriminate in favour of those who are deemed disadvantaged or otherwise deserving, advancing three 'reasons of principle'. These are: that most of the moral arguments are contested and difficult to apply in practice; that (in relation to attempts at 'positive discrimination') it is inappropriate to use the NHS to correct wider social ills; and that, as a long-established institution, the NHS has always provided treatment according to need. They provide an additional 'pragmatic' argument against rationing by just deserts: that the doctors, who still make most of the key decisions, have 'neither the skills, nor always the information necessary to make the kinds of fine discriminatory judgements that would be necessary' (New and Le Grand, 1996, p.64).

■ ■ ■

The main effect of the debate about rationing by exclusion appears to have been to raise the public profile of the issue, and to put rationing on the agenda. While the mean doorkeeper made everybody aware of the problem, his methods of discrimination were too crude and his manner too heavy-handed to offer a satisfactory solution. That required somebody on the inside.

5.2 Rationing by restriction

If it is considered unethical or impracticable to exclude certain people from access to resources, then the next logical step is to restrict the services available to any particular individual. Everybody is allowed in, but they can only have a set menu. There are two broad ways in which the NHS can restrict its menu:

■ it can decide that particular services are *inappropriate,* suggesting that the customer seeks them elsewhere;

■ it can decide that particular treatments are *ineffective* and refuse to provide them (or relatively ineffective and discourage them).

The most important area which the NHS has sought to define as inappropriate is that of long-term residential care for old people and dependent groups. Health authorities have tried to distinguish between continuing medical care and treatment (considered an appropriate deployment of NHS resources) and basic residential care (for which it has referred people to the local authority social services department). In a similar way, the wider development of the policy of community care has transferred many people with mental illness and learning difficulties from long-stay NHS hospitals into various community facilities.

The attempt to redefine the boundary between health and community care has inevitably provoked conflict between health authorities and local social services departments, which have not received adequate additional resources to take up the burden passed on from the hospitals. There has also been a number of cases in which individuals have taken legal action on behalf of family members to compel health authorities to finance continuing residential care.

menu   Some health authorities have also tried to restrict their menu by drawing up lists of treatments they consider an inappropriate use of NHS resources. Top of the list is usually tattoo removal, which is considered a cosmetic treatment of a self-inflicted disfigurement. This is often followed by other cosmetic procedures concerned with enhancing appearance (such as breast reduction or enhancement) as distinct from reconstructive surgery following burns, trauma or removal of malignancy. Gender reassignment surgery is another common exclusion. Treatments for infertility, such as reversal of sterilization or IVF, and, more recently, treatments for fertility, such as vasectomy and female sterilization, have also been restricted. The authorities generally justify excluding these procedures on the grounds that, though the goals of treatment may be desirable to the individual concerned, they are not essential to health, which should be the sole concern of the NHS. They argue that if people wish to pursue these goals, they should do so at their own expense, in the private sector. Furthermore, they cite the results of various surveys and consultation exercises which reveal high levels of public approval for exclusions along these lines.

In addition to excluding treatments deemed inappropriate, the custodians of health service resources have also attempted to push treatments considered ineffective off the NHS menu. This strategy follows the model of one of the most successful rationing initiatives in the NHS – the 'black list' of drugs that could no longer be issued on an NHS prescription. First introduced in 1984, it provoked protests from the pharmaceutical lobby but only muted resistance from doctors, because very few of the tonics and potions and linctuses on the list could be defended from the perspective of rational therapeutics. The list was subsequently extended at regular intervals. The attempt to exclude surgical treatments proved more controversial. This initiative drew authority from surveys revealing dramatic regional variations in the rates at which various operations are performed, which could only be explained by the proclivities of particular surgeons. Furthermore, other research raised questions about the efficacy of time-honoured procedures, such as, for example, the insertion of grommets for glue ear in children and the treatment with dilatation and curettage (D&C) of menstrual disorders in women. Drawing these findings together, some authorities opted to exclude such operations from the NHS menu.

The strategy of excluding specific treatments had, however, only a limited impact. Though launched by some authorities with a fanfare in the early 1990s, the list of excluded procedures remained fairly short, as did the number of authorities imposing rationing in this way (Klein *et al.*, 1996, pp.68–73). One problem was that the number of procedures that could be clearly designated as an inappropriate use of NHS resources was small and hence the financial impact was marginal.

Furthermore, while surveys revealed a majority of the public in favour of such measures, the individuals whose aspirations for NHS treatment were frustrated not surprisingly took a different view. Some even took legal action to compel health authorities to finance particular treatments, such as IVF. Nor were doctors happy with measures which restricted their clinical autonomy:

> Doctors were quick to point out that the case for carrying out specific procedures depended on the particular circumstances of individual patients; that even tattoo removal or gender reassignment could be justified if it meant that the person concerned could, as a result, be enabled to lead a normal life.
>
> (Klein *et al.*, 1996, p.71)

The attempt to rule out surgical procedures judged ineffective raised further difficulties. A survey may reveal that only 30 per cent of patients benefit from a particular operation, leading a health authority to conclude that this is not an effective deployment of resources. On the other hand, any particular individual might calculate that, taking all factors into account, a 30 per cent chance of significant benefit is a chance worth taking. As New and Le Grand (1996, p.37) point out, 'procedures which are ineffective for most people may be effective for a few, and this means that the number of procedures which could be excluded altogether, on the basis that they do *no good to anyone,* is likely to be very small in practice.'

As Klein *et al.* (1996, p.71) conclude, 'outright, explicit denial risked provoking opposition, not only from potential beneficiaries, but (much more importantly) from the medical profession'. As a result many authorities turned away from trying to impose a set menu on their customers to playing the role of *maître d'* and providing them (or at least, their doctors) with discreet **guidelines** recommendations, in the form of clinical guidelines. Instead of banning particular treatments, this approach sought to place them in some sort of order of priority, based on objective criteria of effectiveness. The authorities then attempted, mainly through consultation with doctors, to encourage certain treatment and to discourage others. This approach, which was also pursued in countries such as New Zealand and the Netherlands, promised a much wider scope of application than that of simple restrictions on the menu.

Some commentators, such as New and Le Grand (1996, pp.55–67), rejected the strategy of rationing by restricting the menu in favour of a system which sought to allocate resources according to doctors' assessment of clinical need. In clarifying this approach they distinguished between the allocation of resources according to 'health deficit' and according to 'capacity to benefit'.

1   *Health deficit*
    The most familiar example of the first is the notion that the iller the patient, the more resources they should receive: taken to its conclusion this implies **rescue** the 'rescue principle', that no resource should be spared in the attempt to **principle** save life. It also implies an egalitarian principle, that those in the poorest state of health should receive more care to bring them up to the level of the **health deficit** fittest. The concept of 'health deficit' immediately raises the question of how this deficit is defined, and by whom. Another major problem with this approach can already be seen in the major investment of resources in people who are terminally ill with no realistic prospect of recovery.

2   *Capacity to benefit*
    An alternative approach is to concentrate resources on patients in whom they are likely to have the greatest effect. Often patients who are most seriously ill are those who respond most successfully to appropriate treatment. In such cases rationing according to degree of illness will have the same effect as rationing according to effectiveness. However, in cases where treatment at an earlier stage in a disease is more effective, the principle **capacity to** of allocating resources according to capacity to benefit would favour such **benefit** a patient over one at a later stage whose health deficit is likely to be greater. Cost is another consideration: 'what if, as seems plausible, the more *ill* patients are, the more expensive they are to treat? What if the more *responsive* patients are more expensive to treat?' (New and Le Grand, 1996, p.58). Considerations of cost and effectiveness are brought together in attempts to measure the relative cost-effectiveness of treatment through indicators like QALYs (in section 5.3 below).

Methods of priority-setting or establishing guidelines escaped the problem of declaring explicit bans, but did not resolve the difficulty of making hard choices: they often blurred the boundaries rather than clarifying them. As a result they often also failed to avoid the problems of political controversy and professional resistance that dogged the more explicit approach. Furthermore, all such methods inevitably placed great pressure on the techniques for measuring effectiveness. This is shown in the examples given in the two articles below.

Hospital in cash crisis bars many elderly

David Brindle, Social Services Correspondent

A HOSPITAL has closed its doors to emergency patients over the age of 75 from half its local area in an attempt to survive a 'crisis' in its services.

Hillingdon hospital, in west London, has told family doctors in north Hillingdon that it cannot accept emergency referrals of elderly patients.

The move is the most drastic measure taken in the health service as hospitals prepare for what is widely predicted to be a difficult winter. Doctors are increasingly alarmed.

Dr Mitch Garsin, who chairs the Hillingdon local medical committee, representing the area's general practitioners, said: 'It's looking as though this is going to be an extremely bad winter for Hillingdon, as GPs try to get their patients into beds.'

The development comes days after leaders of Britain's medical consultants warned of hospital services coming 'close to collapse'. The Prime Minister promised to continue above-inflation NHS funding rises, but offered no extra money this year.

Hillingdon hospital trust says its ability to provide acute care has been hit by soaring demand and difficulty in discharging elderly patients.

Hospitals cannot send patients home until social services departments have assessed their needs and arranged services. The problem has been compounded, the letter says, by the unexpectedly high number of admissions of elderly patients from north Hillingdon.

Mount Vernon hospital, in Northwood, helps serve north Hillingdon, but lost its full-scale casualty department in April. Hillingdon hospital says that although this should not have affected elderly care services, it has since been admitting elderly patients from the northern area in 'disproportionately high numbers'.

Philip Brown, the trust's chief executive, said in the letter these were the patients who took the longest to discharge due to the crisis in social services funding putting a huge strain on the rest of the services.

The hospital stopped accepting GP referrals last Tuesday for emergency admission of patients aged over 75 resident in Ruislip, Eastcote, Northwood and Harefield.

Many elderly patients are clinically ready for discharge but awaiting community care arrangements. Mr Brown told the Guardian that 30–35 of his hospital's 300 acute beds were blocked in this way.

The rate of discharges cleared by social services had been almost four times as great last year as now, Mr Brown said:

'We are talking to both social services and the health authority about how we can deal with this situation of acute beds being unavailable to support our accident and emergency department.'

The partial bar on over-75s was regretted and would be lifted as soon as possible. Meanwhile, 'if somebody arrives at our door, we are certainly not going to turn them away'.

The hospital's move has brought an angry response from Hillingdon social services, which claims the community care issue is being used as a smokescreen for NHS problems. Dawn Warwick, acting social services director, said: 'We refuse to be blamed for the difficulties Hillingdon hospital finds itself in.' The real issues were the closure of Mount Vernon's accident and emergency department and a cut in hospital bed numbers.

She said that to ease the difficulties, social services had last week opened extra beds in residential homes and arranged the discharge of seven elderly patients 'over and above our usual quota'.

David Panter, chief executive of Hillingdon health authority, said: 'We are obviously unhappy about the situation, but we understand the pressures on the hospital. We cannot stress too much that we are trying to solve the problems.'

(The Guardian, *14 October 1996, p.3*)

Authority rules out vasectomy ops on NHS

Chris Mihill
Medical Correspondent

VASECTOMIES on the NHS have been ruled out by a health authority in its efforts to make savings.

West Surrey health authority, which faces a deficit of more than £11 million, has cut out the operation in a package of measures to save around £1 million. Vasectomies would be considered 'in rare circumstances if a special case could be made'.

It has called for a 60 per cent reduction in a number of other operations, including those to drain the middle ear – a common condition in children – and tonsils and adenoids, haemorrhoids and varicose veins operations.

Circumcisions, hysterectomies and D and C scrapes for gynaecological problems including terminations, are to be carried out less frequently.

West Surrey plans to spend about £541,000 less on the procedures at its four main hospitals and has asked fund-holding GPs to save about £522,000 on the operations.

It says it wants equitable access for all patients but told family doctors in a letter: 'It is recognized that reducing the amount of activity could lead to longer waiting lists in future years and generate more problems later on.'

It is to issue guidelines on those patients who should get priority for the operations, but 'for vasectomies, the decision is not to purchase any on the NHS,' it said. They cost about £150 at a private clinic.

The cutback list was agreed after discussions with fund-holding GPs, but others have complained that patient health is being jeopardised, particularly that of children needing ear operations.

One GP said: 'Middle ear conditions affect hearing. It's all right for parents with medical insurance who can have the operations done privately, but it means most children will have to wait longer [and] their education will suffer.'

Other health authorities have ordered that elective surgery, such as hip replacements, be performed less frequently, with some budgeting to treat only emergency cases.

The Government has tacitly accepted that waiting lists will lengthen as a consequence of this winter's funding crisis. Stephen Dorrell, the Health Secretary, used evidence of the problem to secure an extra £500 million for the NHS in the Budget.

Many authorities refuse to fund fertility treatment such as in vitro fertilisation, and others have banned 'minor' procedures such as varicose vein or tattoo removal.

● East London and City health authority, which has to save £18 million in the next financial year, is to cut £215,000 from grants to an Aids hospice and a centre for disturbed children, among other spending cuts.

It plans to save £1 million by reducing inappropriate hospital admissions and the time spent in hospital for some cases, and £1.5 million by treating patients locally rather than allowing them to be sent outside the district for operations.

It is to save £280,000 on complementary therapies and some forms of plastic surgery; £2.7 million by ending one-off grants to various bodies, including some voluntary sector services; and £1.5 million by letting waiting lists get longer.

(The Guardian, *27 November 1996, p.12*)

What are the problems of rationing by exclusion or restriction?

5.3   Measuring effectiveness

For any system of rationing health care, the question of the effectiveness of different treatments is of central importance. If resources are being deployed on medications and operations that do not work, then the first step towards rational rationing would be to curtail such spending. If it were clear which medical interventions were more effective than others, then decisions about where to concentrate resources (and where to economize on them) could be made in a way that was both more logical and more open to professional evaluation and public scrutiny. However, the judgement of what is effective depends to a considerable extent on the perspective of the person making the judgement.

From the point of view of the individual, the measure of the effectiveness of any treatment is whether it produces the desired result in terms of relieving symptoms or curing disease. This may be evaluated in purely subjective terms – does the patient feel better? – or by some objective criterion specific to the condition and the treatment, such as whether a drug for diabetes achieves satisfactory control of blood sugar levels. Subjective judgements are, however, notoriously unreliable: remember the consistently high levels of symptom relief achieved by placebos. Further, what produces improvement in one person may not work in another.

In measuring the effectiveness of treatment on a wider scale, from the perspective of the collectivity of people having the same treatment for the same condition, the gold standard is the randomized controlled trial. This method was promoted as 'the key to a rational health service' in an influential book entitled *Effectiveness and Efficiency* by the epidemiologist Archie Cochrane:

randomized controlled trial

> The randomized controlled trial is an experimental design in which people are allocated to two groups at *random*, with one group receiving the new treatment that is being evaluated, and the other (the control group) receiving either no treatment, some inactive substance known as a *placebo*, or the old treatment for the condition. Random allocation should ensure that the two groups are the same in all respects, except for the fact that only one group is receiving the new treatment. Thus any differences in outcomes for the two groups can be attributed to the new treatment rather than any characteristic of the people taking part.
>
> (Cochrane, 1971, p.77)

Randomized controlled trials have proven particularly fruitful in the evaluation of drugs, especially when they are 'double blind', that is when neither the patient nor the doctor knows who is receiving the drug under trial and who is receiving a placebo. However, extending this technique to the evaluation of more complex medical interventions – such as palliative care for the terminally ill – or to long-established treatments or preventive measures, has given rise to methodological and ethical controversies. In terms of the rationing debate, however, the biggest problem is that referred to above: how can the results of epidemiological studies of populations be applied to the treatment of individual patients?

The question of effectiveness acquires a different character when considered from the standpoint of somebody concerned with the allocation of NHS resources who is obliged to take the perspective of society as a whole. Such a perspective inevitably involves an economic aspect: funds allocated to one treatment cannot be spent on another. Its benefits must therefore be measured not only in terms of the improvement in one individual, but also set against the benefit forgone in treating somebody else, the *opportunity cost*. The focus shifts to comparing the increments of benefits yielded by resource allocation decisions: 'it is the value added by intervention – the gain in terms of harm prevented or an improved ability to function – that becomes the principle guiding rationing' (Klein *et al.*, 1996, p.31).

From the point of view of society, the key question is not so much whether a particular treatment is of benefit to a particular person, but whether the same quantity of resources could produce an even greater benefit if deployed on another treatment for another patient. As Smith (1996, p.1553–4) puts it, following a review of a number of effective but expensive treatments, 'the last drops of effectiveness are available at unaffordable costs, which means that decisions must be made to deny some people effective treatments.'

ACTIVITY 2.4

According to Williams (1992), 'anyone who says that no account should be taken of costs is really saying that no account should be paid to the sacrifices imposed on others.' This contradicts the traditional medical view that the doctor should treat the patient strictly on the grounds of clinical needs, regardless of the cost of treatment. What do you think? Is it unethical to ignore costs? Or, conversely, is it unethical to allow considerations of cost to influence treatment decisions?

COMMENT

Perhaps part of the problem here is the conflation of decisions about allocation of health care resources (political) with decisions about treating individual patients (medical). In the past, the politicians decided the framework of the health service spending and doctors worked within these limits. One of the consequences of making rationing more explicit is to encourage doctors to take responsibility for the distribution of resources as well as for treating patients.

quality-adjusted life year (QUALY)

The best known attempt to produce an objective index of the costs and benefits of medical intervention is the concept of quality-adjusted life years, or QALYs (St Leger *et al.*, 1992). The basic unit of the QALY is one year of healthy life expectancy achieved as a result of medical intervention. The predicted life expectancy (or years of benefit attributable to a particular procedure) is multiplied by an assessment of quality of life (on a scale from 0 to 1). The procedure is then costed and divided by the QALY rating to give the cost per QALY, which is taken as an objective indicator of its cost-effectiveness: see Table 2.3.

Table 2.3 Some costs per QALY at 1983–4 prices

Intervention/procedure	*Cost per QALY (£)*
Smoking cessation advice from GP	167
Hip replacement	750
GP control of hypertension	1700
Coronary artery bypass graft for moderate angina with three-vessel disease	2400
Hospital haemodialysis	14000

Source: Moon and Gillespie, 1995, p.223

The QALY is a simple tool for rationing: patients with low costs-per-QALY are given priority over those with higher ones. Concentrating resources on low costs-per-QALY patients frees more resources to treat more patients, thus achieving a higher aggregate health gain. It thus offers an efficient way of improving the health of society and is essentially equitable: it gives each year of life equal weight, regardless of who gets the benefit. It does tend, however, to discriminate against those who need very expensive treatments (who may or may not be very ill) and it may also discriminate against the poor, old people and people with disabilities (Le Grand, 1990, p.59).

The QALY has been subjected to extensive methodological and ethical criticism and attempts to apply it (see the case study of Oregon in section 5.4 below) have produced some highly idiosyncratic results. One set of problems surrounds the question of the quality of life following treatment: does this simply mean the absence of symptoms or suffering or should it have a more positive dimension? Who decides – and at what stage in time? Another is the lack of information about the outcome of particular treatments and the familiar problem of applying the results of population trials to individuals. How is it possible to distinguish between the effects of treatment on life expectancy and quality of life from the effects of other factors, such as an individual's social circumstances, mental state and other incidental influences?

While there have been numerous attempts to perfect the QALY or to devise an alternative index of effectiveness, the most important development in the application of science to rationing in health care in the course of the 1990s has been evidence-based medicine. This approach seeks to use information technology to link the results of research, particularly randomized controlled trials, systematically to the process of clinical decision-making in medical practice. According to Professor David Sackett and his colleagues (1996, p.71), 'evidence-based medicine is the conscientious, explicit and judicious use of current best evidence in making decisions about the care of individual patients.'

The method is described as having five steps:

1   A clear clinical question is formulated from the patient's presenting problem.
2   A literature search is carried out to identify relevant published articles which deal with the problem.
3   The evidence is accessed and evaluated (or critically appraised).
4   Valid and useful findings are implemented into clinical practice.
5   An audit of performance is carried out.

(Evidence Based Medicine Working Group, 1992)

According to one proponent, evidence-based medicine marks a significant advance in the more rational deployment of resources (Sweeney, 1996, p.61). It offers 'the possibility of greater efficiency by identifying which treatments or clinical approaches could be usefully incorporated into practice and which could be excluded.' As a consequence of this, 'improvements in the quality of decisions about purchasing could be made'. Within a short time, numerous treatment guidelines and protocols based on the techniques of evidence-based medicine began to circulate among hospital doctors and GPs, heralding for some a renaissance of scientific medicine.

Others were more sceptical of what one critic dubbed 'the new scientism' (see Extract 2.4). Many commentators have expressed cynicism about ministerial enthusiasm for evidence-based medicine as a device for legitimizing restrictions

evidence-based medicine

on expenditure on health care. Others have raised doubts about the extra bureaucracy required to generate information, disseminate guidelines and monitor compliance. Perhaps most importantly, the proponents of guideline-based purchasing 'may have paid insufficient attention to the uncertainty inherent in clinical practice, with the imposition of a spurious rationality on a sometimes inherently irrational process' (McKee and Clarke, 1995).

Within a few years in the mid 1990s, evidence-based medicine seemed to take the medical world by storm as a wave of books, journals and conferences promoted the new approach. One dissenting voice was that of Professor Rudolph Klein, director of the prestigious Centre for the Analysis of Social Policy at the University of Bath. In Extract 2.4 he outlines his case against what he calls 'the new scientism'.

Extract 2.4 Klein *et al.*: 'The case against the new scientism'

The case for the new scientism is, at first sight, overwhelmingly persuasive. If there is no evidence for the effectiveness of most forms of medical intervention, then it seems reasonable to assume that a great deal of money is being wasted on procedures and treatments that are not doing patients any good: a conclusion reinforced by the fact that there *is* evidence that many clinicians persevere with procedures and forms of treatment long after they have been demonstrated to be ineffective or inappropriate. Similarly, if there are large variations between doctors in the way they use resources, with little evidence that high rates of activity or use of resources lead to better health outcomes for patients, it again seems reasonable to assume that a great deal of money could be saved by bringing practice into line with what the more parsimonious clinicians are already doing.

The logic of this line of argument might even suggest that expenditure on the NHS, far from needing to be raised in order to accommodate the competing claims for extra resources, could be cut. For if demonstrable effectiveness, based on scientific evidence, is to be the only criterion for purchasing, if the onus of proof is to be on doctors to show that their interventions improve outcomes, then most of the existing services provided by the NHS would fail the test and could be scrapped. No wonder ministers and managers embraced the new faith with enthusiasm. For it appeared to offer them the prospect of less pain, less responsibility for taking difficult decisions and a legitimate way of curbing what were often perceived to be the idiosyncratic and extravagant practices of doctors.

Before leaping to this conclusion, however, it is important to recognize the limits, as well as the potentials, of the new scientism ... The new scientism offers great scope for improving the quality of medicine and health care but is not a philosopher's stone for converting scarcity into plenty.

In the first place, the new scientism is not the only source of authoritative knowledge. There is also the experiential knowledge of the medical profession. The point is well caught in the following quotation from the President of the Royal College of Surgeons, Sir Norman Browse, giving evidence to the House of Commons Health Committee (1995):

> There has never been a clinical trial on removing or not removing an acutely-inflamed appendix. You know of the complications which occur if you do not remove it; you know that it is the right thing to do. Just because there have not been double-blind, randomly allocated clinical trials of everything, that does not mean to say that the knowledge which has been accumulated since the Dark Ages finished in about 1415 does not mean anything. You

must not go away with this notion that we are all being ineffective, we do not know what we are doing or, for that matter, that we do not *look* at what we are doing and change if we find something is ineffective. [Browse, 1995, p.72]

Next, consider the notion of effectiveness, which tends to be used as though it were self-evidently unproblematic. This, on closer examination, turns out to be a slippery concept (Blustein and Marmor, 1992). The effectiveness of a medical intervention is a function of its outcome: hence, of course, the current emphasis on research to increase knowledge about outcomes. But rolling back the frontiers of ignorance, however desirable in itself, may turn out to be a Sisyphean task. Even randomized controlled trials (RCTs), which are often seen as the gold standard for evaluating medical innovations, may not be appropriate in all circumstances. Innovation is often a stepwise process, involving the modification of existing procedures over time, and it is not clear at what stage in the process evaluation should take place (Jennett, 1986). Outcomes may, furthermore, be contingent on their setting: the question may often be not how a given procedure works in its place of origin but how it would fare in different environments when applied on a mass production scale by practitioners who may be less skilled in the techniques concerned; the use of keyhole surgery provides a case in point. Lastly, the notion of outcomes is itself contestable (Carr-Hill, 1995). Over what time should outcomes be measured? And whose valuation of outcomes – those of the health care professionals or of patients – should be used? Moreover, the results of scientific trials may not be easy to interpret: at least one study (Fahey *et al.*, 1995) has shown how the way in which the evidence is presented may influence the conclusions drawn.

Assuming that such problems can be overcome – that science can indeed conquer ignorance – some forms of intervention will undoubtedly turn out to be demonstrably ineffective, in which case, of course, the waste involved in their use can be eliminated to the benefit of all (including the patients subjected to the treatment). Some mass screening programmes fall into this category (Russell, 1994). The history of medicine, it has been pointed out (McKee and Clarke, 1995), is full of treatments that were once popular but are now known to be valueless. But more often the evidence may well be more ambiguous and suggest that a given intervention is only selectively effective; that its effects are uncertain and contingent on the circumstances of individual patients. [...]

In the case of life-threatening conditions, moreover, patients may be willing to risk enduring treatment even though evidence of effectiveness may be lacking and the chances of success are extremely slim. They may feel, as in the case of child B [Jaymee Bowen] and of AIDS patients demanding drugs whose efficacy had not yet been demonstrated, that there is nothing to lose by gambling.

References

Blustein, J. and Marmor, T.R. (1992) 'Cutting waste by making rules: promises, pitfalls and realistic prospects', *University of Pennsylvania Law Review*, vol.140, no.5, pp.1543–72.

Browse, Sir N. (1995) Evidence to the House of Commons Health Committee First Report Session 1994–95, in *Priority Setting in the NHS: Purchasing. Vol. II Minutes of Evidence*, HC 134–II, London, HMSO.

Carr-Hill, R. (1995) 'Welcome? To the brave new world of evidence based medicine', *Social Science and Medicine*, vol.41, no.11, pp.1467–8.

Fahey, T., Griffiths, S. and Peters, T.J. (1995) 'Evidence based purchasing: understanding results of clinical trials and systematic reviews', *British Medical Journal*, vol.311, pp.1056–9.

Jennett, B. (1986) *High Technology Medicine: Benefits and Burdens*, Oxford, Oxford University Press.

McKee, M. and Clarke, A. (1995) 'Guidelines, enthusiasms, uncertainty and the limits to purchasing', *British Medical Journal*, vol.310, pp.101–4.

Russell, L.B. (1994) *Educated Guesses*, Berkeley, CA, University of California Press.

(Klein *et al.*, 1996, pp.103–6)

ACTIVITY 2.5

Draw up a list of Sackett's arguments in favour of evidence-based medicine and Klein's criticisms of the concept. Which do you find most convincing – and why?

COMMENT

Much of the controversy around evidence-based medicine may be a result of the application of an approach which is appropriate to a relatively small area of medical practice – for example, to non-urgent surgical procedures or newly introduced drugs – to wider areas of health care, such as routine general practice or care for the dying, where it is not appropriate. The danger of such promiscuous use of the approach is that its inevitable failure may induce a fatalistic attitude towards any attempt at rational rationing.

■ ■ ■

5.4   The Oregon experiment

The debate about rationing in the UK has been heavily influenced by the experience in other countries grappling with similar problems of controlling health care expenditure. As the first attempt at the explicit rationing of health care, the initiative taken in the state of Oregon in the US Northwest in the early 1990s has acquired a mythical status in the international debate about rationing (Klein *et al.*, 1996, p.109). The key features of the Oregon initiative, which was provoked by the crisis of existing system of providing health care for those without insurance, were the attempt to define a basic package of health care and the attempt to engage the public in the rationing process through an extensive consultation process. In Extract 2.5 Dr John Kitzhaber, a physician who, as president of the state senate, was the driving force behind the scheme, outlines its key features.

Extract 2.5 Kitzhaber: 'Prioritizing health services in an era of limits: the Oregon experience'

To answer the question of 'what is covered?' in Oregon, a Health Services Commission was created, consisting of five primary care physicians, a public health nurse, a social worker, and four consumers. The members were appointed by the governor and confirmed by the senate after public hearings. The commission was charged with developing a 'list of health services ranked in priority from the most important to the least important, according to the comparative benefits of each service to the entire population being served' and judged by a consideration of clinical effectiveness and social values.

To carry out the requirement to consider clinical effectiveness, the commission used medical 'condition-treatment pairs' gleaned from two widely recognised classifications of diagnosis and treatment, the Current Procedural Technology (the CPT–4 codes) and the International Classification of Diseases (the ICD–9 codes). Examples of condition-treatment pairs are appendicectomy for acute appendicitis, antibiotics for bacterial pneumonia, and bone marrow transplant for leukaemia. The initial list of nearly 3000 pairs was substantially reduced by combining those for which treatment and outcome were essentially the same …

The determination of clinical effectiveness was based on the input of panels of physicians, who were asked to provide certain clinical information about each condition-treatment pair in their areas of practice. Over 7000 hours of volunteer time was given by Oregon physicians to this effort. We recognise that much of this information represents a consensus by physicians rather than hard empirical outcomes data. None the less, it provided a snapshot on how medicine was currently being practised in Oregon and offered a starting point and a rational framework in which better information on outcomes could be integrated as it became available. It is also important to note that the prioritisation process is dynamic and ongoing. That is, a new priority list is generated each budget cycle to take into consideration new technologies and new information on outcomes.

In addition to considering clinical effectiveness, the commission set up a broad based public process to identify and attempt to integrate social values into the priority list. The statute specified that this public involvement take three forms. Firstly, the commission was required to 'actively solicit public involvement in a community meeting process to build a consensus on the values to be used to guide health resources allocation decisions'. Secondly, the commission was required to hold a series of public hearings around the state and to solicit 'testimony and information' from a full range of health care systems including all recognised advocacy groups for various populations and illnesses and all recognised health care providers. Finally, the legislation required that the Health Services Commission and all of its proceedings be subject to full public disclosure under Oregon's open meetings laws, which govern public bodies.

The Health Services Commission, aware of the importance of public involvement to the success of its work, went well beyond the outreach process required by the legislature. It immediately contacted the various health care interest groups in the state (especially advocates for the poor, the uninsured, and for consumers in general) and enlisted their assistance in generating public participation. By encouraging attendance at Health Service Commission meetings and hearings, and by soliciting testimony, we sought to ensure that the commission received input and information from the broadest possible citizen base. While it is clear that our initial efforts to involve a representative cross section of citizens can and must be improved, the level of public participation in the commission's work was unprecedented, even in a state that prides itself on open and accessible government.

To fulfil the legislative requirement for a community meeting process, the commission turned to Oregon Health Decisions, a grassroots bioethics organisation founded in 1983 by Ralph Crawshaw, a Portland psychiatrist, and Michael Garland, an ethicist at the Oregon Health Sciences University. Dedicated to educating Oregonians on the health policy choices confronting them and on the consequences of these choices, Oregon Health Decisions had been conducting community discussions on a variety of ethical issues for nearly 10 years. Under the auspices of this group the Health Services Commission organised the most extensive town hall meeting process ever conducted in the state. The initial objective was to have at least one town hall meeting in each of Oregon's 30 counties. Not only was that objective met but multiple sessions were conducted in more densely populated areas, bringing the total number of town hall meetings to 47.

After the meetings were completed, the results and opinions of the participants were tabulated and assembled into a report for use by the Health Services Commission and the legislature. The resulting document, *Health Care in Common*, was used extensively by the Health Services Commission in its deliberations and stands as an exceptional example of constructive activism by a dedicated group of citizens.

The first priority list, completed in February 1991, consists of 709 condition-treatment pairs divided into 17 categories. The priority of the categories is based on the commission's interpretation of the social values generated from the public involvement process. Within each category the ranking of the condition-treatment pairs reflects the benefit likely to result from each procedure and the duration of the benefit …

Services in the highest category were those for acute, fatal conditions where treatment prevents death and returns the individual to his or her previous health state (such as an appendicectomy for appendicitis) … Because of the high value placed on prevention by those participating in the community outreach process, the categories of maternity care (including prenatal, natal, and postpartum care) and of preventive care for children ranked very high. Also ranked high as a direct result of the outreach process were dental care and hospice care. At the bottom of the list were categories of services for minor conditions, futile care, and services that had little or no effect on health status.

The final priority list was given to an independent actuarial firm, which determined the cost of delivering each element on the list through capitated managed care. The list and its accompanying actuarial data were given to the legislature on 1 May 1991.

(Kitzhaber, 1993, pp.41–5)

ACTIVITY 2.6

Now consider whether the Oregon model is applicable to the UK. In doing so, you need to concentrate on three issues:

1   Is it relevant, given the differences in health care systems in the UK and the USA?

2   Is the QALY a valid index of need for health care, especially given some of the idiosyncratic results of its use in Oregon?

3   Does its consultation process confer legitimacy, especially when it emerges that 56 per cent of the 600 'citizens' who attended the key public meetings in Oregon were health care workers?

6   Democratic rationing

The NHS is about more than simply producing health; it acts as a mechanism, and a symbol, of reassurance and social stability.

(New and Le Grand, 1996, p.69)

Though the attempts to introduce more formal and explicit mechanisms of rationing health care resources up to the mid 1990s had, by general agreement, only marginal impact, they provoked intense public outrage and controversy. Unlike many health economists and doctors, New and Le Grand took a wider view of the historical standing of the NHS in UK society, recognizing its important contribution to what its founding father Aneurin Bevan described as the 'tranquillity' of the nation. Insisting that the NHS could not be reduced to a company marketing health, they warned the authorities of 'the danger of moving too fast' and emphasized the need to secure popular acquiescence to the more rational allocation of resources that they fully supported.

The very eruption of controversy around issues of rationing revealed the breakdown of the consensus of public approval for the NHS and deference to the medical profession that allowed doctors and administrators to make all the decisions without having to explain or account for them. At a time when people were demanding information, choice and quality, value for money and a high standard of customer care, the authorities were looking to cut costs and raise efficiency. Though doctors continued to enjoy high prestige in society, the fact that they had less power in the health service meant that their status did not so readily guarantee approval of new arrangements in hospitals or GPs' surgeries. The new managerial elite, by contrast, lacked legitimacy either inside or outside   **legitimacy** the health service. The result was that, in a climate of increasing austerity for public health care, the authorities had no alternative but to attempt to construct new links between the public and the health service, in ways that helped to make rationing more palatable.

A number of different mechanisms were proposed to involve the public in the process of allocating health care resources. These included public consultation exercises, a rights-based approach and the restoration of local democracy.

6.1   Public consultation exercises

We have already seen some examples of public consultation exercises in relation   **public** to issues of health care rationing: the public priorities survey conducted by the   **consultation** City and Hackney health authority and the series of public meetings held in Oregon. The media furores around cases like those of Harry Elphick and Jaymee Bowen could also be considered as another mode of public consultation. Indeed it was clear that these cases, and others, were self-consciously pushed into the public realm by doctors and health service managers keen to familiarize the public with issues of health care rationing. The effect of such exercises was to encourage the public to take a degree of responsibility for rationing and its consequences. Once everybody had their say, the public implicitly shared the burden of the decision with the authorities. Both the East London and the Oregon consultations revealed a substantial and, to some observers, an alarming gap between the attitudes of the public and those of health care professionals.

This was reinforced by a survey conducted by Christopher Heginbotham (1993, pp.141–56) in 1992 of more than 2000 members of the public on behalf of the BMA, *BMJ*, the Patients Association and the King's Fund. In Heginbotham's judgement, the public lacked information, and was unduly influenced by 'sheer prejudice' (notably against people with schizophrenia) and by media campaigns (such as for screening for breast cancer). He particularly warned the government of the strength of public approval of 'unlimited' funding for health care and concluded: 'A great deal more work is needed to ascertain the public's awareness about health care priority setting and to ensure that the public is given more information about costs and benefits of different treatments' (p.156). In Heginbotham's view the masses required some intensive tuition before they could be admitted to democratic participation in decisions about the allocation of health care resources.

Two more formal systems of consultation attempted to engage a more enlightened selection of the public: Community Health Councils and citizens' juries.

The *Community Health Councils* were formed as a mechanism for accommodating the upsurge of radical local criticisms of the health service in the mid 1970s. In the late 1970s they became in some areas a focal point of grass-roots resistance to the cuts and closures introduced by the Labour government. After the Conservative government came to power, the CHCs languished in official disapproval and faced repeated threats of abolition. However, in the early 1990s the CHCs underwent a dramatic change in fortunes as an official report entitled *Local Voices* discovered a new role for them in promoting local participation in the process of local 'needs assessment' and 'priority-setting' exercises.

Toby Harris, director of the national association of CHCs, acknowledged that 'the cynical might suggest that it serves the government's purpose if CHCs are implicated in controversial and potentially unpopular decisions' (1993, p.165). However, he argued, 'The responsibility for a decision is not automatically shared by consulting about it'. To which the cynic might reply, 'True, but it helps'. While expressing reluctance about rubber-stamping rationing, Harris welcomed the greater openness in the debate about the allocation of resources and anticipated a 'big role' for the CHCs in this process.

Citizens' juries was an initiative promoted by the Institute of Public Policy and Research, a think-tank loosely aligned to New Labour, and piloted by the Cambridge and Huntingdon health authority in 1996. Anna Coote, one of the leading protagonists of this approach, explained how it works:

> These juries involve small groups of citizens, selected to represent the general public rather than any interest groups, who take part in a fully informed and extended discussion to reach a decision on a specific question or set of questions. They take evidence from witnesses, whom they can cross-examine, and form smaller working groups to deal with particular problems. They deliberate on questions with the help of a moderator and are expected to draw conclusions but not to reach a unanimous verdict. The authority which commissions the jury is expected to publicize the findings and either follow the jury's guidance or explain publicly why it has chosen not to do so.
>
> (Coote, 1996, pp.184–5)

In Cambridge, for example, 16 jurors met over four days and covered three broad questions.

A more experimental approach, also promoted by IPPR, was *electronic democracy* which used new communications technologies to involve the public (Coote, 1996, p.185). Techniques ranged from radio phone-ins to interactive electronic town meetings using cable and computer networks.

6.2 A rights-based approach

Another IPPR initiative – the proposal to establish entitlement to health care as a right – aimed to replace the consumerist approach to health with one based on citizenship (Lenaghan, 1996). Lenaghan acknowledged that to 'earn the trust of the public' the NHS must have a 'rational, equitable and legitimate framework for the allocation of resources'. She rejected the notion of specifying 'substantive rights' to a core package of health care services (which would be rigid and costly), in favour of calling for 'procedural rights' to fair treatment (which would be flexible and cheap): 'If rights to health services are realistically defined, consensually based, broadly understood and consistently enforced, then they can help to mitigate uncertainty, build trust and promote the equitable distribution of resources' (Lenaghan, 1996, p.ii).

The codification of rights in this sense was part of a wider package of reforms to the health service, including the establishment of a national commission to draw up guidelines and codes of practice and citizens' juries as a device for democratic participation.

ACTIVITY 2.7

Which method of consultation do you think guarantees the most democratic process of rationing? Does the fact that the government only appeared to become interested in consultation when its main concern was with curbing public spending on health make you suspicious of these initiatives?

COMMENT

The IPPR's emphasis on procedural over substantive rights carries an unfortunate echo of Mr Major's 'Citizens' Charter' initiatives of the early 1990s (which included the Patients' Charter). These charters offered what appeared to many to be largely token entitlements in the sphere of public services at a time when the availability and quality of such services appeared to be in sharp decline. Though Lenaghan envisaged that the courts would be the last resort in terms of enforcing rights to health care, it was difficult to envisage how else citizens could impose their views in the (highly likely) event of a conflict over the allocation of resources.

■ ■ ■

6.3 A role for local government

Ever since the foundation of the health service, when Bevan established an administrative structure distinct from local government to allay medical fears of political interference, there has been a radical lobby for placing hospitals and surgeries under the control of local councils. Demands for such a reform gathered momentum during the 1980s in response to the replacement, under the auspices of Mrs Thatcher, of local government and labour movement representation on area health authorities, with government appointees of a quite different political complexion. The fact that, whatever the defects of local democracy, councillors were subject to the discipline of the ballot box, had always appealed to those who wished to see more openness and accountability in the administration of the health service. For some, the rise of the primary care team and the advent of locality commissioning (a collective form of GP fundholding) provided an added impetus to an enhanced role for local government in health.

Julian Tudor Hart pioneered a radical synthesis of traditional practice and modern preventive medicine in the valleys of South Wales. On his retirement he continued to campaign for what he considered to be the principles of a democratic and egalitarian health service. These are outlined in Extract 2.6.

Extract 2.6 Tudor Hart: 'Area commissioning and local government'

Strategies for health are a responsibility of government. Electors must choose whether they prefer governments assisted to power by the minorities which profitably sell tobacco, diesel engines, or superfluous medicines, or by the majority which unhealthily consumes them. Implementations of these strategies must depend on people with local knowledge and loyalties, in units that bring people who plan the job together with those who do the job; not forgetting that, as we have seen, the job is done by patients as well as by health professionals. We want planned production with workers' control, the workers including all who contribute to health gain.

Community representatives should be elected by local people, not selected by Ministers from their political networks, so that if they cease to represent the people, they can be got rid of. Where can these elected representatives of the people come from? Unlike Canada and the USA, we have no tradition of local directly elected school boards. We could have directly elected members of Health Boards, sharing in area commissioning of health services at all levels, but this would require invention of an entirely new category of elected local government. The parallel with school governing is apt. Except for parent-governors, local school governing boards are at present appointed, not elected. If there were good evidence of majority participation in elections for parent governors (now exceptional, at least in working class areas) encouraging serious plans for directly elected school boards, there would be a good case for directly elected health boards also. Both the NHS and schools are subjects of intense local interest, and good turnout of voters should be possible for both. However, unless this change occurs, elected local control would have to come from councillors selected (by their follow councillors) for their specific interest in the NHS, but originally elected for the general responsibilities of local government.

Local government responsibility has been opposed on two main grounds. The first is the weakness of local authorities, which have been in perceived decline ever since their heyday at the close of the nineteenth century. Since then central government has been enormously strengthened by changes in communication, and the experience of national mobilisation in two world wars. Fifteen years of Conservative government, steadily stripping out public responsibility for public service and replacing it by opportunities for profitable enterprise, have left councils which started with responsibility for schools, housing, and a wide range of other important local services, either without these functions entirely, or with just enough responsibility to make them credible scapegoats for inevitable failure. The real powers of local government have gone either to private entrepreneurs, or to the 73,000 or so centrally appointed nominees of quasi-non-governmental organizations (QUANGOs), more than twice the number of all elected councillors.

The second justification is the claim that any increase in responsibilities for local government must mean a reduction in responsibility for national government, and that the health service would therefore cease to have a uniform national character. Experience of previous nationally planned but locally applied strategies, for example the 1944 Education Act and the post-war Housing Acts, show that this need not be so. A clear and vigorous central strategy, understood by the mass of the people, not only can but must be applied tactically by local authorities, adapting central plans to local knowledge.

The only shred of support for the contrary view comes from Nye Bevan's unexpected decisions to nationalize all the hospitals in 1948, leaving them with only token elected local control, all of it now gone. As we have seen, this decision was overwhelmingly influenced by a perceived need to secure agreement from the consultants, without whom the NHS could not have gone forward at all. Though Bevan thought this a price worth paying, he never believed this undemocratic arrangement could be permanent, and it is totally irrelevant now.

(Tudor Hart, 1994, pp.96–7)

In parallel with the general demise of left politics in the 1990s, however, voices calling for a revival of local democracy became muted. In its discussion of this option in 1994, the IPPR questioned how democratic local councils now were and warned of the danger of losing the national character of the NHS (Harrison and Hunter, 1994). Most commentators recommended a greater role for some forum to institutionalize the rationing debate at national level, while remaining agnostic about the problem of local accountability (Klein *et al.*, 1996).

7   Conclusion: rationing and the social construction of need

The controversy over rationing health care in the 1990s provides an example of the social construction – indeed, reconstruction – of need in a major sphere of welfare. By making the question of need a public issue, the debate also helped to clarify the distinctive approach to defining and meeting health care needs in the earlier years of the health service. We can now distinguish three phases in the evolution of the health service's approach to need.

7.1   Need collectivized

The post-war NHS was promoted as an institution which met the needs of citizens – comprehensively and, at the point of use, free of charge. It was assumed that these needs were universal and could be met through familiar institutions, hospitals and GP surgeries. The quality of health care received in this way by virtually every individual and every family in the country lay at the heart of the 'social citizenship' which distinguished the post-war UK and ensured its stability. The nature and scale of health care needs was determined by doctors and other experts. The process through which resources were allocated to meet these needs was discreet and opaque.

7.2   Need pathologized

The breakdown from the 1970s onwards of the complex set of settlements upon which the post-war welfare state was based opened up the concept of need to a process of reconstruction. Need – in health as in other areas of welfare – was no longer regarded as an expression of the citizen's entitlement: it was increasingly represented as an unsustainable burden on the state. The drive to curtail public spending and the supply of resources for health care was accompanied by a tendency to discourage and disparage expressions of need. The perception of a deterioration of standards in a health service wracked by strife over cuts and closures, pay levels for nurses and other health workers, and doctors' contracts reflected a wider breakdown in the harmony of UK society.

Furthermore, determination of need by doctors and other professionals was challenged and the process through which decisions over resource allocation were made came into question. Though the structure of the health service remained remarkably stable for the first forty years of the NHS, by the late 1980s its underlying values were in an advanced state of decay.

7.3   Need commercialized

The reform of the health service in the 1990s through the introduction of the internal market and the other measures designed to unleash the spirits of enterprise and competition also accelerated the transformation in the concept of need. As we have seen in Chapter 1, the most significant long-term trend was for the responsibility for meeting welfare needs to shift away from the state onto individuals and families. Thus, while a growing proportion of wealthier people opted to secure their health care needs in the private sector, those who could not afford this were obliged to undergo a more rigorous assessment of need in the health service. Responding to the discipline of quasi-markets, doctors and managers, equipped with quasi-scientific techniques (from RAWP to QALYs to evidence-based medicine), imposed a more austere concept of health care need on the public.

Whereas in the traditional NHS the process of decision-making and resource allocation was opaque, in the reformed health service it was transparent. Mission statements were declared, charters were promulgated, league tables published, complaints procedures were drawn up. Yet though the customer was supposedly 'empowered' by these devices, the 'social citizen' of an earlier era might well conclude that he or she had been disenfranchised.

Further reading

Nicholas Timmins' *The Five Giants: A Biography of the Welfare State* provides an excellent overview of the post-war welfare state; it includes sections on the early days of the NHS as well as the reforms of the 1990s. Perhaps the most thorough treatment of the contemporary debate about rationing is *Managing Scarcity: Priority Setting and Rationing in the National Health Service* by Professor Rudolf Klein, one of the most eminent commentators on health care in the UK, and his colleagues.

Some of the most influential documents in the rationing debate are the pamphlets produced by think-tanks, such as the King's Fund or the Institute of Public Policy Research, or by professional organizations, like the British Medical Association. I would single out New and Le Grand's *Rationing in the NHS* (King's Fund), Harrison and Hunter's *Rationing Health Care* (IPPR) and Wordsworth, Donaldson and Scott's *Can We Afford the NHS?* (IPPR). One of the few comprehensive challenges to these broadly pro-rationing bodies comes from Peter Draper in *Myths about the NHS and Rationing Health Care*, published by the Health Policy Network.

References

BMJ (1993) *Rationing in Action*, London, BMJ Publishing Group.

Bowling, A. (1996) 'Health care rationing: the public's debate', *British Medical Journal*, vol.312, pp.670–674, 16 March.

Cochrane, A. (1971) *Effectiveness and Efficiency*, Abingdon, The Nuffield Provincial Hopsitals Trust.

Coote, A. (1996) 'The democratic deficit' in Mariner, M. (ed.) *Sense and Sensibility in Health Care*, London, BMJ.

Department of Health (1983) *NHS Management Inquiry* (The Griffiths Report), London, HMSO.

Donaldson, C. (1993) 'The economics of priority setting: let's ration rationally!' in *Rationing in Action*, London, BMJ Publishing Group.

Draper, P. (1995) *Myths about the NHS and Rationing Health Care*, Health Policy Network, Banbury, National Health Service Consultants' Association/London, NHS Support Federation.

Evidence Based Medicine Working Group (1992) 'Evidence-based medicine: a new approach to the teaching and practice of medicine', *Journal of the American Medical Association*, vol.268, pp.2420–5.

Ham, C. (1993) 'Rationing in action: priority setting in the NHS: reports from six districts', *British Medical Journal*, vol.307, 14 August.

Harris, T. (1993) 'Consulting the public' in *Rationing in Action*, London, BMJ Publishing Group.

Harrison, S. and Hunter, D. (1994) *Rationing Health Care*, London, Institute of Public Policy and Research.

Health Advisory Service (1983) *The Rising Tide: Developing Services for Mental Illness in Old Age*, London, HMSO.

Healthcare 2000 (1995) *UK Health and Health Care Services: Challenges and Policy Options*, London, Healthcare 2000.

Heginbotham, C. (1993) 'Health care priority-setting: a survey of doctors, managers and the general public' in *Rationing in Action*, London, BMJ Publishing Group.

Hills, J. (1993) *The Future of Welfare: A Guide to the Debate*, York, Joseph Rowntree Trust/LSE Welfare State Programme.

Hunter, D. (1994) 'Managerial challenge' in Gabe, J., Kelleher, D. and Williams, G. (eds) *Challenging Medicine*, London, Routledge.

Kitzhaber, J.A. (1993) 'Prioritising health services in an era of limits: the Oregon experience' in *Rationing in Action*, London, BMJ Publishing Group.

Klein, R., Day, P. and Redmayne, S. (1996) *Managing Scarcity: Priority Setting and Rationing in the National Health Service*, Buckingham, Open University Press.

Le Grand, J. (1990) 'The state of welfare' in Hills, J. (ed.) *The State of Welfare: The Welfare State in Britain since 1975*, Oxford, Oxford University Press.

Lenaghan, J. (1996) *Rationing and Rights in Health Care*, London, Institute of Public Policy and Research.

McKee, M. and Clarke, A. (1995) 'Guidelines, enthusiasms, uncertainty and the limits to purchasing', *British Medical Journal*, vol.310, pp.101–4.

Maynard, A. and Ludbrook, A. (1980) 'Budget allocation in the National Health Service', *Journal of Social Policy*, vol.9, pp.289–312.

Mayston, D. (1996) 'Capital and labour markets for health' in Culyer, A. J. and Wagstaff, A. (eds) *Reforming Health Care Systems: Experiments with the NHS*, London, Edward Elgar.

Ministry of Health (1956) *Report of the Committee of Enquiry into the Cost of the National Health Service*, (C.W. Guillebaud, chair), Cmd. 9663, London, HMSO.

Mohan, J. (1995) *A National Health Service? The Restructuring of Health Care in Britain since 1979*, London, Macmillan.

Moon, G. and Gillespie, R. (eds) (1995) *Society and Health: An Introduction to Social Science for Health Professionals*, London, Routledge.

New, B. and Le Grand, J. (1996) *Rationing in the NHS: Principles and Pragmatism*, London, King's Fund.

NHS Management Executive (1992) *Local Voices*, London, Department of Health.

Powell, J.E. (1976) *Medicine and Politics: 1975 and After* (new edn), Tunbridge Wells, Pitman Medical (first pub. as *A New Look at Medicine and Politics*, 1966).

Sackett, D. *et al.* (1996) 'Evidence-based medicine: what it is and what it isn't', *British Medical Journal*, vol.312, pp.71–2, 13 January.

Sheldon, T. and Carr-Hill, R. (1991) 'Measure for measure', *The Health Service Journal*, 1 August.

Smith, R. (1995) 'Rationing: the debate we have to have', *British Medical Journal*, vol.310, no.6981, p.686, 18 March.

Smith, R. (1996) 'Rationing health care: moving the debate forward', *British Medical Journal*, vol.312, pp.1553–4, 22 June.

St Leger, A.S., Shneiden, H. and Walsworth-Bell, J.P. (1992) *Evaluating Health Services' Effectiveness*, Buckingham, Open University Press.

Sweeney, K. (1996) 'Evidence and uncertainty' in Mariner, M. (ed.) *Sense and Sensibility in Health Care*, London, BMJ.

Timmins, N. (1995) *The Five Giants: A Biography of the Welfare State*, London, HarperCollins.

Tudor Hart, J. (1994) *Feasible Socialism: The NHS Past, Present and Future*, London, Socialist Health Association.

Walley, T. and Barton, S. (1995) 'A purchaser perspective of managing new drugs: interferon beta as a case study', *British Medical Journal*, vol.311, pp.796–9.

Williams, A. (1992) 'Cost-effectiveness: is it ethical?', *Journal of Medical Ethics*, vol.18, pp.7–11.

Williams, P. (1979) *Hugh Gaitskell: A Political Biography*, London, Jonathan Cape.

Wilson, G. (1991) 'Models of ageing and their relation to policy formation and service provision', *Policy and Politics*, vol.9, no.1, pp.37–47.

Wordsworth, S., Donaldson, C. and Scott, A. (1996) *Can We Afford the NHS?*, London, Institute of Public Policy and Research.

CHAPTER 3

Whose Needs, Whose Resources? Accessing Social Care

by Marian Barnes

Contents

`1   Introduction

Unlike social security, which is demand-led, and health care, which since the inception of the NHS has been a universal service, the provision of social care services has always been subject to implicit or explicit assessments of need. There has been a reluctance to establish legal rights to receive social care services, and access is dependent on the judgements of 'gatekeepers'. Although health care is not an individual right, and rationing has always been implicit in decisions about resource allocation, most people can comfortably live their lives assuming that if they get cancer, or if they are injured in a road accident, they will receive treatment without an assessment of their needs or circumstances. However, accessing social care services is rather different. Those seeking support from local authority social services departments have to be seen as 'needy' in order to gain access to a service. Hence they are also seen as objects of pity: 'the elderly', 'the disabled', 'the mentally ill' – people whose personal limitations mean that they are not able to look after themselves and thus need to be cared for (**Hughes, 1998**). They become constructed as members of 'client groups' with needs for support that cannot be met from within personal resources.

This chapter will consider the way in which 'need' is defined in the context of 'social care services'. These services comprise: those intended to assist with aspects of daily living, such as washing, dressing and shopping; services that are intended to provide some form of structured activity, such as day care; assistance with housing or transport; and 'respite care' within a residential unit in order to give family carers a break. The concept of social care is itself a matter of dispute, and this will be addressed during the course of the discussion.

Social care services are delivered within the context of community care policy, which has developed over the last 50 years. However, community care also embraces the way in which families and friends provide support to each other. Thus in order to explore the question of need in relation to social care it is important to look at official policy and at the responses of those whose lives are (sometimes profoundly) affected by this. In this chapter we shall consider:

- The origins of community care policy and the way in which the policy has come to be defined.
- The way in which 'needs' and 'care' have been interpreted in official policy statements, and how this has been implemented in practice by those with the power to assess need and determine whether services are to be provided.
- How carers have articulated and campaigned for their own needs to be recognized and met.
- The questions and challenges raised by organizations of those who have been the objects of community care policy, not only in relation to the way in which services are provided, but also as regards the assumptions of 'need' on which they are based.

The chapter concludes with a discussion of the implications of these alternative perspectives for determining how needs might be defined and met.

2 What is community care?

ACTIVITY 3.1

'Social care' covers a range of very different types of service. Try to identify what social care services might be available in your area for the following people:

■ A woman in her 70s with dementia living with her husband who is about the same age.

■ A young man in his early 20s with a diagnosis of schizophrenia living at home with his parents.

■ A 30-year-old man who has cerebral palsy which affects his speech, mobility and ability to write, and who is studying at university.

■ A 35-year-old woman with learning difficulties who lives with her 75-year-old mother.

COMMENT

The type of help each of these people needs to enable them to live their daily life will be very different. The objectives which each person may seek to achieve through accessing support services are also likely to be different. Who is being supported in each case: is it the woman with dementia or her husband, the woman with learning difficulties or her mother? It will be useful to bear these examples in mind as you think about how the concept of need is defined in the context of social care.

■ ■ ■

The NHS and Community Care Act 1990 consolidated a policy commitment to community care – that is, the provision of care at home or in 'homely' settings, rather than in institutional settings – but community care is not a new policy nor a new experience. Community care would not be possible if parents were not prepared to support disabled children beyond the time at which they might have been expected to leave home, or if adult children were not prepared to support frail elderly parents to enable them to remain living 'in the community' rather than entering residential care. Families were looking after older and disabled relatives long before Sir Roy Griffiths, adviser to the then Conservative government on the implementation of community care policy, said that public policy should start from the position that family care was the best and preferred option (Griffiths, 1988). Some families received help from social services or from health services, while others did not. However, the majority of disabled people were already living in the community, receiving care from families. What the 1990 Act did was to make explicit normative assumptions about where responsibilities for the provision of care lie, and to build a policy based on these assumptions. Thus assessment of a need for social care is not solely a matter of drawing conclusions about individual capacities and worthiness to receive help. It also involves decisions about whether support needs are to be met publicly by the state or from the private resources of families. The quotations below present the official view of the respective roles of families and the state, and provide a backdrop for the discussion that follows.

> Publicly provided services constitute only a small part of the total care provided to people in need. Families, friends, neighbours and other local people provide the

majority of care in response to needs which they are uniquely well placed to identify and respond to. This will continue to be the primary means by which people are enabled to live normal lives in community settings. The proposals take as their starting point that this is as it should be, and that the first task of publicly provided services is to support and where possible strengthen these networks of carers. Public services can help by identifying such actual and potential carers, consulting them about their needs and those of the people they are caring for, and tailoring the provision of extra services (if required) accordingly.

(Griffiths, 1988, para.3.2)

While this White Paper focuses largely on the role of statutory and independent bodies in the provision of community care services, the reality is that most care is provided by family, friends and neighbours. The majority of carers take on these responsibilities willingly, but the Government recognises that many need help to be able to manage what can become a heavy burden. Their lives can be made much easier if the right support is there at the right time, and a key responsibility of statutory service providers should be to do all they can to assist and support carers. Helping carers to maintain their valuable contribution to the spectrum of care is both right and a sound investment.

(Secretary of State for Health *et al.*, 1989, para. 2.3)

Whilst family carers have roles as service providers, they have also come to be constructed as another group with social care needs. The Carers Recognition and Services Act 1995 gave carers the right to ask for an assessment of the care they provide, and to indicate their willingness and ability to continue to provide that care. The implications of this are discussed in more detail in section 4.4. The ambiguous role of carers in relation to statutory services and to those for whom they provide care is another contested area. It has also contributed to the deserving/undeserving distinction that is always present in rationing systems. The potentially competing interests of family carers and those of the direct users of services have also in some instances contributed to the creation of conflict between care recipients and care providers within families.

Who provides and who has access to social care are both subject to considerable negotiation and dispute. More fundamentally, the socially constructed nature of 'social care needs' means that the appropriateness of the concept as a basis for determining access to services is contested. Some disabled people reject an analysis based on 'need for care' and advocate a social rights approach to the provision of personal support services. The all-embracing use of the term 'care' to describe a wide range of needs when applied to older or disabled people has also been challenged. The construction of need as residing in individuals as well as within communities is a further aspect of the contested nature of 'social care needs' that will be considered in this chapter.

3   The origins of community care

Community care policy is intended to provide a structure within which the needs of a number of different groups can be met. The largest group in numerical terms comprises older people, but the policy is intended to encompass services to meet the needs of physically and sensorily disabled people, people with learning difficulties, those experiencing mental health problems, and people living with HIV or AIDS. Whilst the experiences and circumstances of people identified in these ways is very different, they often share experiences of social exclusion. With the exception of people living with AIDS, they also share a history of being the subject of social policies which contributed to that exclusion by physically separating them from the rest of the population in residential institutions. By the start of the post-war period, those policies of institutional care were being questioned and community care policy was starting to be articulated. In order to understand the way in which social care and social need have come to be defined within community care policy, we need to look at the different strands within the development of the policy.

3.1   Community as an object of policy

One thing that becomes obvious as we start to unravel these various strands is that one of the core concepts on which the policy is built – that of community – **community** is rarely defined. The unstated assumption underpinning the way in which the term is used in *Caring for People* (the White Paper which preceded the National Health Service and Community Care Act 1990, hereafter 'the Act') and other policy documents is that community is, quite simply, 'not hospital'. Community, in the terms of the White Paper, is living at home or 'in homely settings' and being in regular contact with family, friends and neighbours. Reference is made to the fact that minority ethnic communities may have different concepts of 'community care', but these are not defined. Community is assumed to apply to locality: community services are 'locally based', in contrast to the 'remote mental hospitals' located geographically separate from the original homes of most of their inmates.

Bulmer (1987), among others, has examined the different meanings attached to the notion of community. He discussed the way in which normative concepts of community may be at odds with people's lived experiences (for example, social relationships between neighbours may be non-existent), and he cautioned against founding a policy on such poorly understood concepts. More recently sociologists and others have explored the significance of variables other than place in defining community identity: gender, sexuality, ethnicity and language are all associated with communities and may have very little to do with where people live. However, the disputed and shifting nature of the concept, evident in much sociological literature that explores both empirical and theoretical aspects of community, is simply ignored in official policy, which takes for granted that everyone knows what is meant by community. In practice the objects of community care policy are disabled people, older people, people with mental health problems, and their families. Community is simply the unexplored context within which families are expected to provide care for their needy members.

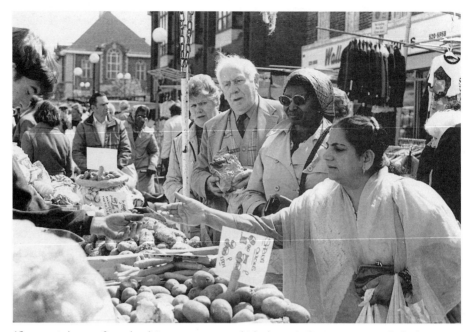

'Community' can refer to localities, or to groups which share similar interests, or which share identities relating to ethnic group, sexual orientation or gender. But is it the community that 'cares'?

ACTIVITY 3.2

To what community or communities do you feel you belong? On what are these based: locality, interest, identity? From which of these communities might you expect to receive the types of 'care' which are the subject of community care policy?

Think about the range of activities which you might need extra help in undertaking if, for example, you were unable to walk following a car accident.

1   From whom would you *want* to receive this type of support?

2   From whom would you consider it acceptable or appropriate to seek help?

3   Who would be available to provide such support?

4   Do you feel the term 'community' describes your relationship with these people?

Although community care is based on a very narrow conception of community, other social policies and practices have been described by reference to community (as defined by locality) and yet focus more clearly on 'the community' as the object of policy.

Community work or community development involves working with people within the communities in which they live in order to support them to define the problems they experience and take action to address them. For example, a common target for community work action has been poor housing conditions, which affect the health and well-being of people living in poverty – particularly families with young children, older people and disabled people. Thus, community work differs from community care in that the objective is to achieve change in the fabric of the communities in which people live, rather than to provide support to individuals.

Community care is based on an assumption that individual unorganized carers (that is, families) will be the major source of care provision outside institutional settings. This differs from community development, which sees active organization on the part of groups of people living within a locality as a source of involvement in determining the nature of problems and needs which are collectively experienced, and the action required to address them. Community development explicitly takes community to be the object of policy, and community groups as subjects in determining the nature of local action. As we shall see later, collective action on the part of organized groups of disabled people, carers and others is starting to impact on community care policy and practice. However, there remains a substantial reluctance among professional social care providers to accept as legitimate the involvement of 'community groups' with *collective* interests, as opposed to input from a series of disconnected individuals whose voices may be listened to as individual consumers of services.

Community social work had a somewhat different emphasis from community work. It was intended as an organizational solution to the problems associated with functional specialism and the large scale of social services departments which created both geographical and bureaucratic problems of accessibility. Rather than organizing workers according to function – day services, social work or domiciliary care workers – the aim was to establish multi-purpose teams on a local basis to enable staff to gain familiarity with the local area and to support early intervention before crises arose. Instead of relying on formal systems, workers were expected to pick up 'referrals' in an informal way through day-to-day contacts in shops, pubs and chats on the street.

Community social work also aimed to mobilize the collective resources of the community in order to provide care. Those resources might be found in churches, working men's clubs or voluntary groups, depending on the nature of the area. It differed from community development in that the objective was not political action by community members, but the provision of care to its members (Hadley and Hatch, 1981).

Neither community development nor community social work was influential in framing community care policy. However, the emphasis within community social work on consolidating voluntary sources of support in order to contain needs for care for individuals within the resources of the community was clearly attractive to the Conservative government in the 1980s. The main pressures for a change in policy came from other directions: first, reaction to poor practice and worse within long-stay hospitals, linked to an individualistic ideology which devalued collective forms of welfare; and second, growing financial pressures caused by the cost of residential care.

3.2 De-institutionalization, 'normalization' and individualism

Early 'community care' White Papers, such as *Better Services for the Mentally Handicapped* (1971) and *Better Services for the Mentally Ill* (1975), promoted the idea that services should be developed 'in the community' rather than being concentrated in residential institutions. This was partly prompted by evidence   **institutions**
emerging from official inquiries into scandals in long-stay hospitals.

87

Extract 3.1 is from the 1971 report of the official inquiry into conditions in Farleigh Hospital, a long-stay institution. It demonstrates the poverty of skills and resources available to provide stimulation for residents, and contains evidence of the violence that could erupt as a result.

Extract 3.1 Farleigh Hospital Committee of Inquiry: 'Institutional "care"'

156. According to Mr Tanner a deputy charge nurse, who has been at Farleigh for the last 12 months and with whose evidence and personal qualities we were particularly impressed, out-breaks of violence amongst the patients in North Ward occur with persistent regularity. This is hardly surprising in view of the high concentration of very difficult patients to be found there ... In 1967–68 the facilities available on that ward were even less than they are today. In particular three crucial needs remained unsatisfied. Staff was short, expert guidance was lacking and the accommodation was unsatisfactory.

157. A visit to the ward by any doctor was a rare occurrence. No informed discussion of the ways in which difficult patients might be occupied and managed was attempted.

158. There were times when three nurses were expected to handle over periods of as long as $11\frac{1}{2}$ hours at a stretch, a group of 40 disturbed, grossly handicapped and epileptic patients.

159. A very few of the patients went for periods of one hour at a time to the occupational therapy department. For the most part all the residents were on the Ward for 24 hours of the day.

160. One charge nurse told us 'when I went to North Ward in 1968 there was virtually no equipment at all to promote play therapy: we managed to collect odd items to keep the patients busy but were handicapped by lack of funds', and again 'my idea was to get the lowest grade of patient doing something. Invariably they were sitting about, there was nothing with which we could amuse them ... I noticed that about five of the very lowest grade were continually noisy and interfering with other patients. This started off a routine hubbub'.

161. Relatives hardly ever came to the Ward. It was usual for the patients to be dressed and taken to meet any visitors in another part of the hospital. It is probable that few people outside the hospital were aware of the conditions in North Ward.

162. The Ward's day spaces were so constructed that to get from one large room to the two small rooms which were also available to patients in a different part of the North Ward Block it was necessary to go out of doors. There were no side rooms or cubicles where a violent patient could be contained. Movement was thus very restricted and nursing supervision almost intolerably difficult.

163. This then was the situation: there were 40 patients in North Ward. Equipment was lacking. Staff were lacking. The patients spent their time cooped up in one large room crowded into close physical contact with each other. In such a situation violence amongst them became contagious.

(National Health Service, 1971, pp.24–5)

Frank Thomas worked for six months as a nursing assistant in a hospital similar to Farleigh. He describes his experience of being acutely aware of the injustice and lack of humanity of institutional life in a book called *The Politics of Mental Handicap*. The introduction to the book quotes a former resident of a long-stay institution:

Being in the institution was bad. I got tied up and locked up. I didn't have any clothes of my own, and no privacy. We got beat at times, but that wasn't the worst. The real pain came from always being a group. I was never a person. I was part of a group to eat, sleep and everything. As a kid I couldn't figure out who I was. I was part of a group. It was sad.

(Ryan and Thomas, 1980, p.12)

Asylums and other forms of residential institution were intended to separate 'abnormal' or 'subnormal' people from the 'normal' population. However, when scandals about what was going on in those institutions started to become public knowledge, it was no longer possible for society to consider its duty had been done by providing 'care' for these needy people out of sight of the rest of us. Breaking down institutional practices and the stigmatization resulting from these was a key strand in the development of professional thinking about community care. Whereas community social work sought to support people in communities by mobilizing the resources of those communities, the de-institutionalization programme sought to introduce *into* local communities people who had been separated from them, sometimes from birth. Those people being moved into communities often needed considerable support in making the transition. They were not always welcomed by those already living in the community, but the major focus of those supporting the transition was not on the development of the community itself, but on the individuals moving into it.

The 'batch processing' models of care predominant within institutions were under attack from an individualist ideology which permeated political as well as professional thinking. Consumer choice was to be stimulated by the development of a 'mixed economy' of care, and professional values emphasized the importance of recognizing and responding to the different needs of individuals. This philosophy was known initially as 'normalization'. It was originally expounded in Canada by Wolfensberger (1972) in relation to people

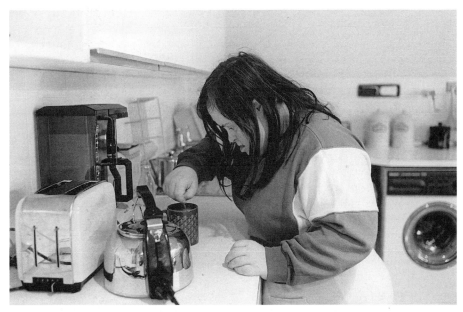

Caring for People *referred to the objective of providing care in 'homely settings'. If that was not possible within the family home, then it could be a small residential unit or group home*

with learning difficulties (then known as mentally handicapped people). The key principles were:

(i)   Mentally handicapped people have the same human value as anyone else and also the same human rights.

(ii) Living like others within the community is both a right and a need.

(iii) Services must recognize the individuality of mentally handicapped people.

(King's Fund, 1980, p.14).

In response to critiques about the objective of making individuals fit with dominant assumptions about what it is to be 'normal', Wolfensberger (1983) later redefined the philosophy as 'social role valorization'. This formulation emphasizes the significance of the extent to which people are valued socially for the self-esteem and social standing of those with stigmatized identities. Thus it recognizes that it is not enough for people to be 'in the community'; rather, their role within the community has to be experienced and recognized by others as a valued one.

These philosophies achieved widespread acceptance during the 1980s as a basis for service developments for people with learning difficulties and other younger disabled adults. However, normalization has not really been applied to the 'care' of older people.

Monolithic and collective forms of welfare provision were becoming unacceptable, so reforming the institutions was insufficient on its own. Dalley (1988) explored the way in which collective forms of welfare provision started to be rejected in favour of solutions based on a familist ideology which located responsibility for welfare within family groups. She distinguished *community*, as used by right-wing thinkers to represent the sum of individuals acting on their own behalf in opposition to the state, from *collective* or *communal* approaches, which she characterized as collective responsibility for all members of the community, with the state at their disposal: 'Responsibility is to be collectivized or socialized rather than privatized' (Dalley, 1988, p.49). However, throughout the 1980s neo-liberal philosophies were emphasizing private responsibilities for care, and it was easy for a rejection of the damaging impact of institutional care to lead to a belief that collective provision was inherently destructive of individual responsiveness. The potential advantages (both material and emotional) to be gained from collective solutions were obscured. By the time community care became a core focus for social policy legislation, community development was largely forgotten and the object of the policy was the individual and her/his carer. The carer was usually a woman and usually a member of the family. Any sense of 'the community' as an object of policy had been lost. Community, in the terms of the 1989 *Caring for People* White Paper, was effectively 'not hospital', and the resource which was to take over from institutions was the family. Care 'in the community' was empirically and normatively understood to be care 'by families'.

3.3   Financial pressures

An ideological rejection of institutional in favour of community-based care was reinforced by a growing awareness of the cost to the state of residential care. The social security budget was being used to pay for private residential care for substantial numbers of older people. The number of places in private homes for people aged 75+ per 1,000 population increased from 7.8 in 1974 to 17.4 in 1984 (Audit Commission, 1986). The Audit Commission pointed out that anyone choosing to live in a residential home was entitled to social security allowances which would meet the full fees of such accommodation up to an amount in excess of the combined attendance allowance and invalid care allowance that was available to those receiving support at home. In addition, stringent conditions had to be met before the latter allowances could be received. This meant that 'less disabled' people were receiving social security benefits to enable them to live in residential homes, whilst 'more disabled people' – including some who would be considered too disabled to be cared for in a residential home – were receiving considerably less in benefits. Actual and projected increases in the cost of residential care being paid for through the social security budget were powerful motivating factors in the change of policy towards community care.

This concern was clearly set out in *Caring for People*. A key objective of the community care reforms was to put a brake on the use of the social security budget to pay for unassessed residential care. A new funding system was central to the proposals:

> The Government proposes to introduce a single unified budget to cover the costs of social care, whether in a person's own home or in residential care or nursing home. The new budget will include the care element of social security payments to people in private and voluntary residential care and nursing homes. Local authorities are to be given responsibility for managing this budget and making the best use of funds available in the light of assessment of an individual's needs. Collaboration between medical, nursing and social services agencies will be essential, particularly when assessing need for nursing home care.
>
> (Secretary of State for Health *et al.*, 1989, para. 8.17)

In spite of professional warnings that community care should not be viewed as a cheap option, community care policy was certainly seen as a financially prudent option, and establishing whether services were giving value for money became a key responsibility of service providers. If the bulk of care was provided by family carers, this would obviously ease the pressure on the public purse. In 1995 The Carers National Association estimated that carers saved the state £30 billion. They estimated that if 10 per cent of carers were to stop 'caring', £2 billion would need to be added to the social security budget to meet the cost of replacement care.

carers

4 Official community care policy and alternative versions

The NHS and Community Care Act 1990 was the first legislative attempt to define the objectives of community care, as well as the institutional arrangements through which it was to be delivered.

ACTIVITY 3.3

Reflect on what you have read so far, and consider the main reasons for the shift in policy away from institutional towards 'community' care. What contradictions do you see as being likely to result from the different influences on this policy shift?

Extract 3.2, from the 1989 White Paper *Caring for People*, sets out the objectives of community care policy. Do they add up to a coherent explanation of community care policy?

Extract 3.2 Secretary of State for Health *et al.*: 'Key objectives of community care'

The Government's proposals have six key objectives for service delivery:

- *to promote the development of domiciliary, day and respite services to enable people to live in their own homes wherever feasible and sensible.* Existing funding structures have worked against the development of such services. In future, the Government will encourage the targeting of home-based services on those people whose need for them is greatest;

- *to ensure that service providers make practical support for carers a high priority.* Assessment of care needs should always take account of the needs of caring family, friends and neighbours;

- *to make proper assessment of need and good case management the cornerstone of high quality care.* Packages of care should then be designed in line with individual needs and preferences;

- *to promote the development of a flourishing independent sector alongside good quality public services.* The Government has endorsed Sir Roy Griffiths' recommendation that social services authorities should be 'enabling' agencies. It will be their responsibility to make maximum use of private and voluntary providers, and so increase the available range of options and widen consumer choice;

- *to clarify the responsibilities of agencies and so make it easier to hold them to account for their performance.* The Government recognises that the present confusion has contributed to poor overall performance;

- *to secure better value for taxpayers' money by introducing a new funding structure for social care.* The Government's aim is that social security provisions should not, as they do now, provide any incentive in favour of residential and nursing home care.

(Secretary of State for Health *et al.*, 1989, para. 1.11)

COMMENT

This list of objectives is a curious mixture of institutional, process and service objectives. With the exception of enabling people to live in their own homes, it has very little to say about the outcomes to be achieved as a result of the implementation of community care policy, an absence which in 1996 was recognized with the launch of a programme of research and development supported by the Department of Health and concerned with 'outcomes of social care for adults'. The extract talks of increasing consumer choice and encouraging private sector development whilst deliberately seeking to curb the use of private residential care. It placed at the forefront of the strategy the assessment of need, both of direct users of services and their carers, without acknowledging the possible conflict between the needs of carers and those for whom they care.

■ ■ ■

In the context of changes throughout the public sector aiming to shift the balance from producer to consumer interests, one of the professed intentions of the community care changes was to give service users and their carers more say in determining the nature of the services they received. The Act sought to achieve this through:

- encouraging user and carer involvement in the process of assessment;
- requiring that social services authorities consult with users, carers, voluntary organizations and others over community care plans;
- the introduction of a complaints procedure intended to introduce an element of independent review to the hearing of complaints;
- the establishment of 'arm's length' inspection units with input from lay members who could be, but were not necessarily, users of services.

The first two of these are of particular relevance and are discussed in full below. First, however, we must consider how, if at all, 'need' and 'care' were defined in official community care policy.

4.1 What kind of needs?

If needs assessment was intended to be a cornerstone of the community care reforms introduced by the 1990 Act, what type of needs were intended to be assessed? How were social care needs constructed by community care policy? Underlying a 'needs-based approach' was the intention that assessment should start from the individual's circumstances and difficulties in order to determine what 'packages' of services were required to meet the needs of the individual, rather than determine whether the individual 'fitted' particular services. Nevertheless, such needs assessment was to be conducted within an overall framework, established by the White Paper and the Act, which set out what services 'social care' was seen to encompass:

> Social care and practical assistance with daily living are key components of good quality community care. The services and facilities, at present largely the responsibilities of social services authorities, which will be essential to enable people to live in the community include help with personal and domestic tasks such as cleaning, washing and preparing meals, with disablement equipment and home adaptations, transport, budgeting and other aspects of daily living. Suitable good quality housing is essential and the availability of day care, respite care, leisure facilities and employment and educational opportunities will all improve the quality of life enjoyed by a person with care needs.
>
> (Secretary of State for Health *et al.*, 1989, para. 2.4)

'Care' is one of those terms which is part of everyday discourse, but which, in the context here, has become the subject of public policy and of rules and procedures determining by whom and how it is to be provided. What do you think are the key components of 'care'?

The term care as used within the *Caring for People* White Paper is often qualified. It is at various points used to mean 'health care', 'social care', or 'residential, nursing or hospital care'. Care may consist in 'looking after those close to them' when it is provided by family or friends, or it may be any one or more of a disparate collection of inputs as indicated by the following description: 'social

'Care' in the context of community care policy often means help with 'activities of daily living'

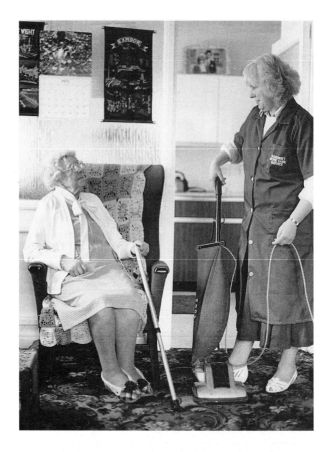

care and support, e.g. for mobility, personal care, domestic tasks, financial affairs, accommodation, leisure and employment'.

The source of care can be another way of defining it: if paid workers are the source then it is 'formal' care; if it is family or friends it is 'informal' care (Thomas, 1993). However, it is not always possible to draw a clear distinction between the motivations of those providing paid care and those of informal carers. For example, home carers often demonstrate a personal concern for an individual which has certain of the characteristics of informal care, whilst some social services authorities have made payments to friends or family members to carry out specific caring tasks.

In spite of evidence that it is difficult to separate caring tasks and caring feelings, one effect of the introduction of markets within social care has been an attempt to commodify care – that is, to make it into a product to be traded. This is evident in the language of *Caring for People*, which, for example, refers to the need to make a 'cost effective care choice' when putting together 'packages of care' (para. 3.4.1) for those whose needs are being assessed. Workers must determine the right amount of care to be supplied to enable people to achieve their full potential (para. 1.8) without encouraging over-dependence. Care has to be applied for (para. 5.10) by reference to the social services 'gatekeepers' to care (para. 6.9). Care can be bought and sold; and it can be managed within a 'care programme' (para. 7.7).

Care can also be contracted to be provided on a 'block' basis, for example the provision of *x* number of places as a source of respite care, rather than in response to an individual assessment. In a study of social care contracts, Smith and Thomas (1993) found that the 'care' being contracted for could consist of quantitative 'inputs' such as the ratio of qualified to unqualified staff, qualitative inputs such as procedures to be followed to ensure safety and security, and occasionally qualitative outputs or outcomes such as privacy, dignity, individuality, consultation and empowerment of residents.

This demonstrates the difficulty of defining exactly what 'care' is within the formal sector of social care provision. The idea that care is something that can be defined in a contract, and which can be exchanged and managed, is very different from lay understandings of care as something that derives from an emotional attachment to another person, or from a sense of personal responsibility for that person. The personal experience of many paid workers also makes it difficult to consider how the care that they show for those who use their services might be specified and quantified within a contract. Defining tasks such as washing and dressing someone and physically supporting them from bedroom to living room, and calculating the time this should take to complete, is only part of the story. During the process of providing such tending care, the worker is also likely to be demonstrating some degree of 'caring about' the person. This could consist of providing emotional support and encouragement, or discussing family members, personal histories or events that are going on in the world outside. It is hard to see how this can be defined in contractual terms.

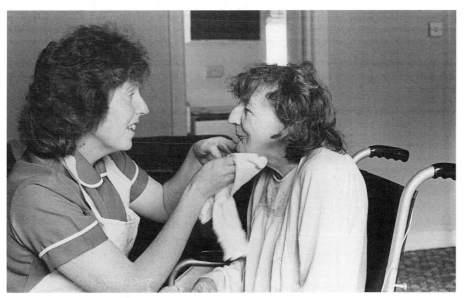

Care may comprise 'tending' or 'caring for' someone. But can effective tending be undertaken without some degree of 'caring about' the person?

4.1.1 Health or social care?

Caring for People concluded that the responsibility for assessing need should lie with social services authorities, who should also have the responsibility for designing and purchasing care packages. The White Paper also discussed the role of health authorities:

Community care is about the health as well as the social needs of the population. Health care, in its broadest sense, is an essential component of the range of services which may be needed to help people to continue to live in their own homes for as long as possible ...

Health authorities will remain responsible for the health care needs of those people who also have a need for social care. Such people may well have special needs for health care, whether for primary care or acute hospital care, or for long-term care. Their handicap or disability may also make them heavy consumers of health care. In some individual cases it may well be difficult to draw a clear distinction between the needs of an individual for health and social care. In such cases it will be critically important for the responsible authorities to work together.

(Secretary of State for Health *et al.*, 1989, paras 4.1 and 4.2)

The penultimate sentence of this quotation can be considered something of an understatement. Not only is the distinction between health care and social care services not clear-cut, but the same service can, at different times, be considered to meet either health *or* social care needs: for example, when is a bath a 'social bath'? A domiciliary care worker employed by the local authority social services department may assist an older person to take a bath as a result of an assessment which indicates a need for assistance with personal care tasks. This may be because of physical frailty or because isolation and depression have led to a lack of motivation to sustain personal care. Following discharge from hospital, a district nurse may visit to assist the same person to bathe because they are considered to have continuing health needs relating to, for example, treatment following a fall. In the first instance the need will be defined as a social need, in the second as a health need. The nature of the service is largely the same, though provided by a different worker employed by a different authority.

Why is this important? It may be important to some recipients of the service who prefer to receive intimate care from a nurse rather than a domiciliary care worker, but the attempt to draw distinctions between health and social needs also has broader implications. There are three aspects that are of particular relevance to this discussion:

1   The distinction between health and social care needs is not solely a matter of institutional responsibilities for service delivery, but also of the way in which disablement, mental distress and learning difficulties are understood. If physical impairment is a problem located in the malfunctioning of particular bodies, then the solution is to adjust those bodies in order to enable them to function as closely as possible to 'normality'. If, on the other hand, the difficulties experienced by disabled people in moving about the communities in which they live are understood as deriving from the fact that the physical environment is designed on the assumption that everyone is perfectly capable of stepping up onto a platform to get on a bus, then the solution lies in the way in which the environment is designed. The implications of this are expressed by a disabled activist involved in a disabled people's coalition:

for example, someone realizes that very small changes in their local environment like the ability to get in a corner shop can make a very significant difference to their lives in that they might not be dependent on people to do their shopping for them – they wouldn't have to wait for their home helps to get basic everyday things that other people get when they want them.

(personal communication to the author)

2 The division of institutional responsibilities and the way in which different agencies work together in meeting need is nevertheless important in the context of objectives relating to the provision of a 'seamless service', as *Caring for People* recognized. Providing the support necessary to enable someone to remain living in their own home can mean that support services are provided by social services, community health and primary care services. At the level of service provision there is a need for both understanding and co-ordination. This is particularly important when people are being discharged from hospital and allowed home because the hospital needs their bed before domiciliary services have been arranged by the social services department. They can find themselves in cold houses, with no food in the fridge and unable to get upstairs to bed.

3 At another level the distinction between different types of need is important in determining whether the care to be provided is a social right of citizenship to be met from publicly funded services (as in the case of health care), or whether it is to be met from private resources (family care), or social care subjected to means testing (such as the domiciliary care provided by most local authorities). This distinction has been spotlighted as the NHS seeks to withdraw from the provision of long-term care for older people.

Some of the issues surrounding the boundaries between health care and social care are highlighted in Extract 3.3, which is a document produced by the NHS Support Federation, an independent pressure group which campaigns to support a fully funded NHS, and the West Midlands Health Research Unit, an independent information service on the NHS.

Extract 3.3 Courtney and Walker: 'Stand and deliver'

The changed role of district nurses is indicative of the retreat from free NHS long term care. Over the last decade many of the caring jobs they previously carried out such as providing catheter care, administering medicines, changing dressings and colostomy bags and bathing people are now carried out by home care assistants under the auspices of social care. The difference being of course that social care incurs a fee.

Christine Hancock, General Secretary of the Royal College of Nursing, highlighted another element of this boundary reshuffle: 'We have some evidence of redesignating what we believe are nursing tasks as social care ... A woman in hospital is suffering from a lot of complications: (she has) severe diabetes (and) ... is on a ventilator with a permanent tracheostomy. The Health Commission is pressurising the district nurses to say that what she needs is social care not health care' (Hancock, 11 May 1995, p.45).

Some of the redesignation of tasks from health care to social care has been centrally led. For example the 1994 NHS Executive document 'Feet First' says health authorities should consider redesignating 'simple' or 'basic' nail cutting from chiropody (health) to a task which can be undertaken by relatives, or other care staff (social).

The association representing metropolitan authorities comments on a further aspect of this redefinition of NHS care: '*health authorities and trusts are defining health care in a very narrow sense indicating acute medical intervention.* The consequence of this is that those patients who fall outside this narrow definition have now become dependent on means tested social services for their continuing/long term care needs' (AMA, 18 May 1995, p.72).

References

Association of Metropolitan Authorities (AMA) (1995) Minutes of Evidence to Health Committee on Long Term Care. Minutes of Evidence House of Commons Session 1994–95, London, HMSO, p.72.

Department of Health (1994) NHS Executive, *Feet First*, EL. (49) (69).

Hancock, C. (1995) Evidence to the Health Committee on Long Term Care, House of Commons, p.45.

(Courtney and Walker, 1996, pp.10–11)

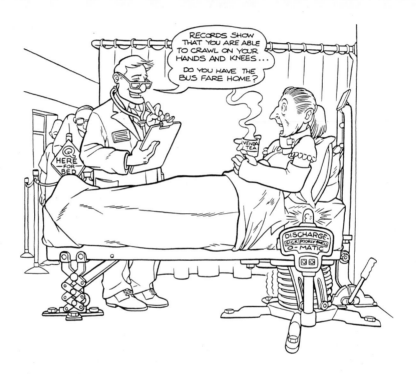

The shifting of boundaries between health and social care opens up another 'perverse incentive': not only to ensure that higher priority is given to meeting needs through accessing social care services via hospital admission, but to define needs as health needs in order to receive 'free' care. Few will mourn the passing of many long-stay geriatric wards in hospitals, and the development of a policy emphasizing care for older people in their own homes is a progressive step. However, if this also means that older people who expected to benefit from health services free at the point of delivery and funded through national taxation for the good of the population as a whole find themselves having to pay for care in the community, then the closure of geriatric wards may be seen as a retrograde step.

4.2 Assessing needs

One of the aims of the NHS and Community Care Act 1990 was that an assessment of individual needs would precede decisions about the services appropriate to meet those needs. The process of assessment was to be separated from that of service provision in order to minimize the likelihood that assessment would be driven by knowledge of, or commitment to, a particular service. For example, rather than a domiciliary care organizer assessing someone to decide whether they should receive home care services, the post of 'care manager' was created in order to assess the range of services necessary to meet the needs of each individual. Assessment was also intended to identify needs which might be met by the provision of services beyond those directly provided by social services departments. The nature of assessment procedures, the criteria adopted to determine what is and what is not accepted as a 'need', and the way in which assessors have gone about their task demonstrate vividly the way in which need is socially constructed.

assessment

4.2.1 Eligibility criteria

Much of the early effort to implement the new legislation within social services departments went into developing procedures and pro-formas for the purpose of assessment. This included developing criteria to allocate individuals to one of a number of pre-determined dependency categories in order to establish whether they were a priority for the receipt of services and, if so, to decide the level of service to which they were 'entitled'. Guidance from the Department of Health stressed that authorities should intervene no more than was necessary in order to foster independence, and that they should concentrate on those most in need. Indeed, as a report produced by the King's Fund (an independent health policy and research organization) made explicit, the assessment and related care management processes introduced by the Act were not solely (or primarily?) intended to enable an understanding of the needs as experienced by the individual referred for or seeking help:

> Assessment and care management will occupy a pivotal position in the new service system. The two processes will mediate between the needs of individual people with disabilities and their carers, and the resources and services for their support in the community or in residential care. In essence, assessments will determine eligibility and establish needs. Care management is a method which social services departments can use to organize the inter-related tasks of needs assessment and the design, management and monitoring of care centred on individual requirements.
>
> As such, assessment and care management are about two distinctly different things. They are about tailoring services around individual needs *and* about resource rationing.
>
> (Beardshaw, 1991, p.7)

Distinguishing between those requiring 'simple' and 'complex' assessments became a way of filtering referrals according to perceived level of need. The term 'targeting' became familiar in the vocabulary of social care workers charged with determining eligibility criteria in the context of resource rationing. Moving from a simple to a complex assessment is often determined by reference to the degree of risk (either to themselves or to others) that the person represents. For example, the King's Fund report quoted above provided details of the three priority levels adopted within Devon Social Services:

- *First priority:* Those people who, without the active involvement of the Department, would be in danger of physical or emotional harm.
- *Second priority:* Those people who, without the active intervention of the Department, would be at risk of losing their independence.
- *Third priority:* Those people who, without the active intervention of the Department, would be unable to maintain a satisfactory quality of life.

(Beardshaw, 1991, pp.15–16)

A report produced by the Department of Health as a result of its monitoring of the implementation of the *Caring for People* reforms throughout 1993/94 identified the difficulties that authorities were experiencing in determining and applying eligibility criteria:

All authorities were struggling with the formulation and consistent application of eligibility criteria. There was often some confusion about different types of eligibility as between:

a the speed of response;
b the level of assessment;
c priority access to services;
d access to particular services.

Furthermore, these different types may be falsely correlated with each other. So, a referral requiring a 'simple' level of assessment might be equated with non-urgent and/or low priority; a distinction not unimportant in the provision of commodes, for example. Alternatively, the assessment of 'simple' needs might be deemed complex if it involved more than one agency. Hospital discharges were another case in point because, whatever the level of patients' needs, most Social Services Departments had undertaken to respond within two or three working days. There was, therefore, a potentially perverse incentive to access care management more quickly through admission to hospital.

(Department of Health, no date, p.30)

4.2.2 Need or risk?

By the mid 1990s social services departments were experiencing severe resource difficulties as a result of the capping of local government expenditure and an increase in the demand for services following the NHS and Community Care Act. Two well-publicized cases highlighted the tension between, on the one hand, a policy which emphasized a 'needs-led' approach to assessment and service provision and, on the other, a context of increasing resource constraint. The 'Gloucestershire case' concerned a disabled man who had been assessed as needing cleaning and laundry services which had been provided. When the authority decided that shortage of funds demanded a reduction in the overall provision of services, the services to this man were withdrawn without a re-assessment of his needs. When the case was referred to the Court of Appeal the decision was that assessment of needs and the consequent provision of services could not be affected by the financial position of the authority. The local authority and the Department of Health took the case to the House of Lords, which found that resource considerations *could* determine whether services were to be provided. This ruling caused considerable consternation to disabled people throughout the country (see Extract 3.4).

Extract 3.4 *Community Care*: 'Law Lords give green light to slash services'

The House of Lords has ruled that cash-strapped local authorities can withdraw community care services, weakening the Chronically Sick and Disabled Persons Act 1970 and leading to calls for a change in the law.

The ruling means local authorities can circumvent their duty under the Act to provide home care services to chronically sick or disabled individuals if they do not have the money.

This would undermine the Act, said Dave Burchell, assistant director of the British Association of Social Workers: 'If we are not going to meet people's needs, then why have the legislation? Parliament should stop passing legislation it is not going to fund.'

Sally Greengross, director general of Age Concern, said: 'No disabled person will ever be able to bank on getting services under the Act or that any services they currently receive will not be cut.'

And despite Gloucestershire Council winning its appeal, social services director Andrew Cozens said the ruling was a victory for no one. The council could not afford to meet the care needs of everyone without extra government funding, he added. He wants 'a new legal framework for community care services for adults'.

Social services directors want a review of community care legislation.

Bob Lewis, president of the Association of Directors of Social Services, said that if Gloucestershire had lost the case, it would have led to local authorities being expected to have an impossible 'open-ended budget'.

'I cannot see that councils will radically change their policies in terms of resourcing because of this ruling,' he said. 'We will continue to spend a lot of money in this area.'

But Karen Ashton, project solicitor for the Public Law Project, which represented Michael Barry, one of the people who brought the case, disagreed: 'Local councils who have been awaiting the outcome of this case may now change their policies.

'There remain many unanswered questions about the obligations of local authorities. Clarification by the courts case by case cannot be the answer. We need a serious debate about the need for law reform,' said Ashton.

Background to the ruling

The House of Lords ruling ends a three-year dispute which began when Gloucestershire Council withdrew home care services from 1,500 elderly and disabled people in 1994, without reassessing their needs, because of a £2.5 million overspend on social services.

In June 1995, four elderly people, including disabled pensioner Michael Barry, challenged the council's action in the High Court. The court ruled that Gloucestershire could use resources as a reason to withdraw services as long as it reassessed need. Barry appealed and the Appeal Court ruled inadequate resources were 'irrelevant' when it came to providing services. Councils must provide services under the Chronically Sick and Disabled Persons Act 1970 once a need had been assessed, it said. Gloucestershire Council and the Department of Health then went to the Lords.

The ruling

Local authorities will not have to provide home care services to chronically sick or disabled people if they cannot afford to after last week's ruling.

The Law Lords' three to two majority verdict in favour of Gloucestershire will allow cash-strapped local authorities to withdraw or reduce services provided under the Chronically Sick and Disabled Person Act 1970 for financial reasons, even when individual needs have not changed.

Reassessments must be carried out before services are withdrawn or reduced because of lack of resources. The ruling affects all local authorities in England and Wales.

Reduced central government funding had left Gloucestershire Council in a 'wretched position through no fault of its own', unable to afford the care it wanted to provide for elderly and disabled people, said Lord Lloyd of Berwick in his dissenting judgement.

Local authorities had been placed in an 'impossible situation' by lack of central government funding and the solution lay with the government, he said. 'The passing of the Chronically Sick and Disabled Persons Act was a noble aspiration. Having willed the end, Parliament must be asked to provide the means.'

Parliament could not have intended the standards and expectations of community care services to differ so much around the country, added Lord Lloyd. Lord Steyn agreed.

But the majority ruling held sway. Lord Nicholls said an interpretation of the law which enabled local authorities to take resources into account would not 'emasculate' the community care legislation.

(*Community Care*, 27 March–2 April 1997, p.1)

The 'Lancashire case' involved a disabled woman who was assessed as needing 24-hour care. The woman concerned wanted to receive this care in her own home, but the authority, taking account of the relative cost of different means of service provision, decided that the care should be provided in a nursing home. In this instance the Court of Appeal accepted that resource considerations were relevant to determining the *way* in which needs should be met. Cost considerations overrode community care objectives of enabling people to remain living in their own homes.

These two examples illustrate how the definition of need remains contingent. Both cases caused social services departments to be extremely cautious in committing themselves to identifying a 'need' for service in the first place. The dangerous word 'need' was to be avoided in setting out the results of an assessment in order to avoid the possibility of legal challenge. Another response was to draw up eligibility criteria to define in what circumstances a person would be assessed as in need of a service. Such criteria could be highly restrictive. The concept of risk came to the forefront in the determination of eligibility criteria.

risk

ACTIVITY 3.4

Extract 3.5 is from a report to Staffordshire's Social Services Committee. In the extract the Director of Social Services talks of the distinction between 'risk of harm' and 'quality of life'. In this formulation the concept of need has been entirely replaced by that of risk. The task of the worker undertaking an assessment is not to assess need, but to assess the risk that the person concerned will experience significant harm if there is no intervention by the social services department. Do you think that this is consistent with the objectives for community care set out in *Caring for People* and quoted in Extract 3.2? The policy change proposed in this report was accepted by the social services committee.

As you read the extract think about how you might react to it if you were:

■ A social services worker responsible for undertaking assessments.

■ A disabled person seeking an assessment of your needs.

Think of people who may seek access to social care services – for example a young adult with learning difficulties, a young mother with severe depression, an 85-year-old man who is a double amputee and who lives alone – and consider some practical examples of the type of harm of which they might be considered to be at risk. How might action to prevent harm be distinguished from action intended to improve quality of life in such circumstances?

Extract 3.5 Staffordshire County Council: 'Report of Director of Social Services'

It is proposed that the general eligibility criteria for access to services should be that:

> The necessity for the provision of services must be evidenced by significant risk of substantial harm if the service is not provided. The risk of harm will generally be to the physical and/or mental health of the person assessed but the risk of harm could be to other people. The service must not be of a type properly the responsibility of health, housing or other agencies.

If the Social Services Committee adopted this statement as its policy, it would not be possible to allocate a service to an individual except where there was a significant risk of substantial harm. This would have the effect of excluding the provision of services on 'quality of life' grounds. For example, it would not be appropriate to arrange for a person with a disability to attend a day centre purely because they would find it an enjoyable activity. It might be a legitimate service to arrange, however, if the person was isolated and there was a significant risk of the person being severely depressed if the service were not provided. It is intended, therefore, for staff undertaking assessments to assess risk faced by the service user, carer and others prior to making any decision on the allocation of resources. In seeking approval to the allocation of resources, staff will need to be able to demonstrate that the anticipated harm is reasonably likely to occur and that provision of the service is likely to result in a significant reduction of the risk.

(Staffordshire County Council, 1996, p.5)

4.2.3 The assessment process

So what information about the circumstances of people referred to social services departments forms the basis of decisions made during the community care assessment process? Departments developed their own forms to guide the assessment process in line with policy guidelines established locally.

ACTIVITY 3.5

Look at the examples of assessment forms shown below. The first is a form used by the Mental Health Division of Shropshire Social Services to assess people with mental health problems. The second is used by Birmingham City Council's Social Services Department in general community care assessments. What do they tell you about the way in which the notion of need is defined for the purpose of assessing whether services are to be provided?

Extracts from a care management and assessment form used by Shropshire Social Services, Mental Health Division

MENTAL HEALTH DIVISION
CARE MANAGEMENT AND ASSESSMENT

These forms are to be completed by the Client, Carer (if available) and the assessing worker.

Client's Name | CRISSP No.

Presenting Difficulties

Reason for referral and Mental Health history; important life events and current network and daily activity). Please include Client's views.

If appropriate include assessment from psychiatrist or previously involved psychiatric pro

Client's Name | MENTAL HEALTH DIVISION | CRISSP No.

Accommodation/Housing Concerns

Include any relevant assessments from Housing Agencies. (To include Suitability: Barriers to Independence; access to Community Services; Transport)
Include comments from Client and Carer.

MENTAL HEALTH DIVISION | CRISSP No.

Client's Name

Mental/Physical Health

If any assessments from GP, Disability Services to include mobility, registration details (eg blind, physical disability), conditions impairing independence and adding to stress or mental health condition. Include comments from Client and Carer.

MENTAL HEALTH DIVISION

Carers Assessment of Client's needs and their own 'needs'.

Recreational/Educational Needs

If appropriate staff from different agencies e.g. day services, colleges, or leisure services should be asked to contribute.
Include comments from client and carer.

...ies involved and contributing to assessment

...act Address | Telephone Number

Financial Help

Have you checked the Client is receiving all the benefits they are entitled to? | YES | NO

Please record financial constraints that might cause difficulty or disruption to implementation of assessment.

Pink

CM4

CM5

104

Birmingham City Council
Social Services Department

Community Care - CR6 - Simple Assessment
(Rev 1. March '95)

Simple Assessment Form

Ensure all sections of CR2 are completed before beginning this form

CIN .... ASSESSOR ....

PERSON'S NAME ....

Details of access to property (inc. keyholders) .... Date ....

ADDITIONAL FAMILY/CARER DETAILS (in addition to CR2)
For emergency contact:

NAME: ....

NAME: ....

ADDRESS: ....

ADDRESS: ....

Post Code: ....

Post Code: .... Tel: ....

Tel: ....

RELATIONSHIP ....

RELATIONSHIP ....

Additional Comments:

INFORMATION

PHYSICAL ABILITY - mobility - any problems?

Inside House ....

Outside House ....

Carrying ....

Equipment used ....

Ability to transfer to bed ....

Ability to transfer to ch

SECURITY - Ability to open/secure door ....

Additional Comments:

Community Care - CR6 - Simple Ass
(Rev 1. N

HEALTH PROFILE

Medical condition if known

Known/acknowledged physical disability/mental health problem/learning disability

Community Care - CR6 - Simple Assessment
(Rev 1. March '95)

Actions needed to maintain/restore independence/self-care

Nursing Service Input Yes ☐ No ☐ If Yes, what tasks undertaken

Additional Comments:

PERSONAL CARE TASKS

Ability to use bath/shower/shave ....

Is commode used? ....

Any Cultural Requirements? ....

Equipment Used ....

Additional Comments: Day/Night/Both ....

SOCIAL CARE TASKS

Collection of benefit/pension ....

Payment of bills ....

Light, heavy, weekly shopping ....

Benefit/Pension Day ....

Details of Cultural requirements for shopping ....

Assistance to budget ....

Getting to Day Centre/Club etc. ....

Travel training ....

Reading/Writing letters ....

Needs Transport to Unit ....

Other (detail) ....

Details ....

Additional Comments: Visiting friends/relatives ....

Social Services Dept.

• 2 •

ARE INFORMATION - CR6 - MODULE 1
Jan '93

Date: ....

Community Care

HOUSEHOLD TASKS:

Light Laundry ....

Heavy Laundry ....

Hot Water Available ....

Equipment Available ....
Is user willing/able to commission laundry service:

YES ☐ NO ☐

Heavy Cleaning ....

Light Cleaning ....

Equipment Available ....

Additional Comments:

DIETARY NEEDS - Please tick

	No Problem	Difficulty	Cause of Difficulty:
Ability to prepare meals	☐	☐	....
Ability to Cook	☐	☐	
Ability to heat prepared food	☐	☐	'Fridge ☐
Availability of gas/electric:	Cooker ☐	Microwave ☐	
Specific Dietary/Cultural Needs			

Additional Comments:

PRESENTING PROBLEMS/CONCERNS - as identified by user / carer / advocate during asse

ANALYSIS OF CIRCUMSTANCES - as identified by Assessor

• 3 •

Social Services Dept.

Means of summoning help?

Is there a telephone?

Any difficulties in making or receiving telephone calls? .... Yes ☐ No ☐

Is the telephone provided by Social Services? .... Yes ☐ No ☐

Who funds telephone? ....

Is there an alarm? .... Yes ☐ No ☐

To where is the alarm linked? ....

Any other communication equipment? Yes ☐ No ☐ Please state

Who provides/funds communication equipment? ....

Are you able to hear door bell/knocker? .... Yes ☐ No ☐

Are you able to answer the door? .... Yes ☐ No ☐

Do you have any concerns about home security? Yes ☐ No ☐

If Yes, what:-

Additional comments or explanations

Extracts from a simple assessment form used by Birmingham City Council

Simple assessments aim to collect very basic information about those aspects of daily living which the person has difficulty with, while complex assessments collect more detailed information, largely about the same things. In both instances the form guides the assessment process along pre-determined paths based primarily on need for support in daily living activities. They do not start from the person's own definition of their 'needs', although they do allow the person who has been referred to make a response to the pre-determined questions. The emphasis is on the person's capacity to undertake practical tasks of self and home care, and on the physical environment within which these tasks have to be carried out. Some questions are asked in order to provide a personal profile: relationships with family, friends, neighbours, education and employment, interests, hobbies, etc., but these are not located within a framework which relates 'needs' to people's need to participate as active members of their community.

Assessments of mental health needs, perhaps more than others, acknowledge the significance of interpersonal relationships in determining needs for support, and thus tend to be less dominated by the assessment of need in relation to 'activities of daily living'. The example included here adopts a more 'open' approach, suggesting a range of headings under which needs might be recorded and allowing for recording of the client's own assessment. This more open approach includes references to needs which might be met by agencies other than social services departments. For example, it recognizes the significance of recreational and educational needs.

■ ■ ■

In the early 1990s Kathryn Ellis undertook research exploring user and carer participation in assessment. This demonstrated the way in which highly structured assessment forms could close down users' own perspectives on their needs. She gave the following example:

> Because pro-formas were designed as much to allocate resources as to involve users and carers in the process, they could disguise users' own priorities. One older woman described how sad she was that failing sight meant she was no longer able to pursue significant leisure activities such as oil painting. As the important consideration for the home care assessor was whether her capacity to care for herself was affected, the pro-forma simply indicated that the woman could 'see with spectacles'.

(Ellis, 1993, p.21)

In her study of the way in which different practitioners within social services departments – social workers, occupational therapists, home care managers and others – carried out assessments, Ellis (1993) looked at the extent to which they were (or were not) responding to the guidance flowing from the Act to ensure that users and carers were participants in the assessment process. She found that many practitioners, regardless of occupational group, were influenced by a medical model of disability which defines needs as those arising from an individual's impaired physical or psychological functioning, rather than from a social and physical environment which excludes disabled people (**Hughes, 1998**). Workers referred to the personal qualities necessary to undertake effective assessment in addition to their formal training. Bureaucratic procedures such as those associated with assessment proformas were sometimes felt to undermine the 'human' aspect of assessment. These 'informal' factors influencing the way in which assessments were carried out could, in some circumstances, mean that the outcome of assessment was influenced by instinct and by moralizing judgements. These findings demonstrate how a definition of need is subject to the judgement of individual workers, as well as the policies of departments.

A major difficulty in ensuring that users can be active participants in the assessment process is a professional belief that getting underneath the 'presenting problem' is central to the professional assessment task and defines the professional skill. This was identified not only by Ellis but also by Marsh and Fisher (1992) in their work exploring 'partnership practice' within social services departments. Ellis found:

> A social worker with the deaf community was unusual in her belief that openly negotiating assessment objectives empowered users. This emphasis on building confidence was not universally shared. One specialist social work team described users as 'passive' and having 'low expectations'. Yet practitioners appeared to take little responsibility for changing that situation. Indeed, their implicit belief in their 'expertise' suggests people were more often expected to accept professional advice than make demands or challenge judgements.
>
> (Ellis, 1993, p.15)

Many of those who were the subject of assessments had approached formal service agencies reluctantly. Many felt they had to reach rock bottom before they should seek help – a judgement which is likely to be reinforced by highly restrictive eligibility criteria for services. In such circumstances many people may find it hard to assert their own view of their needs. Information about the range of services available is often not accessible, particularly to those whose first language is not English. Furthermore, Ellis found some evidence of a deliberate withholding of information by some workers who thought this might overwhelm the user.

Seeking access to formal help often meant renegotiating caring relationships among family members, and some came to feel that seeking to 'interweave' formal and informal support was more trouble than it was worth. In some instances assessors had to adjudicate between the conflicting views and perspectives of users and their family carers. All these factors affected the extent to which the assessment was likely to be experienced as a process in which both users and family carers could participate to achieve a satisfactory outcome. Means testing and rationing also caused some resentment and a sense of injustice that people were being financially penalized as a result of disability.

Although Ellis did find examples of sensitive assessments that resulted in a harmonious view between workers and those they were assessing, her research demonstrates that simply introducing a policy which encourages user participation in this process is not enough. Many of those subject to assessment have not been satisfied that the new procedures enable users' interests to be influential in determining the services to be provided. Thus a number of alternative models intended to strengthen the position of disabled people have been proposed by users and user organizations.

user participation

Becoming your own 'care manager'

When the concept of the case or care manager was mooted, many disabled people argued that the role of assessing need and determining the services necessary to meet those needs was one that they could undertake themselves.

This argument has been persuasive and has led to a number of schemes intended to support disabled people to take on this role and employ their own care assistants. Disabled people's organizations have been prominent in supporting and developing such schemes. For example, the Hampshire Centre for Independent Living produced a *Source Book Towards Independent Living* which contained guidance for disabled people wanting to employ their own care assistants. This included sections on how to write a care proposal, how to advertise for and interview prospective assistants, issues relating to contracts of employment and insurance, and advice on how to live and work together.

Legislation has been necessary to allow social services departments to make direct payments to disabled people to enable them to take on this role within the statutory sector. Disabled people's organizations see this as an opportunity to gain much greater control over both the definition of needs and the way in which they are to be met. Some commentators predict that this will become the predominant means by which disabled people will access personal assistance and support services in the twenty-first century.

Service brokerage

This was introduced into this country from Canada, where it derived from the experiences of parents of people with learning difficulties and their battles with large-scale service systems to obtain the type of services they wanted. Brokers act on behalf of people with learning difficulties to negotiate the services they and their parents decide they need. It is another approach which asserts the rights of individual consumers of services to determine what service they should receive, rather than being dependent on a professional assessment of need. Prior to the introduction of legislation to enable social services departments to make direct payments to service users, there were a few examples of service brokerage schemes operating in this country.

Advocacy

User organizations involving people with learning difficulties and people experiencing mental health problems are developing different models of advocacy. There are also schemes to provide advocacy on behalf of older people who are users of social care services, but these are primarily within the voluntary sector rather than being developed by organizations led by older people. Advocacy can take a number of forms, but what they have in common is the aim of ensuring that the wishes of those who may find it difficult to speak out on their own behalf are represented in their dealings with service providers.

Citizen advocacy involves a partnership between an advocate and a service user in which the advocate speaks as if they were the user themselves: that is, they do not interpret what they feel their partner's needs are, but represent them as their partner would if they had the confidence and communication skills to do this. Where possible, user organizations are supporting people to become self-advocates. An information pack produced by People First, a national organization of people with learning difficulties, describes self-advocacy as follows:

What is self advocacy?

1 Speaking up for yourself.

2 Standing up for your rights.
   - Rights are things that mean you should be treated fairly.
   - Having rights means being the boss of your own life.

3 Making choices.
   - We need information that is easy to understand so we can make the right choices.

4 Being independent.
   - This means doing things for yourself as much as you can, without other people always doing things for you.
   - You can still be independent and have support when you need it.

5 Taking responsibility for yourself.
   - This means looking after yourself.
   - Don't always wait for other people to get things done for you. Get things going yourself.

(People First, no date)

4.3 Planning to meet needs

In addition to encouraging user and carer involvement in assessment, the NHS and Community Care Act placed a requirement on social services authorities to produce community care plans and to consult representatives of users and carers in drawing up these plans. How they should go about this was left to individual authorities to determine. Early studies of the way in which authorities were seeking to consult or otherwise engage with users and carers (separately or jointly) found evidence of good intentions but considerable variation in the way in which they were putting this into practice.

Lindow and Morris (1995) summarized the evidence demonstrating barriers to effective user involvement in service planning. These included:

- Consultation based on 'client group' categories which do not always relate to the way in which people identify themselves and which can be competitive and divisive.

- A tendency to give priority to the views of carers over those of direct service users.

- Some groups are excluded because of a perception that they are not capable of giving an opinion (including people with dementia and people with learning difficulties).

- Other groups are excluded because of the failure of authorities to develop effective means of consulting people from black and Asian communities, and to consult people who use different languages – including deaf people who use British Sign Language.

- Older people constitute the biggest single group of users of social care services, but few are involved in user groups with whom consultations have taken place.

- The agenda is often set by the authority and thus consultation is experienced as a publicity exercise.

Why is it important for users and carers to be involved in discussions about needs at a collective level as well as during individual assessments?

These barriers to consultation indicate at a collective level some of the differences in the way need may be defined by professional and user organizations. Fundamental to these differences is the way in which service organizations allocate people to categories in order to provide a framework within which needs may be defined. Thus physically disabled people are considered to occupy a separate client group category from those with learning difficulties and from older people who also have a physical impairment. Disabled people's organizations committed to a social model of disability emphasize the commonality of experience shared by these three groups that derives from the disabling impact of the physical and social environment in which they live.

Another factor which differentiates many professional approaches to the analysis of need collectively as well as individually is the perceived competence of particular categories of service users to define their own needs. People with learning difficulties may be considered to lack the intellectual capacity to do this, while mental health problems may be seen as resulting in the person 'lacking insight' and being 'out of touch with reality'. Such perceptions are being challenged by user organizations and by some professionals who recognize that the 'problem' may lie as much in difficulties in establishing effective means of communication as in the lack of experience of users in participating in planning processes. Nevertheless, there is a fundamental gap between the perception of the collective views of mental health service users' councils as constituting 'the ravings of mad men' (a psychiatrist quoted in Barnes and Wistow, 1994) and one which recognizes the collective expertise of mental health service users based on personal experience as constituting a necessary input to service planning.

Whilst users are being collectively involved in service planning to an extent which would have been unfamiliar ten years ago, the conclusion of some user organizations is that their energies are better spent in developing their own user-run services, rather than seeking to influence the way in which another day centre may be run. So, for example, mental health service users in Sheffield run their own drop-in centre for younger people with mental health problems who have found statutory services unsympathetic. Disabled people's organizations are increasingly providing similar services to that provided by the Hampshire Centre for Independent Living (see above). Such examples still represent a minority resource, but they provide alternative models of service based on different conclusions about the nature of need experienced by those who are the objects of community care policy.

4.4 A caring resource, or the needs of carers?

Decisions about eligibility for social care services provided through local authority social services departments are also influenced by the availability and capacity of family carers to provide support. Both formal policies and less formalized judgements made by those responsible for making resource allocation decisions reflect this. Indeed, Ellis (1993) found evidence of a degree of 'manipulation' in the way in which assessors sought to explore the availability of informal care:

> a home care manager thought assessors needed to be 'canny' so as not to jeopardise informal support and create 'dependencies'. Assuming most informal carers sought

to withdraw their support, home care managers would establish what carers would provide before explaining what help was available. Both authorities had a policy of supporting carers through the home care service, but one group of managers referred to the 'thin dividing line' they trod between supporting carers and husbanding scarce resources.

(Ellis, 1993, p.21)

The implementation in April 1996 of the Carers Recognition and Services Act meant that carers themselves could request an assessment of their needs. Decisions about the priority to be given to offering a service must take into consideration the impact on the carer of continuing to provide care. However, since eligibility for services is increasingly being determined by reference to risk, the availability of an informal carer is likely to mean an assessment that the level of risk is lower than would be the case if no carer were available.

ACTIVITY 3.6

Return to the notes you made earlier about the key characteristics of care. Consider what this implies for the role of a 'carer'. Draw on your own experiences of family life or friendships to consider the following aspects of 'caring':

1   Can caring relationships exist separately from other types of relationship?

2   Can caring be 'one-way'?

3   Does caring enhance or get in the way of other aspects of a relationship?

4   Who 'cares'?

The Carers Act demonstrates the ambiguous relationship between family carers and statutory services. There are a number of dimensions to this.

Caring and reciprocity

Many caring relationships are reciprocal, but the implementation of the policy requires the construction of one person as the recipient of care, i.e. as the dependant, and the other as the carer-provider. Can a disabled person also be a carer? At what point does a mutually supportive relationship between elderly partners or spouses become unbalanced, identifying one as the care giver and the other the care receiver? Is care giving always in one direction? There are many cases in which those who may be considered 'needy' in one context are also in the position of meeting the needs of others. This may be people with learning difficulties who become partners, older people who provide emotional and at times practical support to younger family members, or a disabled partner helping with the personal care of their spouse.

caring relationships

Friends, families and carers

Caring relationships are usually based in relationships which pre-date the need for 'care', or in which people care about others but may have limited experience of caring *for* them ('tending') – for example, relationships in families between parents and children, husbands and wives or siblings, or between lovers or friends.

Such relationships are often characterized by reciprocity, so that help given by relatives to the older person is considered as an exchange for help received in the past, but there are also examples of previous relationships getting in the

families

Can care recipients also be carers?

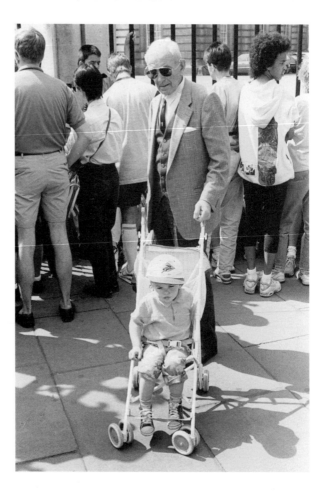

way of good quality care of older parents. In extreme cases this can lead to abuse of the older person by the carer.

In some cases the provision of tending care is given and received as an expression of love within relationships. For others, the provision of personal care can interfere with intimate sexual relations, whilst constant demands for assistance can lead to frustration and anger. Morris (1993) discusses the very different experiences people have of 'caring' within the context of loving relationships:

> Jackie, in describing what were the positive things about receiving personal assistance from someone with whom one has a personal relationship, said, 'I think if you have a relationship with someone you do have a basic recognition of someone as a human being and that makes it alright, that's one of the things. Also there's a lot of trust there, a lot of knowledge and trust … I think there's an absence of embarrassment, you know if you need help in the loo or the bath or around bedtime, you're not likely to be embarrassed with your partner. There's intimacy.'
>
> (Morris, 1993, p.73)

On the other hand, physical dependence on a partner can lead to frustration and anger:

> Catherine explained how certain equipment gave her independence from having to rely on her partner, Robert. A van which she could drive from her electric

wheelchair made a major difference in her life. 'I think there was about six months that we were living here before I got my van, so I was driving to work and someone would help me out of the car at work and someone would help me into the car at the end of the day. And I would come back here and Robert and I had actually negotiated that I wouldn't have somebody in between 5 and 7 because there was one woman who was doing it and she went away and we decided we would try without it for a while.'

She explained why they took this decision. 'It was partly my not wanting to go through the whole interviewing thing again. It was also Robert's very strong tendency to deny the fact that I needed anybody else, you know, he would be able to do everything and there were no problems. I think he … found it really difficult when he was here and I had somebody else here and he would try and … if he was here he would say "oh, don't worry I'll do that, I'll do that" … Anyway we'd arranged that he would be back to help me out of the car, at 5 or 6 o'clock. And the amount of hours that I have spent sitting in the bloody car. I wouldn't sit in this road and I wouldn't drive into our driveway because I was too embarrassed because I knew that neighbours would realise what had happened and they would either come out and ask to help or they'd just stare at me in pity. So I would always park around here and listen to Radio 4 *ad nauseum* until Robert came back. And he used to come back all full of excuses, "it's been so busy at work" and "oh god, I'm sorry". And I would be really angry because he had let me down and if I got angry with him then he would get angrier. We talked about it after I got my van and both admitted how awful it was and he said how awful he felt. He was terrible at time-keeping anyway. But it was a nightmare. It was awful.'

(Morris, 1993, pp.78–9)

In the case of families of people with mental health problems, particularly those with a diagnosis of schizophrenia, there is another important factor affecting the provision of care. Families have, in the past, been implicated if not blamed for the problems of their mentally ill member. Whilst more recent research (Lefley, 1996) has questioned the notion that particular kinds of family relationships can cause schizophrenia, families may not always be the best source of support for those with mental health problems. Family relationships can become severely strained, and in extreme circumstances a wish to exclude the family member can lead to an inappropriate use of compulsory hospital admission to relieve the situation. Here is an example:

Nancy is 53, with a diagnosis of manic depression going back 20 years. She has been a patient continually since 1984 and is detained under Section 3 of the Mental Health Act. Because of this when she goes home she is not discharged but is considered to be on extended leave. The reason for this seems to be that when she 'relapses' or her husband reaches a point where he can no longer cope with her, she can be readmitted to hospital without a reassessment.

There are clearly severe marital problems. Nancy's husband is described by a staff nurse as a man used to having his own way and difficult to deal with. Once Nancy was out shopping with a friend and, on returning later than expected, she found her husband had called the police to find her and ask for her to be readmitted!

(Barnes and Maple, 1992, p.20)

Women and caring

The majority of care within families is undertaken by women family members. Whilst the role of male carers has received attention from those concerned to counteract assumptions that caring is solely a female task (Arber and Gilbert,

The majority of carers are female family members

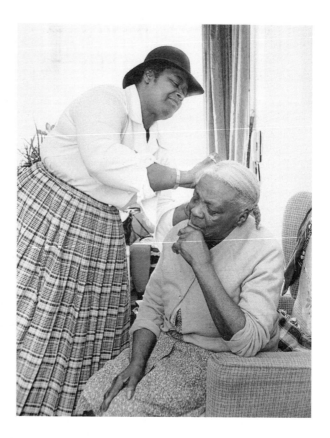

1989; Fisher, 1994), male caring is primarily conducted within spouse relationships and undertaken by older men who have completed their paid working lives. Women carers take on this role throughout their lives. One effect of this is that it reduces their capacity to pursue full-time paid work and thus to develop careers.

Whilst caring may be experienced as both a physical and an emotional burden, it can also form an important part of a woman's personal identity. For such women 'release' from caring may be experienced as a loss of identity rather than freedom to pursue their own interests. The following quote from a woman in this situation provides a graphic illustration. She describes her feelings after the death of her mother, for whom she'd been caring for some years:

> The actual loss of her physically because I'd done so much for her and had so much contact with her physically – made her look nice and brought her clothes and dressed her. And then there was nothing. I remember standing in the front room, not long afterwards, after the funeral and it seemed as though it was the whole world and there was nothing there, just isolation and I did pray to die because she was not there and I wanted to be with her. And the whole routine collapsed. There was nothing to get up for in the morning, she wasn't there to be seen to. I did enjoy doing it once I'd accepted and made the decision for myself to do it – I felt like it was another career.

(quoted in Barnes and Maple, 1992)

Both caring and its loss can negatively impact on the lives of carers, and this impact is disproportionately borne by women. At the same time, demographic changes, shifts in employment patterns, as well as changes in what are perceived to be acceptable divisions of labour between men and women, mean that the availability of female family members who will continue to take on this role cannot be confidently assumed.

'Race', culture and caring

Caring may have a different significance within different communities. Some black women have criticized the analysis by white feminists of caring as constituting a burden on women. Some (for example Graham, 1991) have argued that caring for family members can be experienced as a way of resisting racial and class oppression. Racism, poverty and poor housing conditions may constitute the 'problems' of people's lives, rather than caring *per se*. Attempts to ignore such experiences in order to focus on assessing needs for care as defined within community care policy may miss the point.

At the same time, there is a tendency to assume that caring itself is not a 'problem' within some minority ethnic communities. Stereotypical assumptions about extended families meeting care needs within Asian communities do not reflect the reality of experience and are often an excuse for failing to provide appropriate formal care services.

Different models of health and illness mean that the nature of care provided by family carers may be considered inappropriate or be demeaned by professional workers from different cultures. The following quote, in which an Asian woman talks about her father, provides a particular example of this:

> One of the after-effects of a stroke is an intense headache. They would give him painkillers but they didn't do much. One of the things we do when we are in pain is to give massages. It might not take the pain away, but it helps you to relax. He used to like having his head massaged at that time. The Sister (nurse) used to get really annoyed. She said 'Why are you touching him? All you Asian women mollycoddle your men' ... My mother had become frightened to sit with him or even hold his hand.
>
> (Gunaratnam, 1993, p.119)

Accessing social care can be substantially more difficult for people from minority ethnic communities because of a failure on the part of the service providers to communicate effectively. Simply knowing what question to ask of whom in order to unlock the door to access support is more difficult when people may not even have heard of the existence of 'social care services'.

These different points suggest that a policy built on assumptions that family care is both the best and the preferred option ignores important aspects of interpersonal dynamics as well as structural and cultural factors which affect the availability and capacity of family members to provide care. The nature of services themselves will also affect their accessibility to different groups and thus the potential for interweaving formal and informal support. Future projections of likely levels of need for social care are starting to anticipate the impact of a 'withdrawal' of informal carers from preparedness to continue in this role. One scenario is that the move away from the provision of care in residential units will be halted because of this.

The development of the carers' movement parallels that of the user movement in articulating the experiences of those who are the objects of policy and demanding that their experience in determining their own needs should be recognized. The carers' movement first emerged in the 1950s as a movement of single women providing care for elderly dependants. Throughout its history it has combined campaigning and lobbying at a national level as well as encouraging self-help for carers at a local level (see Extract 3.6).

Extract 3.6 Nancy Kohner: 'A stronger voice'

In 1981, a new organisation was launched. This was to be an organisation of *all* carers, regardless of their sex or age. It was also to be an organisation of carers alone.

Judith Oliver, founder of the Association of Carers and also its first director, was a carer herself. She cared for her husband, who was disabled, and they had a young family. One particular experience motivated her:

> I needed to go into hospital to have an operation. But I was caring for my husband. And the only way I could have that operation was to get my husband up and ready in the morning, get my children off to school, rush off to the hospital, have the operation under a local anaesthetic, and dash back home again so that I was there when the children came in from school and my husband came in from work. At that point I realised that if this was care in the community, then it was nothing.

Judith's awareness of lack of support for carers led her to carry out a small research study, funded by the King's Fund, to find out more about carers' experiences. She interviewed carers around the country:

> What people found most useful in talking to me was that they felt they had been able to speak to someone who was understanding and non-critical and like themselves. And it became clear that what we needed was an organisation through which people could link up.

Judith began to discuss the possibility of setting up an organisation of carers. She wrote to the press, she appeared on television and radio, and like Mary Webster almost twenty years before, she received hundreds of letters in reply, confirming the need for an organisation that would recognise and support all carers – young or old, men or women, married or single.

It was a fundamental principle of the new organisation that carers should not be defined by the disability or illness of the person receiving care. The Association emphasised what was shared by all carers, although this was an idea that was resisted by many professionals at first:

> We found that when professionals became involved in setting up local groups, those groups were always characterised by the condition of the person receiving care. What we wanted was for the professionals to focus on carers *in their own right.*

(Kohner, 1993, pp.8–9)

The carers' lobby became particularly influential in determining national policy on community care during the 1980s. It was clearly in the government's interest to acknowledge the role played by informal or family carers and thus to make a positive response to representations from the Carers National Association (CNA). Jill Pitkeathley, Director of the CNA, was invited to become a member of the group advising Sir Roy Griffiths as he worked on his report, *Community Care: Agenda for Action* (1988), commissioned by the Department of Health. By and large carers were not arguing for the retention of institutional care, but were arguing that the role of carers in delivering much of the support on which community care depended should be recognized and supported. Jill Pitkeathley is quoted as saying: 'I've never known such consensus around a set of proposals as there was around Griffiths. Everyone, on the whole, agreed with the proposals' (quoted in Kohner, 1993, p.20).

Support for carers received legislative recognition when the Carers Recognition and Services Act was implemented in 1996. Also in that year the CNA produced a guide for carers which encouraged them to take advantage of their statutory rights to assessment (see Extract 3.7).

Extract 3.7 Carers National Association: 'What will happen at the assessment?'

An assessment can take different forms, from a simple chat to a detailed assessment. Normally it will be undertaken by one person but where a lot of care is needed, it may be necessary to arrange a meeting between you, the person needing care, a social worker, a doctor and a nurse so that everyone can consider how best to help. The assessment should be carried out in a convenient place for you and the person for whom you care.

The assessment is the chance for you both to tell the social worker what you need and what would make life easier for you. It is important that you both think about the things which you find difficult and the services which could help you …

Try and discuss your views with the person you care for so you can generally agree on what kind of help is needed. However, if you are unable to agree then ask to be assessed independently which will give you both the opportunity to give your points of view. You may find it helpful to make notes before and during the interview so that you don't forget anything.

The social worker is there to help you resolve any problems or disagreements, for example, you may want to carry on doing paid work for as long possible. It is important that social services understand your wishes and provide services to support you. You are entitled to work if you want to.

It can be quite hard to know how to start thinking about what you need and to know what kind of help you would like …

[The following are examples of issues that carers are encouraged to think about in preparing for assessment:]

Do you and the person you care for live together or apart? Is this arrangement satisfactory? If it is not satisfactory then say why.

Does the person you care for have any difficulties in the home? For example, climbing steps and stairs, having a bath – if special equipment can make it easier for the person you look after, then things will be easier for you …

Do you have any health problems? Describe them as fully as possible. For example, if you have a bad back you can get lifting equipment …

Do you feel as though you are suffering from stress or depression?

How many hours a week do you care? This can include the time you spend with the person you care for and the time you spend doing other things for them such as washing, cleaning and cooking. *(List the jobs you do and how long it takes you – it may surprise you!)*

Are there things you find enjoyable and relaxing which you can't do because of your caring responsibilities? For example, you may have given up a hobby or you may want to visit friends.

When was the last time that you had a whole day to yourself to do as you pleased?

(Carers National Association, 1996, pp.6–11)

The Carers Act gave recognition to the needs of carers in their own right and thus suggested that they are another 'client group' who may be recipients of social care. But a carer's assessment must follow an assessment of the person they care for, and it is the provision of care and the capacity and willingness of the person to continue to provide that care which forms the subject of the assessment. For some time prior to the passage of the Act the relationship of 'informal carer' to statutory services had been recognized as ambiguous. Twigg (1989) described three models which provided different frames of reference for the way in which those working in social care agencies understood their relationship with carers. Workers could view carers as resources, co-workers or co-clients.

As resources, carers were seen as another source of support to be drawn on in providing what were not yet then called packages of care. The problem was (and is) that informal carers cannot be 'commanded' in the same way that resources based on formal rules for resource allocation can be. As co-workers, the paid and unpaid carers are colleagues in the 'care enterprise'. Carers are viewed as quasi-professionals with the implication that the direct 'client' occupies a powerless position subject to a caring alliance between formal and informal carer. In the third model, as co-client, the carer is viewed as another person needing help because of the physical burden or emotional stress deriving from their caring role. The prospect of carers becoming co-clients on a large scale is not one which social services authorities view with equanimity: it would represent a substantial new source of need to be met at the same time as removing a substantial caring resource. But nor is the co-client role one that many carers would want to embrace. There is much research evidence to suggest that carers are reluctant to seek help until their physical or emotional distress is nearing breaking point.

So, are carers resources, co-workers or co-clients? Or are they 'caring experts', as more recent research (Nolan *et al.*, 1995) has suggested? Is there necessarily a conflict between enabling people who might be regarded as direct users of services to live in their own or family homes, and ensuring that members of their families are neither forced to take on caring roles, nor exploited if both parties willingly accept such an arrangement?

Whichever of Twigg's three models is dominant among statutory social care providers (and she notes that each is an ideal type, unlikely to be present in 'pure' form in any particular agency), each suggests that there is a strong motivation to ensure that informal carers are recognized, valued and supported. Only in this way will they be likely to sustain a substantial role in providing both practical and emotional support to family members or friends in need of 'care'. It is this that lay behind the passage of the Carers Act.

5   Care, needs or rights?

So far the discussion has focused on definitions and processes associated with obtaining support from statutory authorities with responsibilities for meeting 'social care needs'. At this point, however, we need to step back to consider challenges to the basic concept of 'need for social care'. There are three aspects to the critique of this concept:

- The designation of needs of particular groups within the population as 'special'.
- The question of whether we should be thinking about social rights rather than needs.
- The importance of re-introducing community.

5.1 Special needs?

The term 'special needs' is often used to describe the social care needs of disabled people, older people, people with learning difficulties, and those with mental health problems. The implication is that those needs are different from the needs of 'ordinary' people and that they constitute a problem. However, community care implies that those who were at one time separated from the rest of the population are now living alongside them. An increasing number of people who would previously have been separated from their families within institutions are now living with the families into which they were born. Some are creating their own families (and in so doing confusing further the question of who is the recipient and who is the provider of care) (Booth and Booth, 1994).

In addition, demographic changes mean that the experience of having an older relative who may need extra support for many years is an increasingly

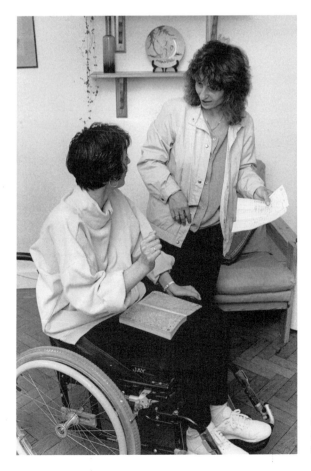

Is 'care' an appropriate way to describe disabled people's needs to be able to travel around the towns in which they live?

119

common one. Families in which caring responsibilities are both more intense and longer lasting than the provision of parental care to children until they reach independence are becoming more 'normal'. 'Ordinary life' often includes living with people with 'special needs'.

If we look at the types of services included within the rubric of social care, we find that many are designed to meet needs we all have for: appropriate accommodation; creative activity and the development of skills which can enhance our capacity to engage in this; transport which enables us to move around; and opportunities to get away from those with whom we live in close proximity from time to time.

One effect of the closure of long-stay hospitals was that those used to having all their physical, social and spiritual needs met within the confines of the institution were discharged into an environment in which the usual practice is for people to seek out for themselves ways in which these varied needs might be met. Since chief responsibility for people with 'special needs' living in the community lies with social services departments, services and resources which most people might expect to receive from housing departments or from employment, leisure and recreational services are accessed through the process of community care assessments. Thus necessities which all of us take for granted and would not consider as comprising 'care' needs come within the notion of social care when the people concerned are disabled, have mental health problems or learning difficulties, or are old and frail.

One effect of this is to maintain the segregation of people: even though they are living within the community, they are not part of it.

5.2 Social care or social rights?

The challenge to producer perspectives coming from within user and carer movements is not just about details of service planning or how assessments should be carried out. It also raises fundamental questions about how needs should be defined, who should define them, and indeed whether need is the most appropriate concept to use. Central to this is the rights versus care debate which has been prominent within the disability movement. Mike Oliver expressed this as follows:

rights

> disabled people are more likely to be out of work than non-disabled people, they are out of work longer than other unemployed workers, and when they do find work it is more often than not low paid, low status work with poor working conditions ... This in turn accelerates the discriminatory spiral in which many disabled people find themselves.

> The majority of disabled people and their families, therefore, are forced into depending on welfare benefits in order to survive ... Further, the present disability benefit system does not even cover impairment related costs and effectively discourages many of those who struggle for autonomy and financial independence. Dependence is the inevitable result and this is compounded by the present system of health and welfare services, most of which are dominated by the interests of the professionals who run them ... and the traditional assumption that disabled people are incapable of running their own lives. Current welfare provision not only denies disabled people the opportunities to live autonomously but also denies them the dignity of independence within inter-personal relationships and the family home.

> (Oliver, 1996, pp.64–5)

This analysis led not only to the successful campaign for legislation enabling social services departments to make direct payments to disabled people for the purchase of their own personal support services, but also to the much broader campaigning for anti-discrimination legislation. The Disability Discrimination Act, implemented in December 1996, was not regarded as having been completely successful in legislating for the rights of disabled people to be free from discrimination in all aspects of their lives, but it marked an important step forward.

Oliver argued against the fundamental notion that 'need' should have a central place in determining welfare policy and provision. He identified an 'unfortunate retreat from active to passive citizenship and from rights-based to needs-based welfare provision' (Oliver, 1996, p.68) at an early stage in the implementation of legislation to introduce a range of welfare provisions at the end of the Second World War. No professionalized service based on the assessment of need rather than on citizenship rights to welfare can redress the imbalance of power between disabled people and service providers, nor ensure that the receipt of support is not dependent on budgetary constraints.

ACTIVITY 3.7

The perspective of Oliver and others who argue for 'rights not care' offers a profound challenge to dominant ways of thinking about the 'needs' of disabled people (which includes people with mental health problems or learning difficulties, as well as people of all ages with physical or sensory impairments). Spend some time thinking about your reactions to this. How would you respond to the following questions?

1   Do people only need to seek access to social care services because of discrimination and exclusion from mainstream social and economic life?

2   Should social care services be available as of right?

3   Is enabling individuals to purchase their own support services a solution to the problems of 'assessment' identified in this chapter?

4   Does 'care' – love, compassion, concern, interest in another person – have anything to do with enabling people to live their lives in the way they choose?

5.3   Independence or participation within a community?

Anti-discrimination legislation addresses people's rights as citizens beyond their status as consumers of services. It seeks to remove barriers to employment, housing, transport, and leisure and cultural facilities which both collectively and individually exclude disabled people. Exclusionary barriers include stigma, ageism, fear or distaste on the part of the 'normal' population, as well as physical barriers. The effects of poverty and poor self-esteem can act on the individual concerned to add to a personal as well as structural experience of exclusion.

If community care policy is genuinely concerned with bringing into communities those who have been physically separated from them, and enabling them to participate in community life (Barnes, 1997), then it should be addressing those exclusionary forces as well as responding to the needs of particular individuals. Oliver (1987) has suggested that rather than spending time counting the numbers of disabled people to help plan services to meet their individual needs, effort should be spent on identifying the disabling effects of local communities in order to take action to remove those barriers which lead to social exclusion. Mental health user groups such as the Nottingham Advocacy Group run regular public awareness campaigns intended to overcome the stigma which excludes many people with mental health problems from community life.

As we have seen, official community care policy has little to say about community. Whilst activists within the disability movement have argued for the need to overcome 'disabling barriers' within communities (for example Swain *et al.*, 1993), much of their recent action has been focused on achieving individual rights to determine and control their own services. Such objectives have little to do directly with community development. What are the implications for communities of including within them people who have previously been excluded? In Derbyshire the local coalition of disabled people is jointly responsible, with the local authority, for the management of a Centre for Integrated Living. They seek to emphasize the objective of integration of disabled people within mainstream society, rather than an objective of independence *per se*. Such an objective implies that 'need' in this context should encompass the needs of the community itself, as well as the individual needs of disabled people, older people and those with mental health problems or learning difficulties, for support to enable them to become effective participants within their communities. Community needs could include investment to ensure that the environment is physically accessible and safe; to provide 'dwellings for life' in which people who become disabled as a result of accident or chronic illness can remain rather than having to move elsewhere; and to ensure that there are community meeting places which can be used by different groups within the local population and thus avoid the separation of, for example, people with learning difficulties within specialist day centres or clubs. Community needs could also include action within the community intended to address directly the potential for stigmatizing those who are 'different' by virtue of disability, mental impairment or mental distress.

6   Conclusion

This chapter has considered the way in which needs for social care are defined in community care policy and practice. It has emphasized the contested nature of the key concepts on which community care policy is based, and considered the way in which decisions about who has access to social care are mediated by financial constraints, personal and professional judgements on the part of gatekeepers, and by the availability of family carers. Although official policy has sought to encourage more active participation by users and carers in the process of determining needs and how they should be met, this objective has been in conflict with a perceived need to maintain control of access to services at a time of resource constraints. This, together with a sense that disabled people should be able to control their own lives and should not be dependent on professional assessment to determine their needs, has led to a number of models of practice which are intended to make fundamental changes in the way in which social care can be accessed.

Some advocates of these alternative practices argue that the concept of 'need' itself should be abandoned and that access to support to enable people to live ordinary lives should be considered as a social right. Similarly, they argue that 'care' is an inappropriate way of viewing the personal support that can enable people to live active lives. This has led in some instances to conflict between disabled people's organizations and those representing the interests of family carers. 'Care' itself is a complex concept that encompasses both emotional and physical labour, given and received within relationships of different types and qualities. Formal policies that rely on the availability and preparedness of family members to take on substantial caring roles for long periods of their lives both exploit family carers and contribute to unwelcome dependence on the part of those receiving care. However, it is neither realistic nor helpful to seek to remove concern, tenderness, love – the 'caring about' aspects of care – from supportive relationships that are intended to enable older people, disabled people and those experiencing mental distress or learning difficulties to sustain and develop social relationships and participate within the communities in which they live.

At the same time, if the objective of community care is to enable community participation, then 'needs' should encompass a broader range of necessities than those usefully considered to comprise 'care'. One important implication of this is that responsibility for the effective implementation of community care policy cannot solely be left to those agencies traditionally considered to have responsibility for social care. The way in which houses are constructed, public transport is provided, and work and education are organized will affect the fundamental question of whether people need to seek access to social care services which might be considered a substitute for participation in mainstream social life.

Further reading

There is a substantial literature on the experience of caring and on the relationship between family carers and formal service providers. Parker (1990) provides a review of research in this area, whilst Twigg and Atkin (1994) report a more recent study which develops the analysis of the way in which carers are viewed by formal service providers. In addition to the work by Oliver (1996) and Morris (1993), key texts articulating disabled people's perspectives on care and rights include Barnes (1991) and Swain et al. (1993). The perspectives of people with learning difficulties are reflected in Segal and Varma (1991) and Ramcharan et al. (1997). From a rather different perspective Prior (1993) considers how the professional organization of services constructs the way in which mental illness is defined and understood, and hence how different professional groups approach the task of 'meeting their needs'. Craig and Mayo (1995) make links between community development and community care.

References

Arber, S. and Gilbert, N. (1989) 'Men: the forgotten carers', *Sociology*, vol.23, no.1, pp.111–18.

Audit Commission (1986) *Making a Reality of Community Care*, London, HMSO.

Barnes, C. (1991) *Disabled People in Britain and Discrimination. A Case for Anti-Discrimination Legislation*, London, Hurst/Calgary.

Barnes, M. (1997) *Care, Communities and Citizens,* Harlow, Addison Wesley Longman.

Barnes, M. and Maple, N. (1992) *Women and Mental Health: Challenging the Stereotypes,* Birmingham, Venture Press.

Barnes, M. and Wistow, G. (1994) 'Learning to hear voices: listening to users of mental health services', *Journal of Mental Health,* no.2, pp.347–56.

Beardshaw, V. (1991) *Implementing Assessment and Care Management: Learning from Local Experience 1990–1991,* London, King's Fund Centre.

Booth, T. and Booth, W. (1994) *Parenting under Pressure,* Buckingham, Open University Press.

Bulmer, M. (1987) *The Social Basis of Community Care,* London, Allen and Unwin.

Carers National Association (1996) *New Rights for Carers: How to Get My Carers Assessment – A Carers Guide,* London, CNA.

Courtney, M. and Walker, M. (1996) *Stand and Deliver: Making Pensioners Pay for Care,* London, NHS Support Federation and West Midlands Health Research Unit.

Craig, G. and Mayo, M. (eds) (1995) *Community Empowerment. A Reader in Participation and Development,* London, Zed Books.

Dalley, G. (1988) *Ideologies of Caring,* Basingstoke, Macmillan.

Department of Health (no date) *Implementing Care for People: Care Management*, London, Department of Health.

Department of Health and Social Security (1971) *Better Services for the Mentally Handicapped,* London, HMSO.

Department of Health and Social Security (1975) *Better Services for the Mentally Ill,* London, HMSO.

Ellis, K. (1993) *Squaring the Circle. User and Carer Participation in Needs Assessment,* York, Joseph Rowntree Foundation.

Fisher, M. (1994) 'Man-made care: community care and older male carers', *British Journal of Social Work,* vol.24, pp.659–90.

Graham, H. (1991) 'The concept of caring in feminist research: the case of domestic service', *Sociology,* vol.25, pp.61–78.

Griffiths, R. (1988) *Community Care: Agenda for Action. A Report to the Secretary of State for Social Services,* London, HMSO.

Gunaratnam, Y. (1993) 'Breaking the silence: Asian carers in Britain', in Bornat, J. *et al.* (eds) *Community Care: A Reader,* Basingstoke, Macmillan in association with The Open University.

Hadley, R. and Hatch, S. (1981) *Social Welfare and the Failure of the State,* London, Allen and Unwin.

Hughes, G. (1998) 'A suitable case for treatment? Constructions of disability', in Saraga, E. (ed.) *Embodying the Social: Constructions of Difference,* London, Routledge in association with The Open University.

King's Fund (1980) *An Ordinary Life,* London, King's Fund Centre.

Kohner, N. (1993) *A Stronger Voice,* London, Carers National Association.

Lefley, H. (1996) *Caregiving in Mental Illness,* Thousand Oaks, Ca., Sage.

Lindow, V. and Morris, J. (1995) *Service User Involvement. Synthesis of Findings and Experience in the Field of Community Care,* York, Joseph Rowntree Foundation.

Marsh, P. and Fisher, M. (1992) *Good Intentions: Developing Partnership Practice in Social Services,* York, Joseph Rowntree Foundation.

Morris, J. (1993) *Independent Lives. Community Care and Disabled People,* Basingstoke, Macmillan.

National Health Service (1971) *Report of the Farleigh Hospital Committee of Inquiry,* Cmnd. 4557, London, HMSO.

Nolan, M., Keady, J. and Grant, G. (1995) 'Developing a typology of family care: implications for nurses and other service providers', *Journal of Advanced Nursing,* no.21, pp.256–65.

Oliver, M. (1987) 'Re-defining disability: some implications for research', *Research, Policy and Planning,* no.5, pp. 9–13.

Oliver, M. (1996) *Understanding Disability. From Theory to Practice,* Basingstoke, Macmillan.

Parker, G. (1990) *With Due Care and Attention: A Review of Research on Informal Care,* London, Family Policy Studies Centre.

People First (no date) People First Information Pack, 207–215 Kings Cross Road, London, People First.

Prior, L. (1993) *The Social Organisation of Mental Illness,* London, Sage.

Ramcharan, P., Roberts, G., Grant, G. and Borland, J. (eds) (1997) *Empowerment in Everyday Life. Learning Disability,* London, Jessica Kingsley.

Ryan, J. and Thomas, F. (1980) *The Politics of Mental Handicap,* Harmondsworth, Penguin.

Secretaries of State for Health, Social Security, Wales and Scotland (1989) *Caring for People. Community Care in the Next Decade and Beyond,* Cm 849, London, HMSO.

Segal, S.S. and Varma, V.P. (eds) (1991) *Prospects for People with Learning Difficulties,* London, David Fulton Publishers.

Smith, P. and Thomas, N. (1993) *Contracts and Competition in Public Services,* paper given at the Association of Directors of Social Services Annual Conference, University of Birmingham.

Staffordshire County Council (1996) *Report of the Director of Social Services to the Social Services Committee,* Staffordshire County Council.

Swain, J., Finkelstein, V., French, S. and Oliver, M. (eds) (1993) *Disabling Barriers – Enabling Environments,* London, Sage.

Thomas, C. (1993) 'Deconstructing concepts of care', *Sociology*, vol.27, no.4, pp.649–69.

Twigg, J. (1989) 'Models of carers: how do social care agencies conceptualise their relationships with carers?', *Journal of Social Policy*, vol.18, no.1, pp.53–66.

Twigg, J. and Atkin, K. (1994) *Carers Perceived: Policy and Practice in Informal Care*, Buckingham, Open University Press.

Wolfensberger, W. (1972) *The Principle of Normalization in Human Services*, Toronto, National Institute on Mental Retardation.

Wolfensberger, W. (1983) 'Social role valorization: a proposed new term for the principle of normalization', *Mental Retardation*, vol.21, no.6, pp.234–9.

CHAPTER 4

Children's Needs: Who Decides?

by Esther Saraga

Contents

1   Introduction

At the turn of the twentieth century, concerns about children are high on the public agenda. They include issues like child abuse, teenage pregnancies, educational standards, drug and alcohol abuse among children, juvenile crime, and the failure of some parents to socialize their children adequately. State concerns have been reflected in a range of important new legislation, including the Children Act 1989 for England and Wales (which was followed in 1995 by The Children (Scotland) Act and The Children (Northern Ireland) Order), the Child Support Act 1991, and legislative and policy changes within the areas of criminal justice and education (see Chapter 5).

Children's rights came to prominence after 1979, the International Year of the Child, leading to the development of a United Nations (UN) Convention on the Rights of the Child, which was adopted in 1989. In the 1980s a number of children's rights organizations were founded in the UK, including The Children's Legal Centre and EPOCH (End Physical Punishment of Children). ChildLine, a national, free, confidential 24-hour telephone helpline for children was set up in 1986, and was soon receiving up to 10,000 calls a day. In 1979 the UK rejected the idea of a UN Convention; it nevertheless ratified it in 1991, one month after the implementation of the Children Act 1989. However, the 1990s witnessed a reaction against children's rights, which were said to undermine the authority of parents and teachers (Franklin, 1995).

It is in this context of rapidly changing and fiercely contested ideas about children and their needs and rights that we shall examine competing constructions of children's needs and the role of parents and/or the state in meeting them. The Children Act 1989 represents a key moment in these debates, as it aimed to strike a new balance between meeting the needs of children and protecting the family from intrusive state intervention. Much of the discussion will therefore focus on this Act and the subsequent similar legislation for Scotland and Northern Ireland. Where the issues apply to the UK as a whole, I shall refer to the 'Children Acts' in general.

The Children Act 1989 was informed by a comprehensive review of child-care law and practice, which was instigated by a range of concerns that had been expressed in the previous two decades, namely:

- The number of children being taken into the care of the local authority, and evidence of the negative effects of care on children's development.
- The increase in the number of reported cases of child abuse.
- Criticisms of the coercive way in which social workers were handling such cases, and of their discretionary powers.

More generally, state intervention was seen to undermine the rights of both children and parents, thereby threatening the sanctity of the family.

A central feature of the new legislation was the duty placed on local authorities (who already had statutory responsibilities in relation to neglected or abused children) to identify all 'children in need' within their area. They were required to plan services to meet those needs so as to promote, as far as possible, the upbringing of children within their own families. In doing so, the welfare of the child was to be paramount. For the first time in UK law, children were recognized as having the right to be consulted and kept informed about all decisions affecting them, there was scope for children to challenge court orders, and complaints procedures for children and young people in care were established.

A fundamental principle of the legislation was that children's needs are best met within the 'family', by parents. In practice, children live within a wide diversity of 'families', but within dominant ideas it is a particular kind of family that is seen as best, or even essential, for both meeting the needs of children and maintaining social order (see **Hall, 1998**; **Lentell, 1998**). The 'family' is seen as a private institution, in which parents have the right, within limits, to bring up their children as they wish without interference from the state. Parents are also seen as having responsibilities towards children. Where these are not fulfilled, the needs of children are cited as the reason or justification for intervening into the family.

Although parental obligations for children are widely accepted, there are very different views on the role of the state. Triseliotis (1993) distinguished five positions:

1   People who choose to have children should be responsible for them; the state is a safety net for cases of serious family failure.

2   The state should intervene only in serious cases, because of the devastating and irreparable psychological consequences for children of separation from their parents.

3   State intervention should be made largely unnecessary, by providing universal, locally based services such as crèches and day nurseries, youth centres, and out of school hours leisure facilities, as well as good income support, adequate housing, and good health and education services.

4   The state should actively intervene to remove children from families that cannot meet their needs, and provide an alternative experience of 'permanent' family life.

5   Children should be granted rights to make their own decisions about their lives, free from adult coercion, including that which is disguised as 'protection'.

The Children Act 1989 perhaps represents a sixth position. By attempting to target all children 'in need' rather than just those 'at risk of harm', it recognized that all families might need support, not just those seen as inadequate, dysfunctional or dangerous. Welfare professionals were to work 'in partnership' with parents, and services should respond, it was argued, to 'the normal vicissitudes of family life' (Aldgate and Tunstill, 1995, p.1).

In all the positions outlined above, it is assumed, first, that we know who 'children' are, and second, in all but position 5, that their key characteristic is dependence on adults. Because of their dependency, children's experiences and their wants and desires are nearly always mediated by adults, who also make the decisions about what is in the best interest of children. But who defines children's needs? Do children themselves have a voice in those definitions and decisions? It will be helpful to keep these questions in mind throughout the chapter.

Section 2 examines the social construction of children's needs within welfare discourses, policy and practices. These needs are largely described as essential and universal, and characteristic of all children. At the same time, some children are seen as 'different' and as having 'special needs', requiring specific forms of welfare intervention.

Section 3 focuses on children at risk of harm within their own family. It examines the tension between the need to protect children and the need to preserve 'the family'.

Section 4 shifts the focus from children to parents, since parents are seen to have the main responsibility for meeting children's needs. It examines ideas on parental responsibility and changing assumptions about gender and parenting.

Section 5 examines discourses on 'children's rights' and the extent to which children can be seen as citizens in their own right, rather than as part of a family, or as apprentice or future citizens.

2   The needs of children

2.1   What is a child?

In order to explore what is meant by the needs of children, we have first to consider how childhood and youth are socially constructed within welfare discourses, policies and practices, and whether it is helpful to see children as a distinct group in relation to welfare.

childhood

Common sense sees childhood as a life stage, distinct from adulthood, from which it is separated by the transitional stage of youth or adolescence. These life stages are generally seen as occurring naturally, with childhood characterized primarily as a time of dependence, in contrast to the independence of adulthood. However, evidence of historical and cultural variations in ideas on childhood suggests that these life stages are not natural, but socially and historically specific – that is, they are socially constructed (Aries, 1962; Goldson, 1997).

Two dominant, but contradictory, essentialist views of children see them either as (a) innocent, vulnerable and in need of protection, or (b) asocial, inherently evil and in need of socialization through firm control and discipline. Children are generally expected to behave better than adults, though other people are frequently allowed to behave less well towards them: for example, children are the only group that it is legally acceptable, under certain circumstances, to hit.

ACTIVITY 4.1

Read Extract 4.1, which is from an academic textbook on social policy in relation to young people. Make notes on what Coles seems to regard as being the central distinguishing features between childhood, youth and adulthood in relation to welfare policy. To what extent is it possible to derive a clear view of children and childhood from this account?

Extract 4.1 Coles: 'Youth and social policy'

Welfare systems designed for children are organized so as to offer opportunities and support for their physical, emotional, social, moral and educational development and to protect them from abuse and exploitation ... Some of this is done indirectly through support for the family, but it also occurs through the direct provision of services for children and young people by agencies of the state ... welfare policy accepts that 'childhood' has a status of 'dependency'. In many societies, and for most children, this dependency is largely provided for within the household and family. Children are expected to be looked after by their families and to be economically dependent upon them. Many welfare systems offer economic and social support to parents with children, together with state support for children who fall outside biological families, because of bereavement or because such families cannot cope adequately with the upbringing. In circumstances such as these ... children are offered surrogate families through fostering, adoption or places in special institutions, such as children's homes ... In Britain and elsewhere, children are also provided with welfare services beyond the confines of the family, through schools, nurseries, medical care and other services based in the community. Where children or young people are regarded as severely disturbed, violent, or potentially 'at risk', they may be catered for in specially designed 'secure accommodation' provided for or paid for by agencies of the state. Children and young people up to the age of 16 are obliged to be educated and to attend school, and legally their parents, or guardians, must ensure that they do so. In most developed welfare systems children are also protected by law from various forms of exploitation. In Britain, children cannot legally engage in sexual activity, and cannot marry or vote ... Nor can they take up many forms of paid employment until a specific age, and then only in limited and controlled circumstances. Children cannot enter into legal contracts or legally own property until the age of majority of 18 in England and Wales, though they can at 16 in Scotland ... Parents are legally responsible for making certain that children are properly cared for, looked after and fulfil all their legal obligations. If children commit criminal offences they are dealt with by special courts, and their parents (as well as the children themselves) can be called upon to answer for their actions, blamed for not exercising proper care and control, and in some cases share in any reparation required by the courts ... Children are, therefore, deemed to be dependent upon adult society, and are nurtured and provided for by both the family and the state. The family is regarded as a natural haven in which protection and dependence can be achieved, but the state acts as guarantor for the welfare and development of all children.

Adults, on the other hand, are accorded different rights and responsibilities. They can marry, vote and enter into contracts, and they are held responsible for their own actions in both the civil and criminal courts. By and large they are expected to provide for their own economic means of support, to engage in paid work, to provide themselves with a living, and to pay taxes towards the cost of general welfare services and the social security of others ... Some adults who cannot find paid work, or who are beyond the age of retirement, receive state support through various forms of social security, unless they are female and living in households, in which case they may be deemed to be financially dependent upon another male wage earner ... In short, adults are treated as full 'citizens' and as such are regarded as independent and responsible human beings ...

Young people are treated neither as children nor as adults ... under the Children Act 1989, they are considered to be capable of making some decisions about their own futures, but are also considered to need both some protection from

131

exploitation and abuse, and some help and guidance in making wise decisions about their own welfare and careers. They are thus regarded, in part, as both independent choice-making human beings, but also as dependent upon other people (and especially their parents) for care, guidance and support. The full rights and responsibilities of adulthood are given gradually, and at different ages, while parents and legal guardians are expected and required to help young people make the transition to full adult status ... Legally, the rights and responsibilities of youth and adulthood present a complex (if not chaotic) picture of the transition to adulthood. In England and Wales, young people can: be at least in part held 'responsible' for crime at the age of 10; undertake part-time employment (between 7am and 7pm) after the age of 13; be liable to pay full fare on public transport (buses and trains) at the age of 14; cease to attend full-time education at 16 and legally engage in heterosexual sex with consent at the same age; vote, be sent to an adult prison, be required to undergo national service and marry without parental consent after the 'age of majority' at 18; ... not legally engage in male homosexual activities until the age of 18; ... and not receive social security at an adult rate in the form of income support if they are unemployed, until the age of 25 ... When they are in the care of local authorities rather than their parents', young people's views must be taken into account in deciding where and with whom they should live, and they may be supported by their local authorities up to the age of 21. If they are homeless and under the age of 16, local authorities must arrange accommodation for them, but after that age, housing may be provided only if they are thought to be vulnerable or at risk ... These and other legal rights help to illustrate that, in legal terms, there is no clear end to the status of childhood and no clear age at which young people are given full adult rights and responsibilities. In short, the legal definitions of childhood, youth and adulthood present a complex array of definitions which have been developed by the different institutions of the state, for different purposes, and at different moments in history.

(Coles, 1995, pp.4–7)

COMMENT

Coles's account demonstrates both the differences in status accorded to children and to adults, and also the lack of clear boundaries between childhood, youth and adulthood. Childhood is viewed as a state of dependence upon adults, with needs being met primarily by parents within families. Some services for children, such as health and education, are also provided by the state, but parents still play a crucial role by ensuring, for example, that their children attend school. It does not seem possible to discuss meeting the needs of children without also considering parents' responsibilities, and whether they are able or willing to fulfil them. The importance of the family for meeting children's needs is reinforced by the attempts that are made to provide an alternative family for children whose biological families cannot care for them.

Young children (under 10 years old) are clearly seen as dependent, needing protection and as requiring decisions to be made for them by responsible parents. They are excluded from the public world of work, and they are asexual. In the public sphere they are primarily visible within education. By contrast, the extent to which children over 10 are seen as dependent and/or responsible for their own actions is much more complicated and contradictory. I noted in particular the contrast between children being held at least in part responsible for their crimes at the age of 10, but not being deemed sufficiently mature to make decisions about engaging in sexual activities until they are 16 for heterosexual activity, or 18 for male homosexuality. (At the time of writing, 1998, the Labour government has stated its intention to allow a free vote in the House of Commons on a proposal to lower the age of consent to 16.)

One central question remains: who has the power to decide when children are capable of deciding for themselves? Clearly, babies and very young children are vulnerable and dependent, though even babies can effectively communicate some of their desires and needs. The adults responsible for them decide which decisions children can make for themselves and how this will change as they grow older; at the same time adults overrule children's wishes when they deem them not to be in the child's best interests. Young children could decide, for example, which clothes to wear, or which toy to play with, but an adult may intervene if a child wants to go outside on a cold day with no warm clothes. One of the characteristics of being an adult is that you are allowed to make decisions that other people might think were not in your best interests, whether this involves the choice to smoke, or for a woman to remain living with a violent partner. In contrast it is widely believed that children should not be allowed to make the decision to smoke or to remain with an abusive parent or parents.

■ ■ ■

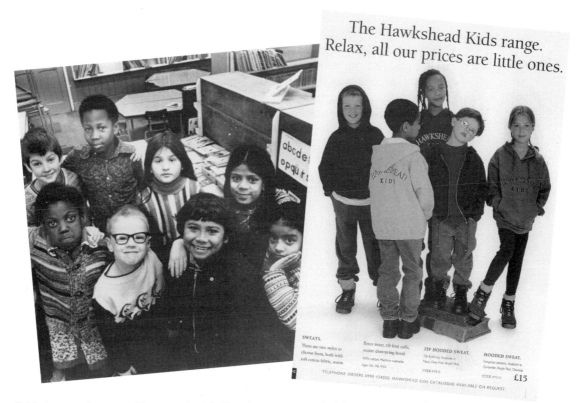

Public images of young children: at school (left) and as consumers (right)

Children are visible within public discourse in fragmented ways: for example, as learners in school, as objects of parental authority and control, as 'victims' of

133

lone parents or family breakdown, as criminals or potential criminals, and as consumers (for example of sportswear). They are rarely discussed in terms of the quality of their childhood experiences, unless these are seen as having an impact on their future as adult citizens. Save the Children (1995) has suggested a number of factors that have contributed to children's invisibility:

- The lack of child-specific information (children are viewed as part of adult categories such as 'family' or 'household').

- Not recognizing children's productive contribution (though many children do paid work, while many work, unpaid, within the home or as carers).

- Not consulting with children or involving them in decision-making (children are seen primarily as passive and dependent, a view which 'enables adults to exercise power over children above and beyond that required to nurture and protect children into adulthood' (p.7).

- The use of a standard model of childhood which is ethnocentric and ahistorical.

The rest of this chapter will be concerned primarily with debates about the needs of children for care and protection. It will be important to keep in mind these questions about constructions of childhood. Chapter 5 looks at the issue of young people in relation to offending and the criminal justice system.

2.2   Changing definitions

children's
needs

Consideration of the ways in which need has been socially constructed is not academic, since they influence the nature of the services provided. Definitions of children's needs and how they should be met, and judgements as to which children are seen as requiring state welfare provision, varies historically and cross-culturally and with socio-economic circumstances.

How would you define the needs of children?

The twentieth century saw the development of psychological discourses: psychologically healthy children were the natural product of normal families. Prior to this parents were more concerned with issues of physical survival and moral growth. For most of human history, and still in many parts of the world, physical survival has been the predominant concern. In the eighteenth and nineteenth centuries in the UK this was combined with moral concerns expressed within religious discourses, such as those of the Evangelical movement, whose main preoccupation was with subjugating children's wills and eradicating the devil (Newson and Newson, 1974).

The early part of the twentieth century was dominated by the ideas of the hygienist movement, who adopted the same moral and authoritarian tones as the Evangelicals, emphasizing discipline and self-control, but expressed now within medical discourses. Their primary concern was the establishment of 'regular habits' during the first five years of life as a foundation for adult physical and mental well-being. Children were seen to have legitimate physical *needs*, which should be met, in contrast to their illegitimate *wants*, or 'pleasure strivings' (Newson and Newson, 1974, p.64). Mothers were expected to make their babies submit to their control, and even physical needs, such as hunger, were to be ignored if expressed at an inappropriate time:

Feeding-times loom large in baby's life, and it is particularly with regard to these that one would urge punctuality ... the normal healthy baby does best on five feeds a day with no night feed ... Baby must be taught the habit of unbroken rest for eight hours at night from the very first.

(Liddiard, 1934, p.42)

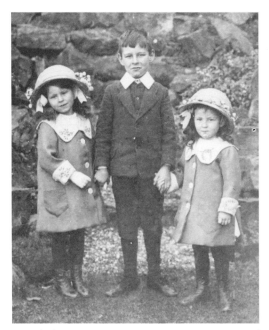 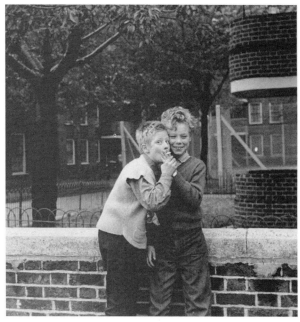

Changing historical images of children: 1904 (left) and 1967 (right)

By the 1950s a dramatic change had taken place. The first five years of life were still emphasized, but normal development depended upon meeting not only physical needs but also legitimate psychological 'wants' or 'desires'. Overwhelmingly, children needed 'mothering'. Although the exclusive focus on mothers was later modified, the dominance of psychological discourses continued.

By the 1970s children were seen as having universal sets of psychological needs. In 1975, Mia Kellmer Pringle, Director of the National Children's Bureau, was asked by the Department of Health and Social Security to produce

a comprehensive document about the developmental needs of all children, about the ways in which these needs are normally met, and about the consequences for the emotional, intellectual, social and physical growth and development of children when, for one reason or another, these needs are not adequately met.

(Kellmer Pringle, 1975, p.13)

Kellmer Pringle (1975, p.15) focused on psycho-social needs, arguing that, 'at present only physical needs are being satisfactorily met, at least to any considerable extent'. Within this framework, children's needs were categorized as:

- the need for love and security;
- the need for new experiences;
- the need for praise and recognition;
- the need for responsibility.

135

The importance of the environment was emphasized, but 'environment' was understood primarily in terms of parents within the family and teachers at school, rather than socio-economic circumstances or the provision of services. Children considered to be 'vulnerable' or 'at risk' included:

Large families with low incomes

Handicapped children

Children in one-parent families (including children born illegitimate and children of divorce)

Children living apart from their families

[Children] belonging to a minority group (including adopted children and coloured immigrant children)

(Kellmer Pringle, 1975, contents page).

Let us now consider changes and continuities in definitions between the 1970s and the 1990s. As we saw earlier, the Children Act 1989 required local authorities to develop services for 'children in need'. This is defined in Section 17 of the 1989 Act as follows:

a child shall be taken to be in need if –

(a) he is unlikely to achieve or maintain, or to have the opportunity of achieving or maintaining, a reasonable standard of health or development without the provision for him of services by a local authority under this Part;

(b) his health or development is likely to be significantly impaired, or further impaired, without the provision for him of such services; or

(c) he is disabled;

and 'family', in relation to such a child, includes any person who has parental responsibility for the child and any other person with whom he has been living.

(Children Act 1989, Section 17, para. 10)

Note that this document, in line with other legal documents, uses 'he' as a generic pronoun to include both girls and boys.

Table 4.1 Number of local authorities (total = 82) using predetermined groups of children for whom social services already have some responsibility to ascertain the extent of need in their area

Predetermined group	No. of LAs (of 82)	% of LAs (of 82)
Children at risk of significant harm	62	76
Children at risk of neglect	61	74
Children in care	60	73
Children accommodated under S.20	59	72
Young people on remand	57	70
Children/young people once in care	55	67
Children in hospital over 3 months	33	40
Privately fostered children	31	38

Note: Predetermined groups are *not* mutually exclusive, so there is the possibility of 100% response rate for each predetermined group.

Source: Aldgate and Tunstill, 1995, p.68

Aldgate and Tunstill (1995) examined how local authorities in England identified the extent of need in their area. On the one hand, most authorities had given priority to those for whom they already had responsibility – that is, those at risk of abuse or neglect. Some also included groups of children identified specifically in the Act, such as disabled children and children leaving care (see Table 4.1). On the other hand, there was much greater variety in the way in which authorities identified other groups of children in the community as 'in need' (see Table 4.2).

Table 4.2 Number of local authorities (total = 82) using predetermined groups of children in the community to ascertain the extent of need in their area

Predetermined group	No. of LAs (of 82)	% of LAs (of 82)
Children with disabilities	56	68
Children with special educational needs	45	55
Children with special health needs	40	49
Young people at risk of criminal acts	40	49
Young people in penal system	36	44
Children with difficult family relationships	33	40
Children at risk/have HIV/AIDS	33	40
Carers with disabilities	32	39
Homeless families	29	35
Drug/solvent abusing children	27	33
Families in bed and breakfast accommodation	24	29
Children excluded from school	24	29
Carers with mental illness	23	28
Children in low-income families	22	27
Children in substandard housing	22	27
Young people in bed and breakfast accommodation	21	26
Children under 8	17	21
Black/ethnic minority children	17	21
School truants	16	19
One-parent families	15	18
Children in specific geographical areas	13	16
Unemployed parents	12	15
Families with utilities cut off	12	15
Children with divorcing parents	10	12
Adopted children	10	12
Children of travellers	9	11
Children with English as second language	7	9
Children in independent school	6	7

Note: Predetermined groups are *not* mutually exclusive, so there is the possibility of 100% response rate for each predetermined group.

Compare the categories used in Table 4.2 with the groups of children seen as 'vulnerable or at risk' by Kellmer Pringle in the 1970s.

1   What are the similarities and differences?

2   What kinds of categories were used in the 1990s to identify children in need? Do any seem to you to be particularly problematic?

3   Are there other needs of children which are not included in either list?

There are both similarities and differences in the descriptions of children in need in the 1970s and 1990s. Certain categories of children were listed on both occasions, though the language used to describe them was sometimes completely different. For example, the terms 'handicapped children' and 'coloured immigrant children' in the 1970s were replaced by 'children with disabilities' and 'black/ethnic minority children' in the 1990s (see **Hughes, 1998; Lewis, 1998a**). Children in one-parent families appeared in both the 1970s and 1990s, though note that in Table 4.2 only 18 per cent of authorities identified them as a group in need, and the term 'illegitimate' was not used in the 1990s.

The groups identified in the 1970s reflected a concern with the way in which the child's 'family' situation deviated from an ideal, white, middle-class norm. By contrast, in the 1990s there was more emphasis on material conditions such as poverty and homelessness, albeit by a minority of authorities. You may recall that Kellmer Pringle started from the assumption that children's physical needs were satisfactorily met.

I also noted the different kinds of categories used in Table 4.2. Some focused on certain characteristics of the children, assuming implicitly they were in need because of who they were: for example, children with disabilities, children under 8, or black/ethnic minority children. Other categories related to children's material circumstances, such as being homeless, living in a low-income family or in substandard housing. A third group referred to social or psychological family circumstances, for example having parents who were divorcing, living in a context of difficult family relationships or being adopted. A final group focused on problematic behaviour of the children, such as drug/solvent abuse, being at risk of criminal acts, truanting from school.

Some of the categorizations did seem quite problematic. I was not sure, for instance, why 'black/ethnic minority children' or 'children under 8' would necessarily constitute groups of children in need. Moreover, 'black' and 'ethnic minority' were used as synonyms for one another, as if only black children have an ethnicity (see **Lewis, 1998a**). I wonder whether you were surprised to see 'children in independent school' included by six authorities. Being 'in need' is not commonly associated with the middle-class children who would most likely attend independent schools.

I thought of the following needs that are not explicitly included in either list:

■   Children who are on the receiving end of racism, or of other forms of discrimination or harassment, because of their 'race', gender, sexuality or disability.

■   Children living in a context of domestic violence (even if they are not direct targets of that violence).

- Children experiencing bullying at school.
- Children living in areas with inadequate health or education services.

You may well have thought of several other groups.

Finally, I was aware that all these categories were defined by adults; there is no evidence of children being consulted in any way.

■ ■ ■

Definitions of 'in need' were also affected by political and financial considerations. Although local authorities had a duty to provide services for children in need, there was no corresponding obligation on central government to give them the necessary resources. Inevitably, therefore, definitions became a way of rationing services. It is interesting to note, in Table 4.2, the small percentage of authorities who included groups of children living in poor material circumstances. Needs were largely defined at the individual level, of the child or family, rather than at a structural level, despite the evidence on links between material circumstances and children's educational attainment and health, as well as their likelihood of entering the care system (Triseliotis, 1993).

The Children Act 1989 has been described as trying to reconcile the irreconcilable:

> it provides for the protection of children but with minimum interference in family life. It avoids structural policy issues by focusing instead on the micro-level of prevention, making explicit reference to support for families of children. Though it would be unrealistic to expect that the Act would tackle wider issues such as employment, income maintenance and housing, nevertheless it was these deficiencies that largely contributed to the failure of previous preventive efforts.
>
> (Triseliotis, 1993, p.10)

2.2.1 Children's own views

Definitions of children's needs in policy are always mediated by adults – more specifically by professional 'experts'. Parents or other adult carers are asked to speak on children's behalf. As Save the Children has pointed out, 'Because all adults have been children once, and because they are felt to understand the "real" needs of children better than the children themselves, the notion of asking children their views directly is rarely entertained and usually seen as unnecessary' (Save the Children, 1995, p.38).

Finding out how children would define their needs is not straightforward. This is not because children cannot tell us, but rather they may not expect to be believed, or they may be fearful of the consequences of speaking about abuse, or of criticizing adults on whom they are dependent. ChildLine has provided one of the few sources of evidence of children's own views. Since the service can, if children wish, be anonymous, children can feel free to speak without fear of the consequences. ChildLine does not pretend that their records constitute representative research into the lives of children in the UK, but what they offer is 'a window into their lives, giving a child's eye view of the problems which afflict them and how they cope' (MacLeod, 1996a, p.6).

ChildLine

Look at Table 4.3, which shows the issues that children called ChildLine about in its first and tenth years of operation.

When you have looked at the evidence, consider whether your ideas about the needs of children have changed.

Table 4.3 Comparison of problem breakdowns for 1986–87 and 1995–96

Type of problem	First year 30 October 1986 – 31 October 1987						Latest year April 1995 – 31 March 1996					
	Girls	%	Boys	%	Total	%	Girls	%	Boys	%	Total	%
Abuser	4	0	17	0	21	0	19	0	52	0	71	0
Being followed	112	1	19	0	131	1	338	0	30	0	368	0
Bereavement	32	0	5	0	37	0	740	1	100	1	840	1
Bullying	437	2	316	6	753	3	8020	11	2180	13	10200	12
Emotional abuse	176	1	58	1	234	1	241	0	59	0	300	0
Family relationship problem	3571	20	1061	19	4632	20	10970	15	2211	14	13181	15
Health	157	1	49	1	206	1	1827	2	366	2	2193	2
Legal	24	0	34	1	58	0	128	0	64	0	192	0
Neglect	144	1	42	1	186	1	100	0	28	0	128	0
Physical abuse	2953	17	1227	21	4180	18	6038	8	2851	17	8889	10
Pregnancy	1129	6	182	3	1311	6	6464	9	317	2	6781	8
Problem with friends	847	5	206	4	1053	4	7371	10	670	4	8041	9
Request for resources	134	1	63	1	197	1	448	1	121	1	569	1
Risk of abuse	591	3	112	2	703	3	463	1	86	1	549	1
Runaway and homeless	260	1	196	3	456	2	1634	2	1010	6	2644	3
School problem	372	2	170	3	542	2	1052	1	390	2	1442	2
Self harm	95	1	40	1	135	1	818	1	30	0	848	1
Sexual abuse	5172	29	1180	21	6352	27	6441	9	1415	9	7856	9
Substance abuse	314	2	172	3	486	2	1419	2	583	4	2002	2
Other	1290	7	567	10	1857	8	18982	26	3737	23	22719	24
Total	17814	100	5716	100	23530	100	73513	100	16300	100	89813	100

Source: MacLeod, 1996a, p.30

COMMENT

Crucially, the table consists of a list of problems defined as such by children. There was an enormous difference in the extent to which boys and girls called the service, suggesting that the needs of children are differentially constructed in terms of gender. Further research by ChildLine shows that, in general, boys find it much harder to talk about their problems (MacLeod and Barter, 1996). There was also a dramatic increase in the number of calls over the ten-year period. One of the most interesting changes was the four-fold increase in the proportion of calls about 'bullying'. This may mean that bullying increased. However, in 1986 bullying was not publicly named as a problem for children; perhaps as it became visible, children were able to give a name to their experience.

■ ■ ■

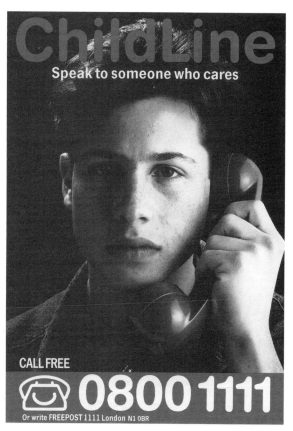

ChildLine: appealing to boys as well as girls

2.3 Universal or special needs?

Most discussions assume implicitly that children have universal needs to be met primarily within the family. Some children are seen to be 'in need' because, for some reason, their needs are not being met; others, such as disabled children, are seen as having 'special needs' because of the particular characteristics of who they are.

universal needs

141

2.3.1   Socio-economic context

Let us consider first the extent to which needs are seen as being dependent upon the wider social and political context. The Children (Scotland) Act 1995 defines 'in need' in a very similar way to the 1989 Act in England and Wales, though it extends the definition to include not only children who are disabled but also those who are *affected* adversely by the disability of another family member. During the parliamentary debates on this Bill, the Scottish Secretary Ian Lang argued that, 'In scope, the Bill goes rather beyond the provisions of the Children Act 1989 for England and Wales. It will provide Scotland with its own Children Act based on Scots law and *Scottish needs*' (*Hansard*, 5 December 1994, emphasis added).

What do you think is meant by 'Scottish needs'?

The phrase 'Scottish needs' suggests that children in Scotland have different needs to children in England and Wales, though no indication is given of what these differences might be, and I found it hard to think of any. By contrast, the Children (Northern Ireland) Order 1995 does not take account of what might be considered to be 'Northern Ireland needs'. It repeats almost word for word the Children Act 1989, but does not consider the impact of the wider social and political context of Northern Ireland. It therefore fails to recognize 'that a significant proportion of the child population experienced multiple socio-economic deprivation … and that all children were having to cope with the rapidly changing nature of modern society and the continuing problem of political violence and social instability' (Kelly and Pinkerton, 1996, p.45).

2.3.2   The social construction of 'special needs'

special needs

The group of children generally associated with the term special needs are those constructed as 'disabled'. But 'special needs' only has a meaning in relation to a conception of the needs of 'normal' children. Discussions of children's needs reveal implicit norms. For example, in a review of the research on residential care for children, Bullock *et al.* (1993, p.15) suggested that: 'The special needs of particular groups, including girls and certain ethnic minorities, are not sufficiently understood'.

Though not labelled as such, children who are black or from so-called 'ethnic minorities' are constructed as children with 'special needs'. Within the Children Acts, local authorities are required to take account of children's religion, racial origin and cultural and linguistic background. This requirement was seen at the time to represent a significant shift in social policy (religion was already part of child-care law). It also appeared to offer positive opportunities (Ahmed, 1991). For example, it allowed challenges and complaints about decisions and services to focus on racial, religious or cultural discrimination, and acknowledged the requirement to provide translations of information and the provision of interpreters when needed. However, within the Acts, 'race' is defined predominantly in terms of identifying some children as belonging to 'ethnic minorities' who are assumed to differ from the majority of white children in terms of their culture, language and religion. Such discourses are problematic: they exclude black children from, for example, Englishness or Scottishness, and they do not allow for 'needs' resulting from structural racism, racial harassment or racial abuse. There is no recognition that either 'race' or 'ethnic minority' are socially constructed categories. For example, in Schedule 2, paragraph 11, the 1989 Act refers to the local authorities' 'duty to consider racial groups to which children in need belong' when making arrangements for day care and fostering, as if such 'racial groups' pre-exist and are easily identifiable (see **Lewis, 1998a**).

The legislation therefore constructs children who are designated as 'ethnic minorities' as different and 'other', and as a homogeneous group with specific sets of needs that are different from those of the normal majority: that is, they are seen as having 'special needs' linked to what is described as their 'culture'. Table 4.2, considered earlier, shows that 17 local authorities in England included 'black/ethnic minority children' as an identifiable group of 'children in need' within the community. This way of constructing 'ethnic minority' children is widespread and taken for granted by most policy-makers and practitioners. For example, a 1996 'handbook for professionals', entitled *Meeting the Needs of Ethnic Minority Children*, includes chapters on topics such as: 'The immigrant (West Indian) child in school'; 'Adoption of children from minority groups'; 'Residential care for ethnic minorities children'; and 'Psychiatric needs of ethnic minority children' (Dwivedi and Parma, 1996).

'Race', 'ethnicity' and 'culture' are characteristics that are applied only to those constructed as different. As Lewis has pointed out, 'An "ethnic minority" is "in" the nation (and may well have been for generations), but not "of" the nation in the way that it is understood as an "imagined community" ' (**Lewis, 1998a, p.22**). However, ChildLine's study of 'children and racism' showed that:

> The overwhelming majority of callers … saw themselves as British, whatever their origin or birthplace. Indeed for some, their problem was fear of being taken away from Britain. Of those who said where they were born, the majority were born in Britain. The overwhelming majority were English speakers with regional accents, only two (refugee children) had difficulty in communicating in English. The picture here was of a group of clearly 'British' youngsters. If most children and adults have a sense of place as part of their identity, for these children, this country is their place.
>
> (MacLeod, 1996b, p.11)

2.3.3 Disabled children

The Children Acts were the first pieces of legislation in which disabled children were identified as a group with special needs that had to be met by local authorities. Local authorities also had to maintain a register of disabled children within their area. To do this requires a definition of disability, and within Section 17 of the 1989 England and Wales Act the following definition is given:

> a child is disabled if he is blind, deaf or dumb or suffers from mental disorder of any kind or is substantially and permanently handicapped by illness, injury, or congenital deformity or such other disability … 'development' means physical, intellectual, emotional, social or behavioural development; and 'health' means physical or mental health.
>
> (Children Act 1989, Section 17, para.11)

The aim of services for disabled children is also set out:

> Every local authority shall provide services designed –
>
> (a) to minimize the effect on disabled children within their area of their disabilities;

and

(b) to give such children the opportunity to lead lives which are as normal as possible.

(Children Act 1989, Schedule 2, para. 6)

Aldgate and Tunstill (1995) found that 'children with disabilities' was the group most commonly included in local authority definitions of need (see Table 4.2). They also found that services and budgets for disabled children had expanded. However, only about half of the authorities gave high priority to services for disabled children, unless they fell into another category as well. More generally there was a debate among policy-makers and practitioners on 'whether disabled children are most appropriately regarded as a "group apart" under arm (c) of Section 17 or whether their needs can be adequately met under the other two arms of need' (Aldgate and Tunstill, 1995, p.35).

Although the needs of disabled children and their right to services were recognized explicitly for the first time, the Children Acts adopted a medical model of disability. In this model disability is constructed as a problem in contrast to the norm of being 'able-bodied', and fails to recognize that definitions of disability are highly contested. Similarly, the goal of services is presented unproblematically as 'normalization'. As Hughes argues, this can nevertheless reinforce the construction of disabled people as 'other':

> The philosophy of 'special needs' was keen to promote the integration of people into ordinary life, to make them more independent and to equip them with various social and practical skills. Critics have pointed out that this approach focused on individual difference and lack of ability, which often meant that provision of services remained separate from the 'mainstream'.
>
> **(Hughes, 1998, p.75)**

3 Children in need of protection

3.1 Children at risk of harm

The Children Act 1989 required local authorities to develop services for all children 'in need' in their area. However, they still had responsibilities to protect children who were at 'risk of harm', and a tension remained between the rights of individual children to protection from harm within their own family, and the continuing promotion of 'the family' as the natural place for raising children, and hence protecting families from state intervention.

risk of harm

What is the difference between being 'in need' and 'at risk of harm'?

This distinction is important, as it marks the boundary between support for families and the requirement to intervene to protect children from their families. Within the 1989 Act, a child is 'at risk' if she or he is suffering, or is likely to suffer, 'significant harm'. This simply shifts the problem of definition to the notion of 'significant harm', with 'significant' being defined as 'substantial, considerable or noteworthy ... significant is a lesser standard than serious or severe' (Hardiker, 1996, p.108). In order to justify intervention, such harm must be seen as occurring in the present or likely to occur in the future; past harm, however severe, is not a criterion for intervention unless the harm is likely to be repeated.

Our concern here is not to try to resolve these problems of definition and assessment of risk or need, but to recognize that they are socially constructed. Deciding whether or not a particular child is at risk, and whether and how to intervene, will always involve complex professional judgements. In deciding when and how to intervene, and whether such intervention can take place on a voluntary basis with the co-operation of the family or requires a court order, social workers are expected to take into account

> a multiplicity of factors. These include the nature of the harm suffered or likely to be suffered, the surrounding circumstances, the parents' willingness to accept responsibility and to co-operate with the helping agencies and, where their care does not meet the child's needs, an assessment of their ability to change.
>
> (Department of Health, 1993, p.13)

The law itself does not create the balance between the state and families; it provides the framework within which professional judgements and decisions are made, and such judgements will always be made in relation to norms of the healthy development of children and of 'good parenting'.

3.2   The rediscovery of child abuse

Since the 1970s new discourses of child abuse and child protection have developed. Child abuse is often discussed as a new social problem discovered in the late twentieth century. However, since the late nineteenth century, the abuse or neglect of children within their families has been visible or invisible, or visible in particular ways, at different historical moments. Professional responses to abuse have also varied, swinging back and forth between measures to rescue children and attempts to prevent abuse through support for families.

child abuse

By the end of the nineteenth century, a problem of 'family violence' had been identified, and this was defined mainly in terms of cruelty to children. It was primarily understood in terms of wider concerns about working-class families and social order in the nineteenth century (see **Hall, 1998**; **Mooney, 1998**). Children were seen as both 'in danger' and 'dangerous', since cruelty to children was assumed to be a major cause of delinquency and social disorder. Voluntary organizations such as the National Society for the Prevention of Cruelty to Children were set up with the aim of protecting children, and their campaigning in the second half of the nineteenth century led to new legislation which for the first time criminalized cruelty, neglect and incest. Opponents of such measures were concerned about the threat to the sanctity of the family and parent–child bonds. The intervention targeted parents (in practice mothers) with the aim of reforming them, and often resulted in women losing their children. Nevertheless, many women sought out such intervention in order to protect themselves and their children from male violence.

In the first half of the twentieth century, all forms of violence in the family were largely invisible, with cruelty and neglect continuing to be subsumed within concerns about delinquency. (Chapter 5 discusses this in more detail, and shows how the 1989 Act finally separated these two categories.) Sexual abuse was constructed predominantly in terms of danger from 'perverted strangers' in 'dirty raincoats'.

The physical abuse of children was 'rediscovered' by doctors in the 1960s. By the late 1980s, a series of scandals surrounding the deaths of children within their families led to a number of public inquiries which criticized social workers for focusing on supportive intervention with parents at the expense of the protection of vulnerable children. Each inquiry led to an increasing use of legal procedures to remove children from their homes. The sexual abuse of children was 'rediscovered' during the 1980s and was associated with a different set of scandals and inquiries. Perhaps the best known of these was the Cleveland crisis of 1987, in which it was claimed that children had been removed unnecessarily from their homes. In these cases social workers were criticized for intervening too intrusively.

The 1990s saw the uncovering of many other forms of abuse that had been 'hidden'. For example, there were increasing revelations of ill treatment and abuse of children within residential homes, sometimes following years of complaints from children that had gone unheard. The extent of abuse in boarding schools, and of bullying in both boarding and day schools, also came to prominence.

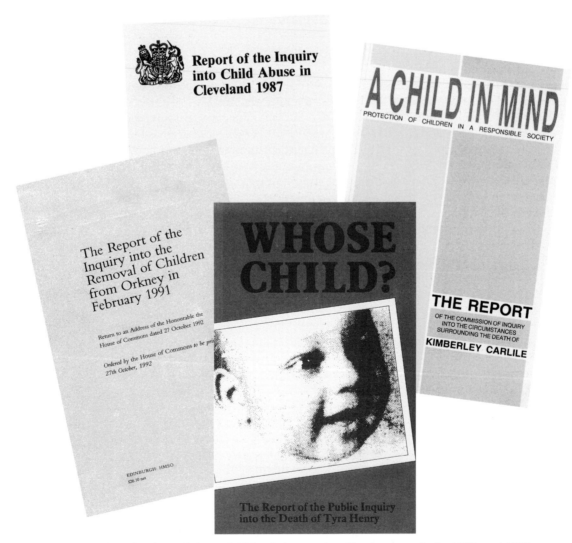

Scandals over the physical and sexual abuse of children led to a series of inquiry reports in the 1980s and 1990s

Although 'child abuse' is generally discussed as if it were a homogeneous category, there were very different public responses to reports of particular forms of abuse. For example, the cases of children who had died within their families were seen as shocking and unacceptable, and led to demands for better professional intervention. In line with the dominant professional discourses, such abuse was seen as something that occurred in 'dysfunctional' or 'dangerous' families. By contrast, cases of sexual abuse occurring within 'normal' families, where in some cases the abuse was 'organized' or involved 'Satanic rituals', were not widely believed. Rather they were seen as the product of the imaginations of over-zealous or interfering social workers, or extreme feminists.

The public inquiry reports did not consider whether or why the abuse had occurred. They focused instead on the lack of clear sets of procedures within social services departments, and their failure to work effectively with other professional groups, in particular the police and the health service. New procedures were introduced to establish multi-agency forms of intervention, now seen in terms of 'investigation'. The inquiries suggested that the welfare of the children had not been seen as paramount, and that professionals should listen to what children themselves had to say. As we have seen, all these concerns informed the new legislation enacted in the late 1980s and 1990s. Subsequent research published by the Department of Health in 1995 suggested that professionals were acting too coercively, invoking child protection procedures in 'minor' cases of abuse. There was a need, it was argued, to shift the balance back once more to 'family support' (**Pinkney, 1998**).

3.3   Contested definitions of abuse

Since the 1980s there have been vigorous debates about definitions of abuse.

ACTIVITY 4.4

Write a list of all the different things that can happen to children which you think constitute abuse.

1   Can you categorize them?

2   Is it straightforward to distinguish between 'normal' experiences and 'abuse'?

3   Can you produce a definition of abuse?

COMMENT

'Abuse' is as hard to define as 'need'. Legal and professional definitions distinguish between categories of abuse, such as physical, sexual and emotional abuse, and neglect. Abuse is commonly seen in individualized terms, as acts of commission or omission by one or more adults. While the most extreme forms of abuse might not be contested, controversies have raged over the boundaries between normal parenting and abuse. Two particular issues caused concern in the public domain in the 1980s and 1990s:

■   The boundaries between discipline and physical abuse, with disputes about the rights of parents and childminders to smack children.

■   The boundaries between physical affection and sexual abuse, with fathers in particular claiming they were frightened to be affectionate towards their children for fear of accusations of abuse.

The failure to consider structural factors is reinforced by the individualizing legal and medical discourses that have constructed abuse. Factors such as poverty, poor housing and unemployment have been discussed as conditions which may create high levels of stress, and hence trigger some forms of physical abuse. Yet it could be argued that living in poverty is in itself abusive to children, since it denies them a range of opportunities that are available to other children. This is particularly significant in the context of huge increases in the numbers of children living in poverty in the late twentieth century (see Table 4.4). Other structural factors that are rarely considered include environmental ones – for example the impact of pollution or food additives. You may well be able to think of more.

■ ■ ■

Table 4.4 **The number and proportion of children living in households on low incomes in 1979 and 1992–93 in the UK**

| | Below 50 per cent of average income[1] | |
	1979	1992–93
Children	1.4m (10%)	4.3m (33%)
All[2]	5.0m (9%)	14.1m (25%)

[1] Income is after housing costs.
[2] 'All' includes children as well as adults.

Source: Department of Social Security, 1995

The simultaneous recognition and marginalization of structural factors which we saw in discussions of 'need' (section 4.2) is illustrated in the report of a National Commission which was set up by the NSPCC in 1994 to consider ways of preventing abuse and neglect in the UK. The Commission adopted what was described as 'a wide definition of abuse', which led to the government and the media dismissing most of their conclusions.

> Child abuse consists of anything which individuals, institutions or processes do or fail to do which directly or indirectly harms children or damages their prospects of a safe and healthy development into adulthood.

> This definition encompasses neglect and abuse in their most direct and acute forms but includes far more. Establishing the full effects on children of poor housing, health care or diet, or the indirect effects of poverty on their well-being would have taken the Commission well beyond its remit; but the effect, both direct and indirect, of these conditions on the families in which children are brought up is damaging. In some instances, it can be profoundly so.
> (National Commission of Inquiry into the Prevention of Child Abuse, 1996, vol.2, p.4)

Criticisms of dominant discourses of child sexual abuse came from feminists. They rejected the idea that it was a 'family problem', emphasizing instead the way sexual abuse was gendered, with men constituting the overwhelming majority of abusers. They saw sexual abuse as an abuse of power, as one aspect of male violence against women and children. In the late 1990s, public discourses of sexual abuse constructed it again as predominantly a problem of perverted men (paedophiles) who sought out children for their own satisfaction, often by taking employment within children's homes or as foster carers. This preoccupation with paedophilia, which resulted in legislation requiring convicted sex offenders to register with the police, also raised concerns for organizations like ChildLine. While welcoming the recognition of the existence of organized paedophile rings, they were also concerned to ensure that 'abuse which happens to children closer to home is not forgotten or overlooked' (MacLeod, 1996a, p.84).

As with definitions of need, children's views are rarely considered when discussing the meaning of abuse. If you look back at Table 4.3 from the ChildLine report (Activity 4.3), you will see how frequently children rang ChildLine in relation to bullying in 1995–96. Other research from ChildLine showed that this was the term that children themselves used for some forms of abuse and assaults: 'Bullying is a word which masks the seriousness of the abuse and assaults that children experience. If these children were adults, they would be complaining of harassment, threatening behaviour, actual or grievous bodily harm, extortion, theft, or criminal damage' (MacLeod, 1996b, p.16).

Research from ChildLine also showed how widespread were the experiences of racism in various forms for some children. Children spoke about: racist bullying at school; racism or prejudice from their parents against friendships which crossed what were seen as 'racial' or 'cultural' boundaries; conflicts between their own desires and parents' expectations which the children described as religious or cultural pressures; physical, sexual or emotional abuse in which racism was a feature; racism or discrimination at school from staff; and street violence (MacLeod, 1996b).

3.4 Professional intervention

Definitions of abuse and neglect are important because their occurrence within families is used as a justification for state intervention into the 'private' domain. As definitions change, so the boundary shifts between perceptions of the need for support for families and the need to protect children from their families.

The intended goals of intervention, and its form, have both varied historically and been highly contested. Since the late nineteenth century, one form of intervention has been to 'rescue' children. During the twentieth century this took the form of local authority social workers using legal processes to remove children from their family and to place them 'in care'. From the 1960s the predominant focus of professional work was on prevention: children were taken into care on what was intended to be a temporary basis, with a view to helping the family to be reunited. However, during the 1970s there was an increasing recognition that prevention was not working, particularly as the majority of children came into care because of the material circumstances of their lives. Large numbers of children were growing up in 'the limbo of unplanned care'; they were described as 'the children who wait' (Thoburn et al., 1986, p.3). The professional view developed that children who could not return home should, if possible, be found new 'psychological parents', to meet the need for 'permanence' in their lives – that is, 'security, stability, the experiences of living as a member of a family; the sense of belonging and being cared about for the foreseeable future; and, for the lucky ones, the experience of loving and being loved' (Thoburn et al., 1986, p.vii).

Until the 1960s, adoption had been seen as a service for childless couples rather than as a resource for children, and most of the children regarded as adoptable were white, healthy babies of unmarried mothers. However, from the late 1960s, the range of 'adoptable' children grew to include, first, all babies, and later children over 5 and disabled children. As adoption became seen as a service for children, the first adoptions were of those children in care whose parents had hoped for adoption, but increasingly the need for permanence was used as a justification also to place for adoption those children whose parents had not requested, or even who had actively opposed, adoption. Evidence for the importance of permanence was drawn from findings that, for example, more than one-third of young prisoners and nearly one-quarter of adults in prison were previously in local authority care, whereas children who were adopted before they were 10 years old fared no worse than the children in the general population (Triseliotis, 1993).

Thoburn *et al.* (1986) saw 1975 as the starting date of the development of the 'permanence movement'. The Children Act 1975 had introduced changes which made the adoption of children from care a more likely option. By the 1990s the pendulum had swung again, and there was a great emphasis on children who were 'looked after' maintaining contact with their family of origin. In addition, 'in care' had come to be viewed as a very stigmatizing status, and the Children Act 1989 referred instead to services of 'accommodation' through which the local authority might 'look after' children, emphasizing that such services should be seen as positive measures of family support.

Residential care and fostering were alternatives for those children who were temporarily 'in care' or awaiting adoption. From the mid 1970s there was a sharp move away from residential care: the number of children in residential placements fell from 60,000 in 1970 to 13,000 in 1990 (Bullock *et al.*, 1993, p.11). Foster care became the preferred alternative, despite the large number of problems and breakdowns in foster arrangements. As a result of the shift to foster care, residential care for children came to be seen as the 'Cinderella' of the social services, or a service of 'last resort', with fewer qualified workers, lower status, worse pay and anti-social working hours. In the 1990s, following the scandals about abuse in residential homes, the subsequent inquiry reports focused largely on staffing. Many of the homes were seen as inadequate, with staff not properly trained, managed or supervised, even though they were dealing with children widely seen as the most difficult in our society. Some children nevertheless preferred residential care to being fostered, as they found it less restrictive and it created less conflict with their own family. However, the consequences for children were often very negative. The experience of going into residential care was often so overwhelming that the initial cause of it was neglected. Furthermore, children leaving care, though identified within the Children Acts as a group of children 'in need', nevertheless frequently experienced homelessness, unemployment and isolation (Bullock *et al.*, 1993).

3.5   Socio-legal discourses: the quest for evidence

Chapter 1 described 'a shift in the emphasis of welfare from care and support towards discipline and surveillance' (p.22). For children at risk, this took the form of a shift from a medico-social construction of child abuse to a socio-legal construction of child protection, with legal rather than medical and psychiatric experts predominating (Parton, 1991). New multi-agency procedures for the investigation of child abuse were developed. Although there was a call in the

child protection

mid 1990s for intervention to shift again to family support, child protection procedures were still invoked for cases of 'severe' abuse.

One consequence of the predominance of socio-legal discourses is that the issues are seen as very simple ones:

> One of the services that the law performs is to transform complex, messy situations involving intricate human relationships and a multiplicity of possible causes into a simple story which makes sense and holds a moral for everyone. The children were abused. The step-father did it. Or the social workers overreacted. The children are returned to their homes. Either way, the social order has been restored. Wicked fathers and step-parents are punished, while children are placed in good stable families. Good parents are rewarded by being reunited with their children. All is well with the world.
>
> (King and Trowell, 1992, p.1)

There are very different criteria for legal or medical/welfare intervention in relation to child abuse. The criminal law is primarily concerned with whether an illegal act has occurred. The 'facts' have to be determined, and the rights of the defendant are balanced against the interests of the child. For medical or welfare professionals, a child's distress or disturbed behaviour may constitute grounds for intervening, with the goal of finding solutions for the child and/or the family (King and Trowell, 1992). This may involve legal proceedings, but civil ones, in which the interests of the child are seen as paramount.

A criminal justice emphasis means obtaining evidence in a way that will secure a conviction in court. In cases of physical abuse or neglect, corroborating or forensic evidence may be available, but the nature of sexual abuse means that these are much less likely to exist. The main evidence available for sexual abuse, if the offender denies it, is the word of the child, and children are generally seen as unreliable witnesses. They are assumed to be highly suggestible, to fantasize, exaggerate, and not to understand the duty to speak the truth. As a result of pressure from many professional and children's rights organizations, attitudes to children's testimony, and the procedures for them in court, have changed. For example, children may be able to give their 'evidence in chief' on video, and to be cross-examined via a live television link, or they may be hidden from the defendant by a screen (Keep, 1996).

Most significantly, the quest for evidence has resulted in clinical interviews with social workers, child psychologists or psychiatrists becoming potential evidence. Welfare professionals are trained to conduct 'disclosure interviews' with children in such a way that the evidence is not 'contaminated' and can be used in court. The focus of such interviews is to establish the 'facts', rather than to help children deal with the emotional consequences of the abuse. Inflexible procedures have developed so that, for example, it has become the norm to have only one interview, even though many abused children (like adults) find it easier to tell their story in parts, over time.

> If ... a child is likely to begin to 'disclose' during the interview ... that interview may well have to be brought to a close in order that the disclosure may be made in front of the video camera ... Yet closing an interview or changing its style may be extremely disruptive for children. Some children also find the technology of video cameras, microphones and one-way mirrors extremely unsettling. It is all too easy too for the interviewer to feel the need to press the child, to play 'hunt the truth' games, searching all the time for more clarification, more details, more confirmation.
>
> (King and Trowell, 1992, p.71)

The consequences for children of this 'search for truth' go still further. Keep (1996, p.31) gives one example: 'Jane and her friend had both been abused by a man known to them, but their evidence was discounted on the grounds that they had talked about it with each other'. MacLeod (1996a, p.72) also points out that 'lawyers commonly advised against therapy for children and usually advised that the parent should not talk to the child about the abuse in case it weakened the case because the child could be seen as having been "coached" '. Yet court delays mean that children may wait for nearly a year for any therapeutic help. Children are constructed here as suggestible and unreliable and consequently treated very differently from adults, whose credibility as a witness is not judged on whether or not they have told their story to anyone. Children phoning ChildLine were very angry that parents and friends were advised not to talk to them about the abuse, and that they were denied therapy.

These interviews, and other aspects of the investigative process such as medical examinations and court experiences, are seen to constitute secondary abuse for children, and evidence from children themselves confirms this view. Many children phoning ChildLine were reluctant to involve social services or other statutory agencies. They did not expect to be believed, and feared the consequences of speaking out: namely that their family would break up, or decisions would be made about them without their involvement. They were also frightened of reprisals from the abuser in the event of an acquittal. Their main concerns were to have someone to talk to, and that the abuse should stop. Those who had counselling or therapy spoke very positively about it.

The criminal justice system is concerned not with child protection, but with the prosecution and punishment of offenders. In practice only a tiny proportion of allegations of sexual abuse come to court, and an even smaller number result in a conviction. The question, therefore, is: 'However outraged we feel at the thought of sex offenders going unpunished ... is the cost of prosecution too high for children?' (Keep, 1996, p.37).

It is clear that children's own views on abuse and on the nature of intervention have not informed policies and practices in relation to child abuse. Other agendas, whether of family privacy or the criminal justice system, may conflict with meeting the needs of children who have been abused.

4   Parental responsibility

parental
responsibility

We saw in Activity 4.1 that it is not possible to explore the construction of children's welfare needs without also examining the responsibilities of parents. In the 1990s, parental responsibility for children became a central feature of New Right rhetoric on the family, and was incorporated explicitly in a range of social policy legislation. It was given new legal status in the UK in the Children Acts, which stressed the importance of professionals working 'in partnership' with parents. The Child Support Act 1991 emphasized that both parents had financial responsibility for their children, whether or not they were living with them (**Cochrane, 1998**). On the one hand, parenting (motherhood and fatherhood) is assumed to be natural. On the other hand, the 1990s saw the increasing development of classes and projects to teach parenting skills to those parents seen as inadequate. Parents were also expected to take on specific responsibilities, for example in relation to their children's education (see the newspaper extract opposite).

Parents told to sign reading pledge

John Carvel, Education Editor

Primary school parents will be asked to sign an undertaking to read with their children at home for at least 20 minutes a day under government proposals for improving literacy, published yesterday.

The parental reading pledge will be included in home-school contracts setting out teachers' responsibilities and parents' contribution towards the good behaviour, attendance and punctuality which will be expected of the children.

(The Guardian, 29 July 1997, p.1)

The rhetoric of the Children Acts broadened ideas about families, recognizing that children live in a wide variety of households, with different kinds of parental figures, or significant adults, who could share parental responsibility with biological parents or at least be involved in decision-making. Coppock (1997) claimed that in practice, however, those who lived in non-traditional families continued to be seen as 'bad parents' or as offering second best to children.

4.1   Parenthood and gender

Common assumptions about the gendered division of labour see women, as mothers, having the prime responsibility for child care. However, in discussions of parental responsibility, 'parent' is used as a gender-neutral term. Within the Children Acts both fathers and mothers automatically have parental responsibility for their biological children if they are married to one another. If they are not married, mothers still have it automatically; fathers can acquire it, but only by agreement with the child's mother or through the courts. Interestingly, within the Child Support Act, unmarried fathers are treated in exactly the same way as married ones. Biological parenthood incurs automatic financial responsibility for children.

What is the significance of the gender-neutral term 'parent'?

The granting of rights and responsibilities to biological fathers, irrespective of their relationship to the child and mother, raised controversy, particularly among feminists. On the one hand, it was seen as appropriate that men should be expected to take responsibility for their biological children. On the other hand, the legislation did not consider the reasons why fathers are not living with their children – it could be because of violence or abuse. Fathers' rights to be consulted about decisions affecting their children may conflict with a mother's and child's right to privacy and their need for protection.

Another consequence of the use of the term 'parent' is that the significance of gender in relation to child abuse has largely been denied or ignored. Most statistics on abuse do not specify the gender of the abuser. In Cleveland in 1987, fathers were overwhelmingly named as alleged abusers (one out of 121 was a woman), but new discourses of 'parents' developed, so that it was parents who

153

were responsible for their children, parents who were seen as the abusers, and the family that was in need of therapy.

Despite the rhetoric of 'parental responsibility', in practice it is women as mothers who are on the receiving end of most social work intervention in relation to their children, because of the social expectations of mothers, because of their greater availability, and also in some instances because of social workers' fear of confronting violent men. Milner (1995) suggests that, as a result, allegations of abuse by fathers are frequently redefined as allegations of neglect by mothers. She concludes: 'the term parenting, although an attempt at gender neutrality, is nothing but an empty gesture. It is impossible to assess "good enough parenting", only "good enough mothers"' (Milner, 1995, p.52).

If child abuse is seen as a 'family problem', then the non-abusing parent (most commonly the mother) becomes equally culpable for her 'collusion' in the abuse or her 'failure to protect' her child. As a result of such assumptions, social workers have often judged women as 'non-protective mothers' or even 'secondary perpetrators', and have withdrawn their support. They then produce exactly the outcome they wanted to avoid:

> some women remade an alliance with the abuser and excluded the child. The conduct of the investigation affected the way in which family members reacted, and to whom they turned for comfort and help. It was, in part, on the basis of these reactions that decisions were made ... about removing the child, prosecuting the abuser and whether a parent-figure – usually the mother – could keep the child safe from harm.
>
> (Farmer, 1993, p.42)

Thus the failure to disaggregate the 'family' into its component parts, to recognize the power relations based on age and gender, and to distinguish between abusing and non-abusing members, has consequences for the meaning of 'family support'. What kind of support is envisaged and for whom?

'Mothering' is defined in terms of caring for children, and results in social work intervention. By contrast, 'Fathering, being ill defined yet of higher status than mothering, is inaccessible to scrutiny in child protection terms' (Milner, 1995, p.52). Expectations of all fathers in relation to child care are very low, and some fathers, especially black fathers of Afro-Caribbean origin and descent, are seen as particularly feckless. However, fathers are seen to have the chief financial responsibility for children and are primarily pursued by the Child Support Agency.

The taken-for-granted assumptions about the 'naturalness' of motherhood and of the role of fathers have such significance for child welfare practices that it is worth looking more closely at how 'good mothers' and 'good fathers' are socially constructed (**Clarke and Cochrane, 1998**).

4.2 The 'good enough' mother

Motherhood is not a natural condition. It is an institution that *presents* itself as a natural outcome of biologically given gender differences, as a natural consequence of (hetero)sexual activity, and as a natural manifestation of an innate female characteristic, namely the maternal instinct. The existence of an institution of motherhood, as opposed to an acknowledgement that there are simply mothers, is rarely questioned, even though the proper qualities of motherhood are often the subject of debate. Motherhood is still largely treated as a given and as a self-evident fact rather than as the possible outcome of specific social processes that have a historical and cultural location which can be mapped.

(Smart, 1996, p.37)

Before the middle of the nineteenth century motherhood had no legal status; only fathers and fatherhood existed in law. Smart (1996) discusses the struggle for motherhood to be recognized, outlining two main influences:

1   Middle-class feminist campaigns on divorce, custody of children and violence within the family, which demanded the legal recognition of motherhood and constructed an ideology of motherhood as caring and the source of special knowledge essential for good child rearing.

2   The work of nineteenth-century philanthropic organizations (**Mooney, 1998**) and later social work, health and psychology professionals, who sought to impose particular standards of motherhood on working-class women.

In section 2.2 we saw that in the 1930s mothering focused on physical care and instilling regular habits. By the 1950s, child psychiatrists were emphasizing emotional care, and the crucial importance of 'mother love' for the normal healthy development of children (Bowlby, 1953). This emphasis on mothers meant that they nearly always gained custody of their children following a divorce, unless they had deviated from normal gender roles, for example by being 'promiscuous' or having lesbian relationships. At the same time 'maternal deprivation' was seen as responsible for everything that happened to children, such as psychological disorders and delinquent behaviour. 'Working mothers' were particularly stigmatized as bad mothers. They tended to be white, working-class women who worked part-time to improve the welfare of their children, or black women who had migrated to the UK, leaving their children behind until they were settled, and who worked long hours for low pay (Williams, 1989). This was in contrast to middle- or upper-class women who employed full-time nannies and/or sent their children to boarding schools; they were rarely publicly criticized.

Later psychological work modified the exclusive focus on mothers, with a shift from concerns about maternal deprivation to identifying the qualities of 'sensitive mothering', which in theory men could also possess. With changes in women's patterns of employment, more women engaged in paid work outside the home, and although it remained an issue of contestation, in the 1990s 'going out to work' was no longer such a clear defining feature of a 'bad mother'. A vocal lobby still suggested that full-time 'working' mothers were neglecting their children, but efforts were made by both Conservative and Labour governments to encourage single mothers into employment.

Under the Children Acts local authorities had a duty to support women who needed help in caring for their children. However, offers of help depended upon the view of a woman's 'mothering' capacity. Women less likely to receive help included those experiencing mental health difficulties, those with drug addictions, alcohol problems or learning difficulties, or those who were in prison. Moreover, women who fell into these categories found that they were not treated as individuals but as part of a homogeneous problem group. By contrast, women seen as deserving of support included those who were blind or with multiple sclerosis (Sone, 1997).

One particular group of women, lone mothers, have always fallen on the wrong side of the boundary between good and bad mothers, though how they are constructed has varied historically. The boundaries between good and bad motherhood were most blurred in the 1970s, when 'illegitimacy' ceased to be seen as a major social problem (Smart, 1996). Since the 1980s, lone mothers have been reconstituted as a burden on the state and re-demonized (see Chapter 6). In addition, requests for support from single mothers, especially if they are black women, are likely to be redefined as child protection matters (Milner, 1995).

Is growing up in a lone-parent family inevitably bad for children?

Lone parents are widely seen as ineffective at bringing up their children:

> On the evidence available such children tend to die earlier, to have more illness, to do less well at school, to exist at a lower level of nutrition, comfort and conviviality, to suffer more unemployment, to be more prone to deviance and crime, and finally to repeat the cycle of unstable parenting from which they themselves have suffered.
> (Halsey, foreword in Dennis and Erdos, 1992, p.xiii)

Such conclusions have been contested, but alternative views have received little publicity. McIntosh (1996) argued that the research quoted in the 1990s was 20 years old, dating from a time when lone parenthood was much rarer and more stigmatized, and that it rarely made distinctions between different groups of lone parents, although the reason for lone parenthood is likely to affect the children. She cited instead other research suggesting that children suffer more from high levels of tension between two parents than from living with one parent, and that many other factors also affect children's development: 'when other parental resources – like income, education, self-esteem and a supportive social environment – are roughly similar, signs of two-parent privilege largely disappear' (Stacey, 1994, p.60).

Thus, ideas on 'good' and 'bad' mothers have changed historically, but at all times dominant views of 'good mothering' have been supported by ideologies of the naturalness of motherhood, and associated with the child-rearing practices of white, middle-class families. They tend to ignore both diversity of family forms and the social conditions under which mothers raise their children.

4.3 The re-emergence of fatherhood

Ideas on good fathers have also varied historically, though contrasts have always been made between irresponsible, feckless or absent fathers and the 'responsible family man'.

Do children need fathers?

In the 1950s fathers' roles were seen primarily in terms of financial and emotional support for mothers. However, by the 1970s, father absence was assumed to mean lack of an authority figure and male role model, resulting in particular in delinquency and inadequate gender role development. Research on 'father absence' took no account of the impact of the reason for the absence. Situations of death, divorce and separation were lumped together as causing concern, while other situations of father absence, resulting from imprisonment or the implementation of immigration laws, were ignored. Very little research has looked at children who have never had a father, so in practically all cases the effects on children are complicated and may be due to loss, change and consequent hardships as much as to the absence of a father.

The re-demonization of lone mothers in the late 1980s coincided with the rise of the men's and fathers' rights movements. Within organizations such as PAIN (Parents Against Injustice) and Families Need Fathers, they campaigned against accusations of sexual abuse and of unfair treatment in relation to the Child Support Agency. More generally, they attempted to challenge men's financial responsibility for their former wives, while increasing their rights over their children. In the new discourses of fatherhood, fathers were not the traditional distant disciplinarian and breadwinner, but emotionally involved and equally as capable as mothers in caring for the children. They claimed, for example, that:

> An active and physically affectionate father can make many positive contributions. He can bring a son to a feeling of 'homosociality', an ability to relate to other men affectionately and communally, as women often relate. A father's affection for his daughter can also break up an identification with motherhood, introducing other forms of identification.

> (Coward, 1996, p.17)

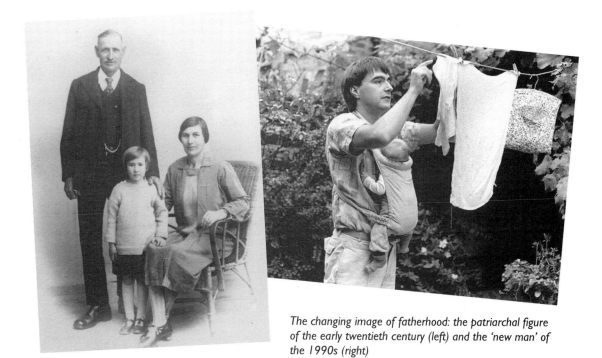

The changing image of fatherhood: the patriarchal figure of the early twentieth century (left) and the 'new man' of the 1990s (right)

In practice, gender divisions of labour within the household persisted, though perhaps in a less extreme form than, say, in the 1950s, and these ideas about the importance of fatherhood for children were highly contested. For example, Smart (1996, p.55) suggested that the reconstitution of fatherhood should not be interpreted as 'a radical reconstruction of men's responsibilities so much as an attempt to demote the significance of the mother who was thought to have become too powerful in the 1970s'.

Given the power of the ideology of the normal family, fathers may also have great symbolic significance for children, so that children brought up without fathers, whether by lone mothers or by two lesbian mothers, may feel different and 'other'. It is also important to recognize that children who have fathers are not a homogeneous group, and have very different experiences of being fathered. Moreover, 'father presence' is never seen as a problem, despite the evidence since the 1980s of the extent of abuse of children by their fathers or step-fathers.

5 Children's rights

The United Nations (UN) Convention on the Rights of a Child had a very significant impact on constructions of children and their needs: first, it established a minimum standard for children's rights around the world; second, an independent body, the UN Committee, was set up to monitor and assess progress on compliance in every country; and third, it became a focus for children's rights campaigners (Franklin and Franklin, 1996).

The Convention includes 54 articles, covering

> a wide range of rights entitlements including the most basic right to life, the right to adequate health care, food, clean water and shelter, rights to protection against sexual abuse, neglect and exploitation, rights to education, privacy, and freedom of association, expression and thought, which are grouped under three broad categories, and labelled the 'three Ps': the rights to provision, protection and participation.
>
> (Franklin and Franklin, 1996, p.102)

5.1 The right to participation

Article 12 of the UN Convention, which is concerned with children's rights to express their own views on all matters affecting them, was particularly important, as it went beyond previous UN declarations on children. Similarly, the Children Act 1989 went further than any previous UK legislation in giving children and young people the right to be consulted.

While this was welcomed by welfare professionals and children's rights campaigners, there were at the same time fears from the New Right that it would undermine the traditional agencies of authority, whether parents or school. The British government was known for its long-standing hostility to the Convention and to ideas of children's rights, particularly the third 'P' of participation. More generally, the government saw children's rights as an issue that was only relevant to so-called developing countries.

children's rights

Criticism of the government came from the Children's Rights Development Unit (CRDU), set up in 1992 to promote the implementation of the UN Convention within the UK, and funded by major charitable trusts and child welfare organizations. In February 1994 the government submitted its first report to the UN Committee, citing the Children Act 1989 as evidence of its compliance with the Convention. The CRDU described this report as complacent, and condemned what it saw as the government's indifference to children's rights: 'whether for reasons of poverty, ethnicity, disability, sexuality, immigration status or geography, many children are denied fundamental rights [listed] in the Convention' (Lansdown and Newell, 1994, p.xiii).

The CRDU's views were endorsed by the UN Committee, which criticized the UK government on many grounds, including: the high numbers of children living in poverty, cuts in state benefits, the number of teenage pregnancies, rising divorce rates, and the prevalence of children sleeping and begging on the streets. Some government policies, such as secure training units for young offenders, were seen as clear breaches of the Convention. The UN Committee also made several recommendations, including: laws to ban the use of physical punishments by parents and in private schools; measures to end health inequalities between children from different social and ethnic backgrounds; and measures to end homelessness.

5.2   The Children Act and children's rights

In order to assess the impact of the Children Act on children's rights, we need to consider first what is meant by 'children's rights' in the context of welfare. Like 'needs', 'rights' is a highly contested concept, particularly when applied to children.

ACTIVITY 4.5

Read Extract 4.2, which is from a social work journal. Then answer the following questions:

1   What different positions on children's rights can you distinguish?

2   What areas of conflict or contradiction are identified?

Extract 4.2 Rickford: 'Right or duty?'

Some commentators have suggested that if we formulate our responsibilities for children in terms of their rights we let ourselves off the hook – that adult duties and children's needs go way beyond any formulation of general rights ...

[The] *Observer* columnist and writer Melanie Phillips ... denounces the promotion of children's rights as harmful to children. 'Children do not have adult "rights" to freedom because they are still life's apprentices. They have needs, not rights. Freedom for them is another word for neglect. They are primarily the recipients of duties because their principal need is to be parented, which means being looked after with love, commitment and discipline. Letting them roam freely with "rights" and "choice" and with no fixed boundaries effectively abandons them to ignorance, error and often harm' [Phillips, 1996].

But there is confusion here about what children's rights as presented in the Children Act and the UN Convention imply, a confusion echoed within the social services world. An appeal to children's 'absolute' right to be protected from abuse or neglect can and has been used to justify over-zealous child rescue practices, while at the same time young people in care have been allowed to kill themselves in car accidents and to prostitute themselves in the name of their 'right' to freedom from restraint or punishment.

The UN Convention and the Children Act both afford children the right to express a view about matters affecting them and have it taken seriously, but neither suggests they should be able to do as they like ... the obligation to consult children is overshadowed by the obligation to promote children's welfare ...

Gerison Lansdown, director of the Children's Rights Office, acknowledges that children have a fundamental need for love which cannot be asserted as a right, but she argues ... 'There are some rights which cannot easily be redefined as needs, such as the right to physical integrity. If you don't assert that right, all sorts of people could interfere in all sorts of ways in the name of it being in the child's best interests. That is why other vulnerable, dependent people have rights, asserted on their behalf by the law ...'

June Thoburn, professor of social work [argues:] 'I think you need both a framework of adult obligations and a set of enforceable children's rights. Children have a right to a decent service ... They have a right to protection, and they also have a right to be consulted.

'We don't say children have rights to decide in child protection cases. Indeed they have to be protected from having to decide. But consulting children is in itself a part of meeting a child's needs, because if we don't listen to them and try to understand how they experience their world, how can we determine what they need?' [Schofield and Thoburn, 1996].

Another objection ... raised to the concept of rights for children is the fact that they depend on the adults who care for them to assert their rights for them – adults who may themselves be infringing those rights. Rachel Hodgkin ... a long-time campaigner for children's rights ... takes a strongly anti-protectionist position, and criticises interpretations of rights that disempower children by treating them ... as 'objects of concern' rather than people ...

'What children hate about abuse is that they are robbed of control, but children are done a further very profound disservice if they are made into victims rather than survivors. They want to be able to talk to adults about things, to get information and to think for themselves how to handle situations.

'Children might want to live with an element of risk in order to do something else, like stay in their family, for example. If child protection procedures take control away from children as soon as they open their mouths, even with the best of intentions, they are echoing the abuse' [Hodgkin and Newell, 1996].

References

Hodgkin, R. and Newell, P. (1996) *Effective Government Structures for Children*, Calouste Gulbenkian Foundation.

Phillips, M. (1996) *All Must Have Prizes*, Little, Brown and Co.

Schofield, G. and Thoburn, J. (1996) *Child Protection: The Voice of the Child in Decision-Making*, Institute for Public Policy Research.

(Rickford, 1997, pp.14–15)

COMMENT

Ideas on children's rights span a wide range, from the view that children have no rights, just needs that adults must fulfil, to the argument that children should have the right to choose even to live in dangerous circumstances. Other positions see children as having rights, but ones that are limited by their vulnerability and dependency. The relationship between 'needs' and 'rights' is a complex one, and in the extract Lansdown argues that in order to try to establish the best services for children it can be helpful to make use of both concepts.

There are tensions and contradictions between, on the one hand, children's rights to freedom, autonomy and involvement in decision-making and, on the other, their right to be protected from harm. Importantly, Rickford distinguishes between the right to be kept fully informed and consulted about decisions and having the right and/or responsibility to make decisions. Indeed, Thoburn suggests that children also have a right to be protected from having to make certain decisions for themselves.

In all the views, except perhaps Hodgkin's, adults are seen to play a central role in both ensuring and limiting children's rights. Hodgkin points out the tension between parents being both children's prime advocates and protectors, and in some circumstances also their abusers.

■ ■ ■

Did the Children Act 1989 represent an increase in children's rights?

The Act has given children a voice in decision-making for the first time. It also established complaints procedures, gave children the right under certain circumstances to their own legal representation, and also gave them qualified rights to refuse to submit to medical or psychiatric assessments or examinations (Sinclair, 1996). However, the rhetoric of 'empowerment' of children within the Children Act, as in the UN Convention, is limited by the requirement to take into account the child's age, maturity and understanding. If the child wants to make a decision deemed detrimental to her or his welfare, that decision can be overruled. As Coppock (1997, p.72) pointed out, 'In other words, the child's capacity to make a decision depends upon an *adult* third party's assessment of the legitimacy of that decision through the same paternalistic mechanism of applying the "best interests" rule'.

In the 1990s, organizations such as the National Association for Young People in Care (NAYPIC) criticized the reports and inquiries into residential care for not paying sufficient attention to the rights of the children and young people themselves. The complaints procedures for children and young people in care established by the Children Acts were often very complex, and were unlikely in themselves to stop abuse, while children who were viewed as troublesome and difficult were less likely to be listened to and taken seriously. NAYPIC argued that more effort should be put into talking to children and young people and involving them in decision-making and drawing up codes of conduct.

The importance of this is reinforced by ChildLine, who found that children in care who contacted them were 'among the most troubled and unhappy children to whom we have talked, and among the most isolated and alone ... They have described ... a story of family dislocation, abuse and several care placements ... A constant theme ... has been their sense of abandonment, unimportance and low self-esteem' (Morris and Wheatley, 1994, p.12). These children felt they had had little say in any decisions, and very little help and support. Many of them were unclear about why they were in care. In addition, a significant minority of the children described experiences of abuse from carers, fellow residents and foster carers. They were also very clear about what they wanted:

> They place enormous stress on their need and wish to have their emotional well-being attended to, but not in ways that they experience as being 'done to'. They want to be involved in both day to day and longer term planning, in ways which

161

allow them to retain some feeling of being in charge of their own lives. They wish to be protected from abuse, but if they are being abused, they want to have some control over measures taken to stop the abuse and offer them protection. In residential homes, protection from other residents is a priority and they want, among other possible options, the freedom to change placements or their key worker.

(Morris and Wheatley, 1994, p.13)

It has also been argued that the Children Acts were more concerned with the rights and responsibilities of parents than with the rights of children, and that the legislation sought to increase parents' rights in relation to the state. The Acts do not address children's rights within the family; for example, there are no procedures for children to complain about their parents. On the contrary, it is argued that parental authority was increased via the development of the notion of 'parental responsibility' and by the expectation within the Acts that the family was 'normally' the best place for children. As we saw in section 4, the use of the gender-neutral term 'parents' has contributed to rendering invisible power relations within families based on both age and gender.

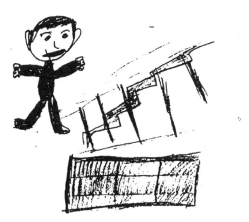

A right to have your opinyon and to argue with your mum or dad with out getting smacked or sent to bed

An unnamed child's drawing from a UNICEF publication on the Children's Rights Development Unit

Finally, it has been suggested that any gains in children's rights within social services were offset by legislation in the 1990s in other fields of welfare – in particular education and criminal justice – which worsened the position of children (see Chapter 5; Sinclair, 1996; **Fergusson, 1998**).

5.3   Children as young citizens

citizenship

If children are to be seen as citizens in their own right, rather than as life's apprentices with needs defined and met by adults, it will require the setting up of appropriate government structures and the provision of direct services for children. In the 1970s the idea was put forward of a Children's Rights Commissioner, who would act as an advocate for children within government, but it was not included in the Children Act 1975. In the 1990s the idea of a national Children's Rights Commissioner was revived and broadened into a possible Minister for Children, following similar developments in countries such as Norway, Israel, New Zealand and Costa Rica (Save the Children, 1995; Hodgkin and Newell, 1996). This was opposed strongly by the Conservative government. Although the 1992 Labour Party election manifesto included the commitment to such a ministerial post, it had disappeared by the 1997 election.

Consultation with children is seen primarily in an individualized way. Since the late 1980s many children's rights officers have been appointed at local level. These are largely concerned with the needs and rights of individual children accommodated by the local authority, but they have also helped children become involved in local decision-making, such as plans to close their residential home (Franklin and Franklin, 1996). Organizations concerned with children's issues are regularly consulted in relation to policy development, but organizations of children themselves rarely are, and certainly not by government bodies. The Children's Rights Development Unit did involve, and consult with, groups of children ranging in age between 8 and 16 years in a variety of circumstances and settings. These included schools and youth clubs, young people looked after by the local authority or who were leaving care, children who had been abused, children who were carers, and children who were homeless (Lansdown, 1995). Extract 4.3 shows how even young children can take part in decision-making.

Extract 4.3 Langley Children's Project: 'Children taking part in decisions'

One of the objectives of the Langley Children's Project near Manchester ... is to develop effective means to enable children and young people to directly express their views and needs, both within the project and more generally.

The project – based on a housing estate with high levels of poverty, unemployment, crime, drug abuse and health problems – operates an under-fives service with four crèches, a parent and toddler group, a mini gym and a toy library. Children between the ages of 5 and 13 ... also benefit from an after school play scheme, an out of school collection scheme, holiday playschemes and a girls' group ...

The project has developed several areas in which children participate in decision-making:

- a Children's Forum which has a formal place in the management of the project
  ...
- under-fives are offered a range of choices;
- over-fives have an evaluation session at the end of each play session;
- the girls' group, which works on developing confidence through issue-based work.

The Children's Forum, which is run by children and young people, has been meeting since the project was set up. The members discuss issues that concern them, look at how the services of the project are developing and are consulted on new procedures and systems. They are involved in influencing play and care initiatives on Langley and have started to develop contacts with other children's groups. Recently, the Children's Forum was involved in the recruitment process for two new staff for the project.

One of the children commented: 'I was glad to be part of the interviewing and glad to be part of the Children's Forum because we can make things happen for children on Langley'.

Another child said that being involved with the Children's Forum 'makes me feel that I have my own opinions'.

(Langley Children's Project, 1994a and 1994b)

5.3.1 Direct services for children

ChildLine has argued that, if children are young citizens, then more services should be available directly to children, rather than indirectly as members of their family. The rapid growth of ChildLine showed that children will make use of a service that they can go to themselves. ChildLine started in response to concerns about child abuse, but we saw in Table 4.3 that although thousands of the 600,000 children who contacted ChildLine in its first ten years phoned about abuse, there was a wide range of concerns:

> What made ChildLine unique was not only its direct accessibility to children ... but also that children *wanted* to use it. These have made the service what it is: the only national mental health and child protection service children access directly themselves.

> For perhaps the first time children became users of a service rather than recipients of services. Prior to its existence, children were elected for 'help' when adults noticed – or decided – that something was amiss. But here was a place they themselves could elect to approach. Changing the nature of the relationship between children and 'help' is one of ChildLine's greatest achievements ...

> Despite all the advances in child care and welfare, children are the group least able to ask for help and draw attention to their views about the help they require. They use ChildLine because it offers them a way of talking which works for them. This allows us to identify what children 'need' before they can 'go somewhere'. The medium of the telephone offers some absolutely key defining features which children desire.

> First, it is free and accessible at home and in public.

> Secondly, children can call anonymously and need never give their name ... Children want confidentiality too [and] we can respect children's wishes in the main ...

> Thirdly, children and young people see the organisation as being theirs ...

> Fourthly, communication on the telephone is limited to voice and ear ... a limitation which also offers children freedoms, and safety in its broadest sense – they are safe from physical abuse or interference from the adult with whom they talk. But they also benefit from a sense of not having to be responsible for the adult ... Perhaps most importantly, the medium offers invisibility. Children are not looked at, not the object of anybody's gaze or touch ...

> Finally ... the telephone also provides callers with more control over the process, timing and pace of the 'help' they ask for.

(MacLeod, 1996a, pp.13–17)

Direct services for children are not seen as an alternative to care for children by their families or by other significant people in children's lives: 'Talking to child callers only confirms how blessed are children with loving families. One of our main aims ... has always been to build a bridge between children and their families, so that they can, wherever possible, seek help and support there' (MacLeod, 1996a, p.14).

6   Conclusion

In this chapter we have explored changing and contested constructions of childhood and the needs of children, and their consequences for welfare organization, policy and practice. At the turn of the twentieth century, debates about children's needs and welfare interventions have taken place in the context of fears about the decline of the traditional family, and of new discourses of children's rights, which have raised a series of tensions and dilemmas.

Children, the family and the state

It is widely assumed that children fare best within stable two-parent families. A central dilemma for state intervention has been how to intervene to support traditional families and to regulate deviant or dysfunctional ones without transgressing family privacy and undermining parental responsibilities for children. There is a tension between the recognition of abuse within families and an acceptance of the value of family life (in all its varied forms) for most children. The impact of gender and age-related power relations within families means that there may be conflicts of interest between different members of a family.

State intervention has also been affected by financial considerations, with definitions of 'need' being used to ration services. Crucially, there is a tension between the recognition of the effects of material circumstances and general social provision on children's lives, and the dominant construction of welfare policies and practices in an individualized way, targeted at specific children or families.

Diversity and differences among children

Children are predominantly viewed as a homogeneous group with universal needs, resulting from their natural dependency. They are therefore seen as apprentice adults, and this standard model denies the impact of gender, 'race', class, disablement, geography and social and material circumstances on the experience of childhood. Children as a general category, however, are seen as subordinate to adults, while, within this category, it is white, middle-class, able-bodied children who are seen implicitly as the 'norm'. The power of this norm means that children, families and lifestyles that are 'different' are seen as abnormal, and the justifiable targets of intervention (Save the Children, 1995). Some groups of children are consequently seen as 'other', as 'in need', or as having 'special needs'.

Contested views on children's rights

The Children Act legislation in the UK and the UN Convention on the Rights of a Child represented a major shift in thinking about children, from 'objects of concern' to people with rights. Rather than adults acting 'in their best interests' the legislation 'intended to acknowledge and concede children's abilities as autonomous decision-makers' (Franklin, 1995, p.3).

However, consultation with children and their involvement in decisions is complex and contradictory, and even within policy rhetoric, let alone actual practice, is applied inconsistently across different fields of welfare. There is frequently no reference to children's changing competence to make decisions as they get older, thus avoiding the difficult question of who decides, and on what basis, that children can decide for themselves. There may also be conflicts of interest between adults and children, in particular in relation to criminal prosecutions of abusers.

The challenge for those concerned with the quality of childhood experiences in the present, rather than in terms of producing future adult citizens, is to imagine the implications of viewing children as citizens in their own right, and not just as members of family units. The experience of ChildLine as a direct service for children demonstrates not only that children would use such services, but that it is possible to construct children as welfare users rather than simply as recipients of welfare that someone else has decided they need.

Further reading

Discussion of welfare services and legislation for children in the UK and in Ireland can be found in Hill and Aldgate (1996). Children's rights are discussed by Franklin and Franklin (1996), and in the edited collections by Pilcher and Wagg (1996) and Scraton (1997). Save The Children (1995) offers a radical look at the global implications of a 'new agenda' for children. Ideas on 'mothering' and the re-emergence of 'fatherhood' are discussed in Silva (1996). ChildLine publishes a series of pamphlets about what children tell them about their experiences; see in particular MacLeod (1996a).

References

Ahmed, S. (1991) 'Routing out racism', *Community Care*, 27 June.

Aldgate, J. and Tunstill, J. (1995) *Making Sense of Section 17, A Study for the Department of Health: Implementing Services for Children in Need, Within the 1989 Children Act*, London, HMSO.

Aries. P. (1962) *Centuries of Childhood*, London, Cape.

Bowlby, J. (1953) *Child Care and the Growth of Love*, London, Penguin.

Bullock, R., Little, M. and Milham, S. (1993) *Residential Care for Children: A Review of the Research*, London, HMSO.

Clarke, J. and Cochrane, A. (1998) 'The social construction of social problems', in Saraga (ed.) (1998).

Cochrane, A. (1998) 'What sort of safety net? Social security, income maintenance and the benefits system', in Hughes and Lewis (eds) (1998).

Coles, B. (1995) *Youth and Social Policy*, London, UCL Press.

Coppock, S. (1997) '"Families" in "Crisis"', in Scraton (ed.) (1997).

Coward, R. (1996) 'Make the father figure', *The Guardian*, 12 April, p.17.

Dennis, N. and Erdos, G. (1992) *Families Without Fatherhood*, London, Institute of Economic Affairs.

Department of Health (1993) *Children Act Report*, London, HMSO.

Department of Health (1995) *Child Protection. Messages from Research*, London, HMSO.

Department of Social Security (1995) *Households Below Average Income: A Statistical Analysis 1979–1992/93*, London, HMSO.

Dwivedi, K.N. and Parma, V.P. (1996) *Meeting the Needs of Ethnic Minority Children: A Handbook for Professionals*, London, Jessica Kingsley Publishers.

Farmer, E. (1993) 'The impact of child protection interventions: the experiences of parents and children', in Waterhouse, L. (ed.) *Child Abuse and Child Abusers: Protection and Prevention*, Research Highlights in Social Work, no. 24, London, Jessica Kingsley Publishers.

Fergusson, R. (1998) 'Choice, selection and the social construction of difference: restructuring schooling', in Hughes and Lewis (eds) (1998).

Franklin, B. (1995) 'The case for children's rights: a progress report', in Franklin, B. (ed.) *The Handbook of Children's Rights*, London, Routledge.

Franklin, A. and Franklin, B. (1996) 'Growing pains: the developing children's rights movement in the UK', in Pilcher and Wagg (eds) (1996).

Goldson, B. (1997) '"Childhood": an introduction to historical and theoretical analyses', in Scraton (ed.) (1997).

Hall, C. (1998) 'A family for nation and empire', in Lewis (ed.) (1998b).

Hardiker, P. (1996) ' The legal and social construction of significant harm', in Hill and Aldgate (eds) (1996).

Hill, M. and Aldgate, J. (eds) (1996) *Child Welfare Services: Developments in Law, Policy, Practice and Research*, London, Jessica Kingsley Publishers.

Hodgkin, R. and Newell, P. (1996) *Effective Government Structures for Children*, London, Calouste Gulbenkian Foundation.

Hughes, G. (1998) 'A suitable case for treatment? Constructions of disability', in Saraga (ed.) (1998).

Hughes, G. and Lewis, G. (eds) (1998) *Unsettling Welfare: The Reconstruction of Social Policy*, London, Routledge in association with The Open University.

Keep, G. (1996) *Going to Court: Child Witnesses in Their Own Words*, London, ChildLine.

Kellmer Pringle, M. (1975) *The Needs of Children*, London, Hutchinson.

Kelly, G. and Pinkerton, J. (1996) 'The Children (Northern Ireland) Order 1995: prospects for progress?', in Hill and Aldgate (eds) (1996).

King, M and Trowell, J. (1992) *Children's Welfare and the Law*, London, Sage.

Langley Children's Project (1994a) *Annual Report 1993–94*, Langley, Langley Children's Project.

Langley Children's Project (1994b) *Evaluation Report Year One*, Langley, Langley Children's Project.

Lansdown, G. (1995) 'The Children's Rights Development Unit', in Franklin, B. (ed.) *The Handbook of Children's Rights*, London, Routledge.

Lansdown, G. and Newell, P. (1994) *UK Agenda for Children*, London, Children's Rights Development Unit.

Lentell, H. (1998) 'Families of meaning: contemporary discourses of the family', in Lewis (ed.) (1998b).

Lewis, G. (1998a) 'Welfare and the social construction of "race"', in Saraga (ed.) (1998).

Lewis, G. (ed.) (1998b) *Forming Nation, Framing Welfare*, London, Routledge in association with The Open University.

Liddiard, M. (1934) 'General management of the child from birth to five years', in Arbuthnot Lane, Sir W. (ed.) *The Hygiene of Life and Safer Motherhood*, London, British Books Ltd.

MacLeod, M. (1996a) *Talking with Children about Child Abuse*, London, ChildLine.

MacLeod, M. (1996b) *Children and Racism*, London, ChildLine.

MacLeod, M. and Barter, C. (1996) *We Know It's Tough to Talk: Boys in Need of Help*, London, ChildLine.

McIntosh, M. (1996) 'Social anxieties about lone motherhood and ideologies of the family: two sides of the same coin', in Silva (ed.) (1996).

Milner, J. (1995) 'A disappearing act: the differing career paths of fathers and mothers in child protection investigations', *Critical Social Policy*, no.38.

Mooney, G. (1998) '"Remoralizing" the poor?: gender, class and philanthropy in Victorian Britain', in Lewis (ed.) (1998b).

Morris, S. and Wheatley, H. (1994) *Time to Listen: The Experience of Young People in Foster and Residential Care*, London, ChildLine.

National Commission of Inquiry into the Prevention of Child Abuse (1996) *Childhood Matters*, London, HMSO.

Newson, J. and Newson, E. (1974) 'Cultural aspects of child rearing in the English-speaking world', in Richards, M.P. (ed.) *The Integration of a Child into a Social World*, Cambridge, Cambridge University Press.

Parton, N. (1991) *Governing the Family: Child Care, Child Protection and the State*, London, MacMillan.

Pilcher, J. and Wagg, S. (eds) (1996) *Thatcher's Children? Politics, Childhood and Society in the 1980s and 1990s*, London, Falmer Press.

Pinkney, S. (1998) 'The reshaping of social work and social care', in Hughes and Lewis (eds) (1998).

Rickford, F. (1997) 'Right or duty?', *Community Care*, 9–15 January, pp.14–15.

Saraga, E. (ed.) (1998) *Embodying the Social: Constructions of Difference*, London, Routledge in association with The Open University.

Save the Children (1995) *Towards a Children's Agenda: New Challenges for Social Development*, London, Save the Children.

Scraton, P. (ed.) (1997) *'Childhood' in 'Crisis'*, London, UCL Press.

Silva, E.B. (ed.) (1996) *Good Enough Mothering? Feminist Perspectives on Lone Motherhood*, London, Routledge.

Sinclair, R. (1996) 'Children's and young people's participation in decision-making: the legal framework in social services and education', in Hill and Aldgate (eds) (1996).

Smart, C. (1996) 'Deconstructing motherhood', in Silva (ed.) (1996).

Sone, K. (1997) 'The right stuff', *Community Care*, 13–19 March.

Stacey, J. (1994) 'Scents, scholars and stigma: the revisionist campaign for family values', *Social Text*, no.40, pp.51–75.

Thoburn, J., Murdoch, A. and O'Brien, A. (1986) *Permanence in Child Care*, Oxford, Blackwell.

Triseliotis, J. (1993) 'The theory continuum – prevention, restoration and permanence', in Marsh, P. and Triseliotis, J. (eds) *Prevention and Unification in Child Care*, London, Batsford.

Williams, F. (1989) *Social Policy: A Critical Introduction*, Cambridge, Polity Press.

CHAPTER 5

'Give 'em What They Deserve': The Young Offender and Youth Justice Policy

by John Muncie

Contents

1   Introduction

This chapter focuses on the particular case of young people who find themselves in trouble with the law. At first sight this may appear an odd example to use to illustrate how 'needs' are defined and met by social intervention. A common belief is that young offenders should forfeit all their rights to welfare, or other support, once they have broken the law. In this view, what is paramount is not 'meeting individual needs' but ensuring public protection and maintaining social order – or, rather, meeting a public 'need' for safety takes precedence over addressing whatever 'needs' the offender might have for 'justice' or 'rehabilitation'. In practice, however, things are not so simple.

The juvenile justice system (since the early 1990s more commonly referred to as the youth justice system) has evolved since the nineteenth century as a mechanism to afford young people a separate and different kind of justice to that meted out to adults. There is an assumption that young people should not always take full responsibility for all their actions. For example, a 'broken home', a 'deprived neighbourhood' or a 'disordered personality' may be considered as contributing to their law-breaking. In such cases it makes little sense to use the full weight of the law to punish offenders. Furthermore, it is sometimes assumed that criminalizing the transgressions of the young may only succeed in cementing 'criminal careers' and propel young people into a 'life of crime'. The youth justice system provides a good example of how these contradictions between the need to punish and the need to provide support and protection operate in practice.

The chapter examines four competing strategies for dealing with young offenders:

- Welfare-based interventions designed to help young people in trouble and to secure their rehabilitation and reintegration into mainstream society.

- Justice-based interventions designed to give young people the same legal rights as those afforded to adults.

- Diversionary interventions designed to prevent young people offending and to keep them out of court and custodial institutions.

- Custodial interventions designed to punish offenders and prevent further offending through punitive deterrence.

The aim throughout is to explore whose needs are addressed and how far they are met through each of these strategies. In particular, the chapter illustrates how the definition of 'need' varies considerably when the meeting of 'need' is the province not only of welfare institutions, but also of the criminal law. In both spheres, 'need' may not necessarily be something that individuals actively pursue, but something that is imposed from above. For example, the 'need' for care and removal from home may be defined as being 'in a child's best interests', although such a definition may not be shared by the child or its family; or the 'need' for control may be defined in terms of a social requirement for safety, in which a young offender's simultaneous 'need' for help, justice, rehabilitation or support to prevent re-offending may be given little or no priority. In these circumstances it often appears as if some higher authority – welfare professionals, magistrates, the government – knows best. We are told what we need, whether we like it or not.

Above all, the arena of youth justice is one of continual contestation. None of these four strategies is ever hegemonic or exists in pure form. From the early nineteenth century, when the troubled and troublesome among the youth population were first thought to require a different response to that afforded adults, youth justice has been riddled with confusion, ambiguity and unintended consequences.

This chapter is designed to assess the relative impact that these competing strategies have made on youth justice practice, focusing in particular on developments since the 1960s. It is predominantly a history of political and professional debate, in which the diverse and competing discourses of justice, custody and diversion have come to do battle with that of welfare over the management of the 'delinquent body'. Although the debates are presented in a chronological fashion, it would be misleading to view the developments as one of a unilinear shift, say from custody to welfare to justice to diversion, and so on. These strategies (and the discourses surrounding them) may have different histories and may have surfaced and achieved ascendancy at particular moments, but they all have a contemporary presence and relevance.

2   The welfare imperative

The key principle underlying all work with young offenders is that their general welfare must be ensured. The Children and Young Persons Act 1933 established that all courts should have primary regard to the 'welfare of the child'; this has since been bolstered by the 1989 Children Act's stipulation that a child's welfare shall be paramount. Similarly, the UN Convention on the Rights of the Child requires that in all legal actions concerning those under the age of 18, the 'best interests' of the child shall prevail (Association of County Councils *et al.*, 1996, p.13).

ACTIVITY 5.1

Reflect on the two phrases 'welfare of the child' and 'best interests'.

1   What do they suggest to you?

2   At what age should a person be considered 'adult' and be held fully responsible for their actions?

3   Why should the principle of 'best interests' be considered more appropriate than, say, 'full responsibility' or 'just deserts' when dealing with young people who find themselves in trouble with the law?

COMMENT

The principle of welfare in youth justice has proved to be consistently controversial. Yet since the early nineteenth century most young offender legislation has been promoted and implemented on the basis that young people should be protected from the full weight of the criminal law (see Chapter 4). It is widely assumed that below a certain age young people are *doli incapax* (incapable of evil) and cannot be held fully responsible for their actions. In England and Wales this presumption dates back to the fourteenth century.

doli incapax

However, the age at which such responsibility begins differs markedly across Europe. In the Republic of Ireland the age of criminal responsibility is 7, in Scotland and Northern Ireland 8, in England and Wales 10, in France 13, in Germany 14, in Spain 16, and in Belgium and Luxembourg 18. This alerts us to the fact that how certain age groups – child, juvenile, young person, adult – are perceived and constituted in law is not universally agreed upon. Each is a socially and historically specific *concept*. As such, each is also liable to review and change.

In England and Wales, whilst the under 10s cannot be found guilty of a criminal offence, the law presumes that those under 14 are also incapable of criminal intent. To prosecute this age group the prosecution must show that offenders were aware that their actions were 'seriously wrong' and not merely mischievous. During the mid 1990s the principle of *doli incapax* came under attack from both of the main political parties in the UK. The doctrine was placed under review by the Conservative government following a High Court ruling in 1994 that it was 'unreal, contrary to common sense and a serious disservice to the law'. Three years later the Labour Home Secretary, Jack Straw, announced that the principle would be abolished in order to 'help convict young offenders who are ruining the lives of many communities' on the basis that 'children aged between 10 and 13 were plainly capable of differentiating between right and wrong' (*The Guardian*, 21 May 1996; 4 March 1997). In addition, a Conservative Green Paper, *Preventing Children Offending* (Home Office, 1997a) and a Labour consultative document (Home Office, 1997b) both suggested that some children *below* the age of 10 should be placed under night curfew orders on the assumption that they were *at risk* of becoming persistent offenders. In some respects this might be construed as evoking the principle of acting 'in a child's best interests', since early intervention was assumed to be influential in preventing future offending. However, it was also driven by a desire to impose a greater control over parents to ensure that their children behaved responsibly. The proposal was also noteworthy because it would enable the criminal law to be used even when no offence had been committed. Neither of these notions was new. The very origins of youth justice can be traced back to the early nineteenth century as an instrument to deal not only with those convicted of crime, but also those who were homeless, vagrant or 'unnaturally independent'. Indeed, the principle that some young people should be removed from their home and placed in care 'for their own good' has been pivotal in youth justice policy throughout much of the twentieth century. From the outset, then, it is important to note that the youth justice system is not only concerned with the *control* of offenders, but also with the *care* of offenders and those considered 'at risk'. As a result there is a persistent confusion in its fundamental rationale and purpose, which raises questions such as:

- How far should the law penetrate family life?
- Who defines what is in a child's 'best interests'?
- On what basis are such decisions made?
- What are the implications of such decisions for that child's future involvement with professional and institutional bodies?

■ ■ ■

2.1 Victorian legacies: care and control

The idea that young people, in certain circumstances, should be subject to different forms of intervention to that afforded adults first surfaced in the early nineteenth century. Until then child offenders were not only punished with imprisonment, but were subjected to transportation or the death penalty. The modern concepts of 'delinquent', 'young offender', 'juvenile' or 'adolescent' did not exist. Children did not live in a separate world, dress differently or behave differently to adults, but quite 'naturally' drank alcohol, gambled and engaged in work activities that we would now describe as adult and likely to 'contaminate young minds'. The age of criminal responsibility was 7. The laissez-faire ideology of this period could not countenance the notion that children should be spared from the full application of the law merely on account of age. Neither could it accommodate the idea that the homeless or vagrant should automatically be able to look to the state for support (see **Mooney, 1998**).

Legal recognition that juveniles were in some way different from adults first emerged in the field of penal reform. Although the introduction of the penitentiary and the reform of local prisons in the early nineteenth century did not entail any special differentiation on the basis of age, the emphasis placed upon separation, classification and categorization highlighted age differentials and led to various conclusions being drawn about the position of the young. For example, The Society for the Improvement of Prison Discipline and the Reformation of Juvenile Offenders, established in 1817, was convinced of the need to separate juveniles from the hardened adult criminal in order to avoid their moral contamination. The Society advocated the establishment of separate but highly controlled institutions in which young offenders could be reformed and reclaimed. As May (1973, p.12) has recorded, 'cellular isolation clearly revealed the mental and physical differences between children and adults', and she notes how this led prison inspectors to conclude that 'so marked is the distinction in the feeling and habit of manhood and youth that it is quite impractical to engraft any beneficial plan for the lengthened confinement of boys upon a system adapted to adults'. Thus the early period of modern imprisonment permitted the apparently unique needs of the young to be recognized. Through refinements in prisoner classification the concept of juvenile delinquency was created.

juvenile delinquency

In 1838 the first penal institution solely for juvenile boys was opened at Parkhurst. Yet as Weiner (1990, p.132) has noted, its regime was hardly less repressive than that endured by adults. It was 'decidedly of a penal character' and its founder assured the Home Office that there was 'no reason to doubt that a strict system of penal discipline is quite compatible with the means requisite for the moral and religious improvement of the offender'. Prisoners were manacled and confined to their cells except for brief periods of exercise and religious instruction. Yet this severity was viewed as philanthropic. Parkhurst's governor claimed that 'every punishment is a weapon drawn from the armoury of truth and love ... and directed for their real happiness' (cited by Weiner, 1990, p.133). However, Parkhurst did little to undermine the prevailing view that *all* offenders should be held fully responsible for their actions. Long before its conversion to a women's prison in 1864, its administration had ceased to speak of its role as one of reformation and rescue.

Pressure to develop separate institutions (other than prison) for the delinquent young was also developing from voluntary organizations such as the extravagantly titled Philanthropic Society (for the Prevention of Crimes and the Reform of the Criminal Poor; by the Encouragement of Industry and the Culture of Good Morals, among those children who are now trained up to Vicious Courses, Public Plunder, Infamy and Ruin). Founded in 1788, the Philanthropic Society aimed to reform the delinquent *and* the destitute child by establishing a separate 'asylum' to rescue children from the 'vices of the street' by providing religious and industrial instruction.

By the turn of the eighteenth century these early initiatives began to flounder, but they were revived and augmented by the reformatory movement of the 1840s. Inspired by the establishment of the Mettray reformatory in France, which had instituted a regime of strict self-denial, religious zeal and continual exercise for delinquents and vagrants, the Philanthropic Society established its own agricultural farm at Red Hill in Surrey in 1849. Lauded as a great success, the cause was subsequently taken up by such philanthropists as Mary Carpenter, the daughter of a Unitarian minister. A forceful critic of penal regimes such as at Parkhurst, Carpenter was convinced that reformation depended on meeting the perceived needs of children for care and support as well as overt discipline. The causes of crime were seen to lie firmly in deficiencies in working-class family life, in the low moral condition of parents, and in parental neglect. Preventing the contamination of youth and restoring their moral guardianship in the family were to serve as the principles for 'humanitarian' reform:

reformation

> The child ... must be placed where the prevailing principle will be, as far as practicable, carried out – where he will be gradually restored to the true position of childhood ... He must perceive by manifestations which he cannot mistake, that this power, whilst controlling him, is guided by wisdom and love; he must have his affections called forth by the obvious personal interest felt in his own individual well being by those around him; he must, in short, be placed in a *family*.
>
> (Carpenter, 1853, p.298)

Carpenter's language was notably gender-specific, but concern was directed as much at girls as boys. Whilst boys were considered at risk of offending, girls were viewed as particularly vulnerable and susceptible to prostitution and immorality. Indeed, Carpenter herself argued that criminal women and girls were especially depraved: 'they are, as a class, even more morally degraded than men' (cited by Gelsthorpe, 1984, p.2).

Carpenter labelled the destitute as the 'perishing' class and the delinquent as the 'dangerous' class. Advocating industrial schools for the former and reformatories for the latter, her initiative was to gain legal status in the Youthful Offenders Act 1854 and the Industrial Schools Act 1857. Whilst boys were put to work in manufacturing, girls were employed in mending clothes and cleaning, and often endured a higher degree of control in which the smallest details of their everyday life were subject to regulation (Weiner, 1990, p.140). By 1860 there were 48 certified reformatories holding about 4,000 young offenders. The development of industrial schools was slower, but by the end of the century reformatories and industrial schools held more than 30,000 inmates. The state had come to assume the responsibility of parents for one in every 230 of the juvenile population (Radzinowicz and Hood, 1990, p.181).

These initial movements to recognize the 'welfare of the child' were by no means universally accepted. Traditional advocates of the principles of punitive justice argued that age could not be taken as a sufficient index of responsibility,

punitive justice

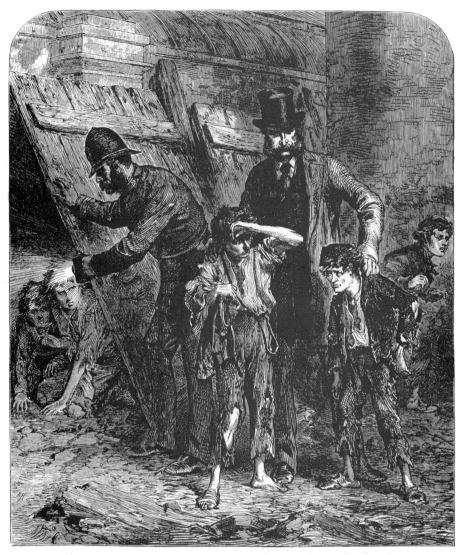

Discovering the young offender: deprived, depraved or delinquent? An engraving from the
Illustrated London News, *1871*

and that *no* circumstances should preclude the necessity of punishment in
dealing with all offenders, whether juvenile or adult, male or female. In contrast
to the reformist discourse of welfare and rescue, May (1973, p.25) has noted a
continuing and influential body of opinion that punishment should fit the crime
and not be mitigated by personal circumstances; that juveniles should be treated
as all other offenders; and that 'the idea of pain might be instantly associated
with crime in the minds of all evildoers'. As a result of these influences,
Carpenter's proposals were subject to legislative compromise. Before entering
a reformatory, a 14-day prison sentence had to be served. Moreover, the 1854
Act was only permissive, so magistrates could continue to send juveniles to
prison if they deemed this preferable. The reformatory system was thus grafted
on to the existing institutions of punishment and justice and did not replace
them.

Such tensions between reclamation and punishment for the destitute and delinquent alike have continued to impact on the rationale and practices of a separate system of justice for juveniles. Significantly, it was only through the initiation of such disputes that the concepts of the 'young offender' and 'juvenile delinquent' achieved both public and political recognition, and thereafter their own legal status. Before the reformatory movement of the 1840s it was impossible to talk with any precision of the existence of delinquency and the *young* offender.

How was the 'problem' of juvenile delinquency created through the institutions and legal powers of the emergent youth justice system in the mid nineteenth century?

2.2 Welfare legislation

The argument that age and the neglect and vice of parents should be taken into account when adjudicating on juveniles in court may have been partial and contested, but it opened the way for a plethora of welfare-inspired legislation in the twentieth century. Moreover, as Clarke (1975, p.12) has argued, it created a 'hole' in the principles of traditional punitive justice 'through which subsequent armies of psychiatrists and social workers have run and thoroughly confused the law's focus on criminal responsibility'.

juvenile courts The Children Act 1908 established the principle that young offenders should be dealt with separately from adults by way of juvenile courts. These differed from their adult counterparts in that the public were excluded, there was no jury, and there was no right to legal representation. They were empowered to act upon both the criminal offender *and* the 'delinquent' child who may have been found begging, vagrant, in association with reputed thieves, or whose parents were considered to be unworthy. As such, the categories of delinquent (the troublesome) and destitute (the troubled) were conflated. Moreover, as the conditions constituting neglect were so broad, the court and the state were able, in the name of welfare, to intervene more directly into any element of working-class community and family life which they deemed to be immoral or unruly.

Nevertheless, as Morris *et al.* (1980, p.21) have noted, the juvenile courts remained essentially criminal courts. The idea that the child was a wrongdoer prevailed, and despite a new range of sentences from fines, discharge and probation to committal to industrial school, whipping and imprisonment (if over 14), the procedures for dealing with adults were usually thought to be the most appropriate for dealing with children. Although imprisonment for children under 14 was abolished, the Crime Prevention Act 1908 set up specialized detention centres where rigid discipline and work training could be provided in a secure environment. The first of these was at Borstal in Kent.

By the time of the Children and Young Persons Act 1933 assumptions about delinquency and neglect were thoroughly conflated. In deliberations before the Act, the 1927 Home Office Departmental Committee on the Treatment of the Young Offender had argued:

> there is little or no difference in character and needs between the neglected and the delinquent child. It is often a mere accident whether he is brought before the court because he was wandering or beyond control or because he has committed some offence. Neglect leads to delinquency.
>
> (Home Office, 1927, p.6)

As a result, the 1933 Act directed magistrates to take primary account of the 'welfare of the child'. In this, considerable responsibility was given to probation officers (recruited in the main from charitable societies) and social workers (recruited from the Charity Organisation Society).

Whilst the goal of 'delivering welfare' through the 'personal influence' of 'professionals' was heralded as an important victory for the welfare lobby, it was to provide the juvenile justice system with a fundamental contradiction which is still being grappled with today. The two philosophies of criminal justice and welfare remain incompatible, because while the former stresses full criminal responsibility, the latter stresses welfare and treatment to meet the needs of each individual child. Moreover, the definition of what constitutes 'need' was, and remains, problematic. For example, through the 1933 Act, the court was empowered to act *in loco parentis*, establishing itself in law as *the* responsible body capable of adjudicating on matters of family socialization and parental behaviour, even when no 'crime' as such had been committed.

By the 1950s a system had emerged in which the remit of juvenile justice stretched from dealing with the neglected by way of some form of welfare assistance, such as receiving children into local authority care (empowered by the Children Act 1948), to providing attendance centres (run by local authorities and the police) and detention centres (run by the prison service) expressly designed to 'retrain' the offender through hard labour and punitive military drill (empowered by the Criminal Justice Act 1948).

As Alcock and Harris have argued,

> By now the situation had reached a new level of confusion. The disposition of the 'deprived' and the 'depraved' was the subject of two different pieces of legislation, and the measures available and personnel involved reflected the muddled reasoning which sought to provide in different ways for young people with all kinds of perceived problems. Thus whether to 'punish' or 'treat' children and young people in trouble was a question which was for the time being suspended in favour of a kind of continuum involving, at one end, social casework within the family for the deprived and at the other 'short sharp shock' methods for the depraved hard cases. In the centre, the notions of 'punishment' and 'treatment' were merged into the ambiguous notion of 'training'.
>
> (Alcock and Harris, 1982, p.95)

Such confusion was to become most prominent in the spate of committees, recommendations and Acts concerned with the control and treatment of juveniles that characterized the 1960s. These culminated in the highly controversial Children and Young Persons Act 1969 in England and Wales and the Social Work Act 1968 in Scotland. Both advocated a rise in the age of criminal responsibility and sought alternatives to detention by way of treatment, non-criminal care proceedings and care orders. It was one element in the Labour Party's vision of a society based on full employment, prosperity, expanded educational opportunities and an enlarged welfare state which would overcome social inequalities and thus remove a major cause of young offending (Pitts, 1988, p.3). Moreover, the prevailing political view of the late 1960s was that young offending was largely trivial and transient in nature and above all was so commonplace that the full weight of the law was unjustified and counter-productive. In England the 1968 White Paper *Children in Trouble* argued that: 'It is probably a minority of children who grow up without even behaving in ways which may be contrary to the law. Frequently such behaviour is no more than an incident in the pattern of a child's normal development' (Home Office, 1968, pp.3–4).

In Scotland the Kilbrandon Report described delinquency as a 'symptom of personal or environmental difficulties' (cited by Morris and McIsaac, 1978, p.26). Young offending was seen as an indication of maladjustment, immaturity or damaged personality, conditions which could be treated in much the same way as an illness or disease. The report advocated the abolition of the juvenile court and its replacement by a welfare tribunal. In England the White Paper advocated a range of interventions intended to deal with offenders through systems of supervision, treatment and social welfare in the community rather than punishment in custodial institutions. Central to both was the increased involvement of local authority social workers. Their role was to prevent delinquency by intervening in the family life of the 'pre-delinquent'; to assess a child's needs; and to promote non-custodial disposals. A significant reduction in the number of young people appearing before the courts was envisaged, with offenders, in the main, being dealt with under care and protection proceedings or informally. The perceived need was to keep young people out of court altogether. When court action was unavoidable, civil proceedings leading to care orders implemented by the local authority were to replace criminal proceedings leading to custodial orders. Attendance centres and detention centres were to be phased out in favour of either community-based intermediate treatment (IT) schemes, which would offer supervised activities, guidance and counselling, or residential care in local authority-run Community Homes with Education (formerly known as approved schools). Magistrates were no longer to be involved in detailed decisions about appropriate treatment; this too was to be the province of social workers and social service professionals (Morris and McIsaac, 1978, p.25).

intermediate treatment

These proposals, which were to inform much of the Children and Young Persons Act 1969 and the Social Work (Scotland) Act 1968, were thus quite explicitly based on a social welfare approach to young offenders. Authority and discretion were notably shifted out of the hands of the police, magistrates and prison department and into the hands of the local authorities and the Department of Health and Social Security. As Thorpe *et al.* (1980, p.6) declared, 'the hour of the "child-savers" had finally arrived'.

However, in England and Wales during the 1970s, vital elements of the Children and Young Persons Act 1969 were never implemented. The Act had consistently attracted criticism during its draft stages for being too welfare-minded and permissive (Bottoms, 1974). The new Conservative government that came to power in 1970 almost immediately declared it would not implement those sections of the Act which were intended to raise the age of criminal responsibility from 10 to 14 years and to replace criminal with care proceedings. The Conservatives essentially objected to state intervention in criminal matters through a welfare rather than a judicial body. Likewise, magistrates and police responded to the undermining of their key position in the justice system by becoming more punitively minded and declining the opportunity to use community-based services on a large scale. Above all, rather than replacing the old structures of juvenile justice, the new welfarist principles were grafted on to them. The treatment/punishment continuum was merely extended. Intermediate treatment was introduced but detention centres and attendance centres were not phased out. Community Homes with Education arrived but retained the character of the old approved schools. Care proceedings were made in criminal cases but, as it was still possible to take criminal proceedings against children under 14, the former were only occasionally used (Thorpe *et al.*, 1980, p.22). When care orders were used, they were largely targeted at girls, on the grounds of 'moral danger' and for 'status offences' – running away from home, staying out late at night, and so on – which would not be punishable by law if committed by an adult and rarely considered as 'serious' if committed by boys.

In practice traditional principles of punitive justice were never seriously undermined by the 1969 Act. The new welfare elements of the system were generally employed with a younger age group of, for example, low-achievers at school, 'wayward girls' and truants from 'problem' families designated as 'pre-delinquent' – the domain of social workers. The courts meanwhile continued their old policy of punishing offenders – the magistrates' domain. Whilst ideologically opposed, 'the two systems have in effect become vertically integrated and an additional population of customer-clients has been identified in order to ensure that they both have plenty of work to do' (Thorpe *et al.*, 1980, pp.22–3).

Why do welfare reforms in youth justice always appear to face opposition from advocates of punitive justice? What are the unintended consequences of welfare-based initiatives?

2.3   Children's hearings and family group conferences

In Scotland a different outcome emerged from the welfare/punishment debates of the 1960s. The sheriffs, probation officers and police associations gave way to the advocates of reform. The Social Work (Scotland) Act 1968 established new social work departments, gave local authorities a general duty to promote social welfare for children in need, and established the children's hearing system (which came into operation in 1971).

children's hearings

Children's hearings are not criminal courts but welfare tribunals serviced by lay people from the local community. Before cases reach a hearing, they are referred to a reporter from a range of bodies including education authorities, social work departments, the police and procurators fiscal. The role of the reporter is to sift referrals and decide on a future course of action. In the early 1980s around half of all referrals were considered unworthy of future action, 5 per cent were referred on to a social work department, and the remainder were passed on to children's hearings. The main grounds governing such action are when the child:

- is beyond the control of parents;
- has fallen into bad associations and is exposed to moral danger;
- is subject to lack of parental care, causing suffering or ill health;
- has committed an offence;
- has been the victim of a sex or cruelty offence;
- lives in a household where there is, or is likely to be, the perpetrator of such an offence;
- has failed to attend school regularly.

On its inception a majority of the grounds for referral were for offences. By the 1990s, however, non-offence grounds predominated, which was reflected in a rise in the number of girls referred for care and protection reasons. Reporters are thus endowed with considerable discretionary power. Initially they do seem to have been influential in reducing the numbers facing processing and adjudication. Between 1969 and 1973 a reduction of 39 per cent was achieved, whereas in England and Wales the numbers considered by the juvenile court increased by 4 per cent (Morris and McIsaac, 1978). However, rates of referral have increased in the 1990s (McGhee *et al.*, 1996, p.62). When a case reaches a hearing it is deliberated upon by three lay members of a panel, the parents or guardians of the child, social work representatives, and the child him/herself. Legal representation is not allowed. The hearing cannot proceed unless all parties understand *and* accept the grounds for referral. Unlike the English youth court, the hearing does not determine guilt or innocence (it can only proceed if guilt is admitted) and is solely concerned with deciding on future courses of action. Before reaching any decision, reports on the child from the social work department are heard. In a review of the hearings' more positive features, Dickie concluded:

> The system encourages communication and collaboration between the relevant professions and permits a flexibility in the provision of services appropriate to the child's changing needs. Above all, perhaps, is its capacity to focus on the interests of the individual child and to tackle problems in a manner which encourages the family to participate and retain its self respect … a system which has such inherently strong welfare values must appeal to social workers.
>
> (Dickie, 1979, p.68)

Following a hearing, one of three decisions is made: to discharge the referral, to make a supervision order, or to make a residential supervision order. The most frequent (and increasing) disposal is a social work supervision requirement. About 15 per cent result in residential supervision. The latter usually involves committal to a list D school (the equivalent of an English Community Home with Education). However, it is also worth remembering that whilst over 15,000 children are referred to a hearing each year, there are also another 700 or so whose offences are considered so 'serious' that the hearing system is bypassed and they are referred directly to the adult sheriff and High Court system (Gill, 1985). In this respect Scottish welfarism is reserved only for less serious offences, and some routes into adult justice have remained unchallenged. Moreover, the hearings system only deals with those up to the age of 16. Whilst in Scotland there are almost no penal options for those under the age of 16, custodial institutions still exist for those over the age of 16, and their regimes are far removed from the promotion of welfarism. In 1985 the only custodial centre for young people at Glenochil, Alloa came under increasing criticism following a sequence of suicides unparalleled in the custody of young people. As in England, some of Scotland's most punitive systems still appear to be reserved for its young. The goal of welfarism also appears to be consistently prey to shifts in the broader political climate. As McGhee *et al.* concluded,

> Nearly 25 years later the gap Kilbrandon tried to close between the needs of children in trouble with the law and children in need of care is beginning to open … this change in outlook is reflected both in the United Kingdom and abroad and is likely to pose a serious challenge to the philosophy which lies behind the Children's Hearings System. Increased public pressure to make children accountable for wrong

doing, plus a growing concentration on the needs of victims, have contributed to the public focus shifting from the welfare of the child to offending behaviour and its consequences.

(McGhee *et al.*, 1996, pp.68–9)

Nevertheless, the Scottish hearing system is frequently invoked as a model for the reform of judicial-based systems. In the 1990s reformers also looked at the experience of family group conferences (FGCs), an approach pioneered in New Zealand and based on traditional systems of conflict resolution within Maori culture. FGCs involve a professional co-ordinator, dealing with both civil and criminal matters, who calls together the young person, their family *and* victims to decide whether the young person is 'in need of care and protection' and, if so, what should be provided. According to NACRO (1995), FGCs have proved to be remarkably effective in dealing with young people of all races. Since their introduction in New Zealand in 1989, there has been an 80 per cent reduction in the number of those in care for welfare or criminal reasons. Nearly all FGCs reach agreement and are able to advise on an active penalty – usually community work, an apology or reparation. Furthermore, it is argued, FGCs act as an effective forum for enabling the participation and strengthening of families whilst respecting the interests of victims (Hudson *et al.*, 1996, p.234). In England and Wales in 1995, despite increasing interest, FGCs only operated in child abuse and child protection cases, and then on an experimental basis involving five social services departments and one voluntary agency. However, as NACRO (1995) argues, there exists a potential to introduce family conferencing and decision-making at various points in the judicial process, including caution/prosecution, bail/remand, social work reports and following release from custody. Indeed, in October 1996 Hampshire police, working with youth and social services, initiated a two-year experiment to assess whether FGCs involving offender, family, friends and victims would be successful in diverting young offenders away from crime at an early age.

family group conferences

2.4 'In a child's best interests'?

Welfare in youth justice is predicated on the assumption that all intervention should be directed towards meeting the needs of young people, rather than responding to their deeds. Historically, therefore, it has tended to see little differentiation between offending and non-offending troublesome behaviour: both are symptomatic of a wider deprivation, whether it be material neglect or lack of moral guidance. As a result, it is capable of drawing many more young people into its remit than it would if it was solely concerned with matters of guilt or innocence. Remarking on the impact of the Children and Young Persons Act 1933, Springhall (1986, p.186) argued that there was 'abundant evidence' to show that rather than diverting youth from court, the Act positively encouraged it. Because of the 'welfare' focus of the Act, there was an increased willingness to prosecute on the assumption that care and treatment would follow. Similarly, because delinquency has been ill-defined, there has been little or no control over who might be considered deserving of intervention. The persistent critique of welfarism (which gathered pace in the 1970s – see section 3.2 below) is that its rhetoric of benevolence and humanitarianism often blinds us to its denial of legal rights, its discretionary and non-accountable procedures, and its ability to

needs/deeds

impose greater intervention than would be merited on the basis of conduct alone. As Hudson (1987, p.152) has said, 'identifying needs amounts to listing reasons for intervention', which often leads to young people being drawn into the justice system at an earlier age and for relatively innocuous offences. In particular, welfarism seems to encourage greater intervention into the lives of young women on the grounds of 'moral danger' and on presumptions of being 'at risk'. Consequently, 'wayward' girls may find themselves committed into the residential care of the local authority, and thence into stigmatizing institutions, without having committed an offence (Gelsthorpe, 1984, p.2).

ACTIVITY 5.2

Read through the ten major assumptions of welfare-based strategies as detailed by the report of the Black Committee in Extract 5.1. The Committee was established in Northern Ireland in the late 1970s to overview youth justice practice and to suggest proposals for reform. You will find it useful to make notes on this extract. As you do so, pay particular attention to the following:

■ the causes of offending;

■ the purpose of intervention;

■ who might be the key agencies and personnel involved;

■ the central characteristics and objectives of welfare strategies.

Use the grid below to record your own summary of the extract. It will prove useful when we compare welfare with other youth justice strategies in the remainder of this chapter.

Assumptions of welfare strategies
Causes of offending:
Purpose of intervention:
Key agencies:
Key personnel:
Key characteristics:
Objectives:

Extract 5.1 Black Committee: 'Assumptions of welfarism'

(a) delinquent, dependent and neglected children are all products of an adverse environment which at its worse is characterized by multiple deprivation. Social, economic and physical disadvantage, including poor parental care, are all relevant considerations;

(b) delinquency is a pathological condition; a presenting symptom of some deeper maladjustment out of the control of the individual concerned;

(c) since a person has no control over the multiplicity of causal factors dictating his delinquency he cannot be considered responsible for his actions or held accountable for them. Considerations of guilt or innocence are, therefore, irrelevant and punishment is not only inappropriate but is contrary to the rules of natural justice;

(d) all children in trouble (both offenders and non-offenders) are basically the same and can be effectively dealt with through a single unified system designed to identify and meet the needs of children;

(e) the needs or underlying disorders, of which delinquency is symptomatic, are capable of identification and hence treatment and control are possible;

(f) informality is necessary if the child's needs are to be accurately determined and his best interests served. Strict rules of procedure or standards of proof not only hinder the identification of need but are unnecessary in proceedings conducted in the child's best interests;

(g) inasmuch as need is highly individualized, flexibility of response is vital. Wide discretion is necessary in the determination and variation of treatment measures;

(h) voluntary treatment is possible and is not punishment. Treatment has no harmful side effects;

(i) the child and his welfare are paramount though considerations of public protection cannot be ignored. In any event, a system designed to meet the needs of the child will in turn protect the community and serve the best interests of society;

(j) prevention of neglect and alleviation of disadvantage will lead to prevention of delinquency.

(Black Committee, 1979, pp.32–3).

3 Justice-based initiatives

During the 1970s, faith in social work's ability to diagnose the causes of delinquency and to treat these with non-punitive methods came to be increasingly questioned. The discretion of social work judgements was defined as a form of arbitrary power. Many young people, it was argued, were subjected to apparently non-accountable state procedures and their liberty was often unjustifiably denied (Davies, 1982, p.33). It was argued that the investigation of social background was an imposition, and that social work involvement not only preserved explanations of individual pathology, but also undermined a young person's right to natural justice. It may also have placed young people in double jeopardy – sentenced because of their background as well as their offence – and unintentionally accelerated movement up the sentencing tariff. On the experience of the 1970s, in which the numbers of custodial sentences increased dramatically, a 'back to justice' approach argued that a return to notions of due process and just deserts was called for.

3.1 The opposition to welfare

The critique of welfare had three main elements. Each came from markedly divergent political positions. From the Right, welfare and rehabilitative systems were condemned as evidence that the justice system had (once again) become too 'soft on crime'. Second, radical social workers argued that the 'need for treatment' acted as a spurious justification for placing considerable restrictions on the liberty of young people, particularly girls, which were out of proportion either to the seriousness of the offence or to the realities of being 'at risk'. Third, civil libertarians and liberal lawyers maintained that welfarism denied young people access to full legal rights and that their 'cause' would be better served by restoring due process to the heart of the justice system.

In England and Wales, the numbers sent to youth custody increased dramatically during the 1970s. This was in direct contradiction to the intentions of the 1969 Act. The re-commitment to custody was based partly on the popular belief that the 1970s witnessed a rapid growth in juvenile crime, characterized by a hard core of 'vicious young criminals'; partly on a tendency by magistrates to give custodial sentences for almost all types of offence (particularly if the offender was already subject to a welfare-based care or supervision order); and partly on the role of welfarism in drawing juveniles into the system at an increasingly earlier age. Rather than acting as a check on custodial sentencing, these developments acted collectively to accelerate the rate at which a young

net widening

person moved through the sentencing tariff – a process known as net widening. As a result, the number of custodial orders rose dramatically. As a 1981 Department of Health and Social Security report concluded, the number of juveniles sent to borstal and detention centres increased fivefold between 1965 and 1980. Less than a fifth of this rise could be attributed to increased offending. Rather, the increase in incarceration was believed to reflect a growing tendency on the part of the courts to be more punitive (Department of Health and Social Security, 1981).

Much of this new authoritarianism coalesced with a highly public debate in the mid 1970s about the supposed criminality of black youths and their involvement in street crimes such as 'mugging'. Police/black youth relations deteriorated rapidly. Landau and Nathan's (1983) study of the Metropolitan Police area showed that for particular offences – violence, burglary, public order – black youths were treated more harshly than their white counterparts: they tended to be charged immediately rather than have their cases referred to a juvenile liaison bureau for a decision about whether to caution or not. Afro-Caribbeans make up about 5 per cent of the population in London, but 17 per cent of the people arrested. Black youths tend to enter the system at an earlier age and more often than whites. In court they are less likely to be given a non-custodial sentence, and young black males receive longer custodial sentences despite fewer previous convictions (Fitzgerald, 1993). In 1987, 9.8 per cent of the under 18s received into custody were from ethnic minorities compared with their representation in the general population of no more than 5 per cent

(Children's Society, 1989, p.10). In the early 1980s, in the borstals and detention centres of the South of England, black youths often constituted over a third of the inmates (Kettle, 1982, p.535).

While magistrates were committed to incarcerating the young offender, social workers extended their preventive work with the families of the 'pre-delinquent'. Ironically, this development meant many more children were under surveillance, the market for the courts was widened, and more offenders were placed in care for relatively trivial offences. In practice, preventive work meant that children were being sent to institutions at a younger age. As in the past, new institutions which were supposed to reform youth instead created new categories of delinquency. As Thorpe *et al.* have remarked, the liberalism of the 1969 Act produced a judicial backlash in which popular wisdom about juvenile justice and its actual practice became totally estranged:

> The tragedy that has occurred since can be best described as a situation in which the worst of all possible worlds came into existence – people have been persistently led to believe that the juvenile criminal justice system has become softer and softer, while the reality has been that it has become harder and harder.
>
> (Thorpe *et al.*, 1980, p.8)

Such arguments appeared all the more pertinent when applied to the situation of young women. Young women were frequently brought into court for offences which might be dealt with informally or ignored if committed by adults or young men. Frequently their offences were (and remain) related to behaviour regarded as sexually deviant and promiscuous, or to a perceived need for their 'protection'. Here a moral evaluation of what constitutes 'need' is much stronger. Whilst cultural codes of masculinity, toughness and sexual predator are the norm for young men, there is little or no conception of 'normal' exuberant delinquency for young women. Consequently when young women appear before the court they are likely to be viewed as 'abnormal' – they are not only breaking the law, but also the rules of how they should behave. Because of the statistically exceptional nature of their criminality, female delinquency tends also to be seen as a perversion of, or rebellion against, their 'natural' feminine roles. As Hudson (1988, p.40) argues, a predominantly treatment- and welfare-focused paradigm adjudicates as much on questions of femininity as it does on matters of guilt or innocence:

> when white male youth commit criminal offences they are not usually seen as intrinsically challenging normative expectations about behaviour for young and adult men ... rarely is there any suggestion that male delinquency is incongruent with masculinity ... Young women, however, are predominantly judged according to their management of family, sexual and interpersonal relationships ... they are subject to a double penalty: firstly because they have broken the law and secondly because they have defied social codes which prescribe passivity for women.
>
> (Hudson, 1988, pp.39–40)

The end result of such gender-specific modes of social control is that young women tend to be drawn into the youth justice system for reasons wholly unrelated to the commission of offences (Casburn, 1979); they are less likely to be fined and more often placed on supervision or taken into care than young men (May, 1977); and they are more likely to be ordered to be removed from home on 'care, protection and control' rather than 'offence' grounds (Shacklady Smith, 1978). As Harris and Webb (1987, p.154) concluded, 'whether the overt

Young women: doubly deviant?

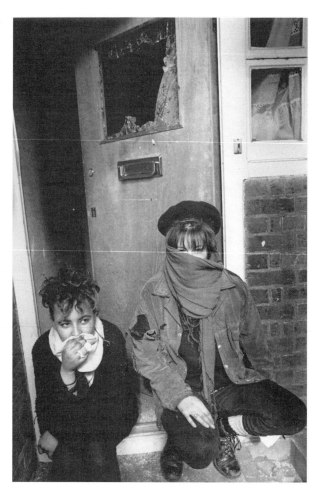

intent of the courts and the experts is to monitor girls' behaviour or whether such monitoring is rather the effect of an almost complete dearth of ideas as to what is to be done, the effect of these processes is a disproportionate exercise of power over girls'.

This critique of the gender-specific nature of youth justice also coalesced with a critique of welfare and rehabilitation in general. In Britain, Clarke and Sinclair (1974, p.58) argued that 'there is now little reason to believe that any one of the widely used methods of treating offenders is much better at preventing reconviction than any other'. They questioned the notion that delinquency and crime were symptoms of individual pathology and instead advocated interventions based on the assumption that crime was *rational* action performed by ordinary people acting under particular pressures and exposed to specific opportunities. Crime, they argued, could best be controlled by making targets harder (for example through improved security measures) rather than by trying to identify and tackle any presumed underlying causes. The most devastating critique of welfare, however, came from Martinson's (1974) analysis of 231 studies of treatment programmes in the USA. He concluded that 'with few and isolated exceptions the rehabilitative efforts that have been reported so far have had no appreciable effect on recidivism' (Martinson, 1974, p.25). This conclusion was widely received as 'nothing works': that it was a waste of time and money to devote energy to the treatment of (young) offenders.

Finally, liberal lawyers and civil libertarians maintained that welfare, rather than being benevolent, was an insidious form of control. Young offenders were considered to need protection not only from the Right's punitive justice, but also from welfare's 'humanitarianism'. As Taylor *et al.* noted,

> Under English law the child enjoys very few of the rights taken for granted by adults under the principles of natural justice. The law's reference to the child's 'best interests' reflects the benevolent paternalism of its approach. Essentially as far as the courts are concerned, the 'best interests' principle empowers social workers, psychologists, psychiatrists and others to define on the basis of their opinions what is good for the child … [the law] does not require that the experts should substantiate their opinions or prove to the court that any course of action they propose will be more effective in promoting the best interests of the child than those taken by the parent or by the child acting on his own behalf … a child may find that his/her arguments against being committed to care are perceived as evidence of their need for treatment, as a sign, for example, that they have 'authority problems'.
>
> (Taylor *et al.*, 1979, pp.22–3)

Similarly Morris, commenting on the Scottish hearing system, argued:

> Euphemisms are frequently used to disguise the true state of affairs, to pretend that things are other than they are. Courts become tribunals, probation becomes supervision and approved schools are renamed residential establishments. But few are deceived by these verbal devices.
>
> (Morris, 1974, p.364)

Underlying this critique is a scepticism towards the value of treatment, welfare and therapy and their ability to provide justice for children. For example, Morris argues that the introduction of compulsory treatment measures has been purchased at the expense of other values such as individual liberty, natural justice, due process and fairness. As 'treatment' is the key term which characterizes the procedures and disposals of welfare systems, most critiques of welfarism have drawn attention to the inappropriateness of using such medical terminology to describe law-breaking. The Kilbrandon Report indeed made extensive use of such medical terms as 'symptom' and 'diagnosis' and compared its own recommendations to those of medical practice. The implications of this approach to understanding delinquency are far-reaching. In particular, Kilbrandon defined the 'problem' in terms of individual pathology and maladjustment rather than, for example, a 'problem' arising out of the social, economic and political condition of young people (factors such as poverty, unemployment, irrelevant schooling, housing redevelopment, or lack of recreational amenities). As a result, juvenile justice in Scotland in particular became dominated by the jargon and practices of the child-saving ideology – 'at risk', 'prevention', 'disturbance', 'deprivation', 'personality disorder', 'treatment', 'cure' – which act to reconstitute a child's identity as deviant and pathological. Such 'character assassinations', it has been argued, legitimate greater incursion into a child's life than could be provided by simply concentrating on the circumstances of the act of misconduct (Morris *et al.*, 1980).

3.2 The justice model

In the wake of these wide-ranging criticisms of welfarism, a new justice-based model of corrections emerged. Its leading proponent, Von Hirsch (1976), proposed that the following principles be reinstated at the centre of criminal justice practice:

- Proportionality of punishment to crime, or the offender is handed a sentence that is in accordance with what the act deserves.
- Determinacy of sentencing and an end to indeterminate, treatment-oriented sentences.
- An end to judicial, professional and administrative discretion.
- An end to disparities in sentencing.
- Equity and protection of rights through due process.

'back to justice'   Proponents of 'back to justice' argued that determinate sentences based on the seriousness of the offence, rather than on the problems of individual offenders, would be seen as 'fair' and 'just' by young people themselves. A greater use of cautions by the police for minor offences, they argued, would help to keep young people out of the courts. When in court, closer control over social workers' social inquiry reports would ensure that intermediate treatment (IT), care orders or other forms of welfare intervention would only be used in the most serious cases. The role of social work, it was maintained, would be to offer supervision schemes only in those cases when custody was being suggested. Social work should only be involved at the 'heavy end' of offences. Above all, a greater promotion of community-based interventions by government and social services departments should be promoted. Leading proponents of this philosophy, such as Morris *et al.* (1980) and Taylor *et al.* (1979), maintained that a social work understanding of delinquency and assessments of 'best interests' only reinforce the principle of individual pathology and the need for the working-class delinquent to adapt to and accept a position of material and social inequality. Furthermore, they condemned the fact that since the 1908 Act the fate of juvenile offenders had been increasingly dictated by the discretionary and arbitrary powers of individual social workers and magistrates. Children's rights, they argued, would be better upheld by returning to the principle of equality before the law.

In some respects such arguments marked a return to the early nineteenth-century approach of viewing the juvenile as a young adult. However, they were complemented by proposals for law reform which would decriminalize such juvenile crimes as drinks and drugs offences, and homosexual or heterosexual behaviour under the age of consent, and would remove the force of law from misdemeanours such as truancy and running away from home.

In this way it became possible to raise the issue of the 'rule of the law' as a progressive demand. Furthermore, proponents such as Taylor *et al.* (1979) argued for the right to legal representation and legal aid in the juvenile court and for it to be accepted that the proceedings were injurious. The 'back to justice' approach thus advocated reform of both the English and Scottish systems of youth justice so that the court's role as an administrator of *justice* would be reinstated.

This activity is in two parts. First, read through the nine major assumptions of justice-based strategies outlined in Extract 5.2.

Second, complete the following grid. To help you, the categories for welfare strategies (see Activity 5.2) have already been completed.

	Assumptions of welfare strategies	Assumptions of justice-based strategies
Causes of offending	Multiple deprivation/ neglect/lack of parental care	
Purpose of intervention	Treatment/rehabilitation	
Key agencies	Social work/children's hearings	
Key personnel	Welfare professionals	
Key characteristics	Care proceedings Indeterminate sentencing	
Objectives	Respond to individual needs	

Extract 5.2 Black Committee: 'Assumptions of justice-based strategies'

(a) delinquency per se is a matter of opportunity and choice – other factors may combine to bring a child to the point of delinquency, but unless there is evidence to the contrary, the act as such is a manifestation of the rational decision to that effect;

(b) insofar as a person is responsible for his actions he should also be accountable. This is qualified in respect of children by the doctrine of criminal responsibility as originally evolved under common law and now endorsed by statute;

(c) proof of commission of an offence should be the sole justification for intervention and the sole basis of punishment;

(d) society has the right to re-assert the norms and standards of behaviour both as an expression of society's disapproval and as an individual and general deterrent to future similar behaviour;

(e) sanctions and controls are valid responses to deviant behaviour both as an expression of society's disapproval and as an individual and general deterrent to future similar behaviour;

(f) behaviour attracting legal intervention and associated sanctions available under the law should be specifically defined to avoid uncertainty;

(g) the power to interfere with a person's freedom and in particular that of a child should be subject to the most rigorous standard of proof which traditionally is found in a court of law. Individual rights are most effectively safeguarded under the judicial process;

(h) there should be equality before the law; like cases should be treated alike;

(i) there should be proportionality between the seriousness of the delinquent or criminal behaviour warranting intervention and the community's response; between the offence and the sentence given.

(Black Committee, 1979, pp.33–4)

3.3   The justice vs. welfare debate

The practical result of this resurgence of legalism and 'back to justice' was predictably complex and contradictory.

In 1979 the Conservatives launched a strong attack on delinquency in the run-up to the General Election, and throughout the early 1980s condemned the 'soft' way that 'dangerous young thugs' were dealt with. Through the liberal use of terms such as 'wickedness' and 'evil', delinquency once more became a moral issue. Many Conservatives attributed the increase in delinquency to the supposed permissiveness of the Children and Young Persons Act 1969 and to liberal child-rearing practices of the 1960s (Morgan, 1978). Margaret Thatcher, the incoming Prime Minister, attacked those who had created a 'culture of excuses' and promised that her government would 're-establish a code of conduct that condemns crime plainly and without exception' (Riddell, 1989, p.171). The search for individual or social causes of crime – personality disorders, unemployment, social deprivation, lack of opportunity – was to be abandoned. The rhetoric of treatment and rehabilitation was to be replaced by the rhetoric of punishment and retribution. Welfarism was to be replaced by the rule of law, while the language of 'rights' was supplanted by one of self-responsibility and obligation (Anderson, 1992, p.xviii).

In October 1979 it was announced that new 'short sharp shock' regimes would be introduced into detention centres. In 1982 a new Criminal Justice Act gave magistrates powers to sentence young offenders directly to youth custody centres (previously they were limited to making recommendations to the Crown Court for borstal training). Those parts of the 1969 Act which had advocated a phasing out of custody were officially abandoned. It seemed as if there was going to be a considerable increase in the number of juveniles facing incarceration (McLaughlin and Muncie, 1993, p.176).

However, the 1982 Act also endorsed the expansion of schemes to *divert* juveniles from custody, and introduced strict criteria before custody and residential care could be considered. The justice model had already cast the relative indeterminacy of care orders in a particularly negative light. When the

1982 Act made 'criminal' care orders harder to recommend, the result was a massive contraction of the residential care sector. The number of young people in Community Homes with Education (CHEs) declined from 7,500 in 1975 to 2,800 in 1984, while the number of CHEs fell from 125 to 60. By the late 1980s the use of care orders in criminal cases had become so insignificant that they were abandoned. It no longer became possible to commit offenders to residential care on the grounds that they were in 'need' of welfare. Equally it was hoped that by granting magistrates more powers to attach specified activities to supervision orders, to make community service orders available to 16 year-olds, and to fine parents rather than the young offender, the numbers eventually received into custody would be reduced. Early research (Burney, 1985) showed that such reductions were not forthcoming, but gradually case law, on what amounted to an offence to be considered sufficiently 'serious' to warrant custody, became more tightly defined. Lawyers in certain areas began to use the law to protect juveniles from unwarranted or premature custody.

Under the Criminal Justice Act 1988 the criteria for custody were further tightened and restricted. The aim of diversion – both from court and custody – **diversion** was repeatedly affirmed in criminal justice consultative documents and circulars. Prosecution was to be used as a last resort and replaced by formal police cautioning. Furthermore, Home Office circular 14/1985 encouraged the use of informal warnings in order to keep juveniles off the criminal statistics altogether. Indeed, the result from the mid 1980s was a marked reduction both in prosecutions and in the rate of known offending (Gelsthorpe and Morris, 1994, p.977). It appeared as if justice-based principles of proportionality in sentencing or 'just deserts' had provided a more visible, consistent and accountable decision-making process which, despite the law and order rhetoric, was also able to make a significant impact on the numbers of young people in custody (see section 4.1 below). Nevertheless, as Clarke (1985) pointed out, the staking out of 'justice' as a strategy for reform has allowed the proponents of law and order to recruit the arguments of 'natural justice' for their own ends, although the former is more concerned with retribution and the latter with judicial equality and consistency. Within the political climate of the early 1980s, notions of 'justice' and 'anti-welfarism' were politically mobilized by the Right. Doubt was increasingly cast on the ability of the 'back to justice' movement to reorganize this arena politically. In these circumstances it was not surprising to find that some political credibility returned to those who wished to reassert the principle of welfare in the processing of young offenders.

Davies (1982), for example, argued that the failures of welfare were due in the main to partial implementation and lack of financial backing. Whilst the call for greater judicial safeguards for young people in court was lauded, it was argued that this should not preclude a determined defence of welfarism's central 'caring' practices. Similarly, Cullen and Gilbert (1982) maintained that welfarism remains the only route through which the state can be forced to recognize that it has an obligation to care for an offender's welfare and needs. Expunging it completely will only produce more repressive and punitive outcomes.

Whilst this welfare vs. justice debate dominated the early 1980s, it also came to be viewed by some as particularly sterile. Asquith, for example, argued that the 'back to justice' conception of law as due process makes it inattentive to the inequalities that are built into the formulation of law and its operation in a class-divided society:

Policies which ignore the social and economic realities in which children find themselves, while promoting greater equality and justice within formal systems of control, may not only ignore, but may compound the structural and material inequalities which have been historically associated with criminal behaviour.

(Asquith, 1983, p.17)

To those who clung to welfarism as a solution to the problems of juvenile justice, Thorpe *et al.* had this to say:

Rather than arguing about the relative merits of 'justice' and 'welfare' we ought perhaps to take a step backwards and survey the framework which effectively supports them both. The beads may be of different colours and situated at opposite ends. But they are on the same thread.

(Thorpe *et al.*, 1980, p.106)

Should young offenders be dealt with by strict legal procedure or by social service casework? In what ways might both of these strategies fail to meet the needs of young people?

4 Diversion and community corrections

One of the cornerstones of youth justice is that young people should be protected from the rigours of adult justice. This has meant that a range of diversionary strategies have been employed, including:

- Diversion from crime: typically this involves various methods of crime prevention which can range from improved security ('target hardening') to skills training and education.

- Diversion from prosecution: since the early 1970s the police have increasingly adopted a system of cautioning minor offenders through formal warnings rather than seeking prosecution. About 60 per cent of young offenders are dealt with in this way, but there are wide and fluctuating regional variations.

- Diversion from custody: whilst alternatives to adult prisons have existed since the mid nineteenth century, the notion of custody, in any form, being harmful and counter-productive gained prominence first in the 1960s and again in the mid 1980s. Community-based programmes have increasingly been promoted as viable alternatives to custody. In 1995 about 40 per cent of those convicted were dealt with by such means.

4.1 Alternatives to prosecution and custody

Contrary to the predictions of many commentators, both the youth crime rate and the youth custody rate declined dramatically during the course of the 1980s. Indeed, the late 1980s has been proclaimed as amounting to a 'successful revolution' in criminal – particularly juvenile – justice policy (Allen, 1991). In contrast to media and political discourse, criminal statistics released by the Home Office indicated that the numbers of young people aged 17 or under convicted or cautioned decreased from 204,600 in 1983 to 129,500 in 1993. The number of young offenders sentenced to immediate custody also fell significantly. In 1983, 13,500 males aged between 14 and under 18 were sentenced to immediate custody for indictable offences, compared to 3,300 in 1993. This represented a fall from some 15 per cent of all court dispositions to 11 per cent (see Table 5.1).

The precise reasons for these dramatic – and largely unexpected – reductions remain contested. One factor was a 19 per cent fall in the overall juvenile population in this period. However, another explanation refers both to the stricter legal safeguards against custody introduced under the 1982 and 1988 Acts and to the impact of the Department of Health and Social Security's Intermediate Treatment Initiative of 1983. Under the Initiative, the DHSS financed the establishment of 110 intensive schemes in 62 local authority areas explicitly to provide alternatives to custody (Rutherford, 1989). Intermediate treatment practitioners were required to evolve 'new justice-based styles of working' which focused less on the emotional and social needs of juveniles and more on the nature of the offence. Intermediate treatment was to be restricted only to those offenders who were at risk of custody. Through such means it was hoped that magistrates would be persuaded that intermediate treatment was no longer a 'soft option', but a 'high tariff' disposal.

Table 5.1 Number[1] and percentage of persons aged between 14 and under 18 sentenced to custody for indictable offences, England and Wales, 1983–95

Year	Number sentenced to immediate custody		Percentage sentenced to immediate custody of all those sentenced for indictable offences	
	Males	*Females*	*Males*	*Females*
1983	13,500	–	15.3	–
1984	12,000	200	14.4	2.5
1985	11,500	200	14.7	2.6
1986	8,900	200	14.0	2.5
1987	8,200	100	14.0	2.5
1988	7,300	100	13.7	2.6
1989	4,700	100	11.7	2.1
1990	3,600	100	9.5	1.7
1991	3,500	100	9.9	1.9
1992	3,300	100	10.4	1.7
1993	3,300	100	11.1	2.6
1994	3,600	100	11.1	2.8
1995	4,200	100	12.0	3.0

Source: adapted from *Criminal Statistics for England and Wales 1995*, Table 7.9

[1] Numbers rounded to nearest 100.

A strong 'alternatives to custody' ethos was developed within many social work departments and supported by campaign groups such as the National Association for the Care and Resettlement of Offenders (NACRO), the Association for Juvenile Justice and The Children's Society. They argued that custody fails to prevent re-offending, does little to meet the needs of victims, and is less effective than community-based programmes. Extract 5.3 outlines many of these arguments.

Many also agreed with the critiques of the welfare approach and the coercive role that social workers had played previously, and in doing so developed a justice-based approach as self-styled youth justice workers: 'The once ambiguous, if not ambivalent, attitudes about custody held by social workers during the early 1980s have been replaced by unequivocal opposition' (Rutherford, 1989, p.29).

Extract 5.3 Children's Society Advisory Committee: 'The case against custody'

Penal custody is the most severe sanction society has available for adults. We also use it for juveniles. Indeed the only deliberately punitive institutions (detention centres) within the prison system were *reserved* exclusively for its youngest inmates. The Committee believe that this situation cannot be justified.

There is an expectation that custody will *prevent re-offending* by the young person concerned. Yet there is comprehensive and emphatic information on the failure of custody as an individual deterrent. The reconviction rates are well established and if anything are worsening. For those released from detention centre the rate has risen from 50–60% in the 1960s to over 70% now. Nearly 84% of those sent to youth custody re-offend within a two year period from release.

It is difficult to assess the value of custody as a more widespread *deterrent*. Custody is a fairly remote concept for most young people; it often seems to practitioners that paradoxically, it is those who do know friends who have been to custody who seem most likely to follow suit. There is also some evidence emerging – e.g. from Northamptonshire – that where custody is reduced the crime rate is actually falling. Certainly there is no evidence in those areas where alternatives to custody are operating with considerable success that there is an increase in offending. A report by the Home Office Psychological Unit in 1984 into the operation of the 'short, sharp, shock' found that there was no deterrent effect in the catchment areas of the Detention Centres studied; neither the general levels of crime nor the numbers of young males appearing in court were reduced.

A juvenile in custody is making no restitution or *reparation* to the victim for the offences. On the contrary, the offender continues to take very considerable resources from the community provision of high security institutions and the employment of security and allied staff. At no time does the victim of the crime feel directly compensated or even acknowledged.

With regard to *public safety* it is self-evident that prisons provide society with immediate 'protection' from the offender. The Committee does question the overall protection which is offered by custody; it is clear that the great majority of juveniles sentenced to custody pose no serious risk to the community and indeed they may become a significantly greater danger on their return. Custody may suppress the individual into temporary conformity until the point of release but this period of containment is spent exclusively in the company of other offenders. Society is best protected by responses which reduce levels of offending in the longer term.

Penal custody can never *re-integrate* young people into the communities against which they offend and where, ultimately, they must learn to live. Youth custody centres have limited training facilities and staff are not trained or employed to work with young offenders on programmes for reducing further offending. Detention centres have never had a semblance of a rehabilitative function. They have always been based on the premise that short, sharp structured regimes can shock children out of delinquency. Removal to penal custody leads to broken links with family, friends, education, work and leisure and causes stigmatisation and labelling. This in turn results in increased alienation, attention from statutory agencies and greater risk of further offending. Even when prison department institutions do attempt a more rehabilitative function, they have few links with the child's community. They are not in a good position to phase out institutional control and reintegrate the child with community support ...

The Committee are convinced that penal custody for juveniles should be phased out at the earliest opportunity.

(Children's Society, 1989, pp.12–13)

Many social services departments began to construct their policies on the basis of minimum intervention, maximum diversion and underpinned by justice as opposed to welfare principles. A range of community-based alternatives to custody were also created to deal with more serious offences. The use of community service orders increased, and new requirements were attached to some supervision orders to enhance their credibility with magistrates. Magistrates were able to specify the nature and type of programme rather than leave it to the discretion of the supervisor. As Rutherford (1989, p.29) argued, 'By providing constructive and credible alternatives to custodial sentences, projects were able to effectively intervene at the sentencing stage ... Given the recognition that there is a viable local resource, custody ceases to be an acceptable option in all but exceptional cases'.

A further possible explanation for the decline in youth custody lies in efforts to divert juveniles from court (through the increased use of informal police cautioning) as opposed to diverting from custody once in court (as the intensive intermediate treatment schemes were designed to do) (Gelsthorpe and Morris, 1994, pp.976–7). Home Office circular 14/1985, for example, encouraged the police to use 'no further action' or 'informal warnings' instead of formal action. Until a reversal of the policy in 1994, the number of juveniles brought into the system did decline. The practice varied regionally, but in Northampton in 1985, for example, 86 per cent of juveniles who came to the notice of the police were either prosecuted or formally cautioned; by 1989 this had been reduced to 30 per cent.

A major aim of all such developments also appeared to be a reduction in court processing and custody on grounds of expense and effectiveness. In 1990–91, it was estimated that keeping an offender in custody for three weeks was more expensive than 12 months of supervision or community service. Furthermore, 83 per cent of young men and 60 per cent of young women leaving youth custody were reconvicted within two years, whilst the reconviction rate of those participating in community-based schemes was assumed to be substantially lower. NACRO's (1993) monitoring of the Intermediate Treatment Initiative indeed found reconviction rates of between 45 per cent and 55 per cent, but subsequent research funded by the Home Office and the Department of Health could find no clear evidence to suggest that community penalties held more than a modest advantage over custody in preventing re-offending (Lloyd, Mair and Hough, 1994; Bottoms, 1995).

4.2 Punishment in the community

punishment
in the
community

The Criminal Justice Act 1991, heralded as a significant move in policy away from custody, attempted to provide a national framework in which to build on the success of local initiatives and to expand the use of diversionary strategies to include young adults (17–21 year olds). The Act's anti-custody ethos – 'prison is an expensive way of making bad people worse' (Home Office, 1990, para. 2.7) – was justified through the promise of more rigorous community disposals. These were not to be considered as alternatives to custody, but as sentences in their own right. Significantly, both custody and community alternatives were now justified in terms of their ability to deliver punishment. When custody was not considered suitable, the alternative lay in a variety of means of delivering punishment in the community through attaching conditions to supervision, introducing curfew orders (with or without electronic monitoring), combination orders and community service. It was further evidence of the diminution of the principle of meeting individual needs in youth justice policy and practice.

'Punishment in the community' was formally established as the favoured option, but as a corollary this required a change in focus for the juvenile court and the practices of probation and social work agencies. For the latter it meant a shift in emphasis away from an approach of 'advise, assist, befriend' and towards tightening up the conditions of community supervision and community service work (see **McLaughlin, 1998**). For the former it meant the reorganization of the juvenile court system (which had previously dealt with criminal and care cases) in order to create youth courts and 'family proceedings' courts to deal with such matters separately. The Children Act 1989 had already stipulated that care orders should no longer be available in criminal proceedings, thus cementing the principle of determinant sentences and sentencing solely for offences, rather than on grounds such as lack of parental control. After more than 130 years of confusion, the way in which the 'deprived' and the 'delinquent' were dealt with was finally to be separated. To do so meant formally removing the goal of welfare from youth criminal justice policy.

ACTIVITY 5.4

Refer back to sections 4.1 and 4.2 and consider the possible reasons why custody rates for young offenders declined during the late 1980s and early 1990s.

1   How important was the introduction of new forms of community sentencing?

2   Can you think of any reasons why community sentences, on their own, might fail to divert offenders from custody?

COMMENT

The discussion in these sections suggested a number of reasons why the numbers of 14–18 year olds sentenced to custody declined from approximately 13,000 in 1983 to 3,500 in 1993. These include:

■   A decline in the number of juveniles in the population at large.

■   A decline in the juvenile crime rate.

■   The introduction of stricter criteria for custody.

■   The introduction of intensive intermediate schemes.

- Support for alternatives to custody from magistrates.
- The increased use of informal warnings by the police.
- The proven failure of custody to prevent re-offending.
- The cost of custody.
- The diminution of social work's 'welfare' role.
- The expansion of social work's 'justice' role.

It is difficult to disentangle any one of these 'causes' as being the key influence. Rutherford (1989) emphasizes the role of youth justice practitioners in developing 'viable' community packages, whilst Gelsthorpe and Morris (1994) stress the pivotal role of the police in diverting offenders away from the system altogether through the use of informal warnings. However it is explained, the period proved to be one of the most remarkable in youth justice history. It suggested that the use of custody could be reduced to minimal levels without increasing crime rates or placing the public in greater danger. Nevertheless, many researchers and commentators have been sceptical of the ability of community programmes, on their own, to achieve the often stated aim of diversion from custody (for example Cohen, 1985; Hudson, 1987; Muncie, 1997). Rather, the 'movement to community' is likely to produce a series of negative effects, including:

- Up-tariffing: the tendency for community corrections to be used instead of lower tariff disposals, such as fines, supervision and probation.
- Lack of purpose: the contradiction between the punitive, reparative and welfare aims of community-based programmes.
- Jeopardy: the risk of accelerating routes into custody through breaches of the conditions of community sentences.
- Contamination: the inability to prevent re-offending through the re-establishment of deviant identities and careers.
- Political vulnerability: a failure to recognize and respond to the broader social context of both offending and criminal justice reform. Whatever progressive elements are present in an anti-custody ethos, they are forever prey to knee-jerk and reactionary overhaul.

■ ■ ■

In contrast to such scepticism, however, evidence has slowly accumulated that, despite the 'nothing works' pessimism that had pervaded youth justice for two decades, some forms of community intervention can be successful in reducing some re-offending. These include behavioural and skills training, training in moral reasoning, interpersonal problem-solving, skills training, and vocationally oriented psychotherapy (McGuire, 1995).

In a review of over 400 research studies on the effectiveness of such 'treatments', Lipsey (1995) argued that when intervention is focused around behavioural training or skills issues and sustained over a period of at least six months, a 10 per cent reduction in re-offending can be expected. Similarly, initiatives in caution-plus and reparation schemes have reported positive effects. For example, Northamptonshire's Diversion Unit deals with young offenders who have already been cautioned and brings offender and victim together to discuss compensation. Following such reparation, 35 per cent re-offended, compared to over 80 per cent of those leaving youth custody (Hughes *et al.*,

1998). The HALT programme in Holland had similar results, with cautioning being supplemented by work relevant to the offence, payment of damages and an educational component. Both schemes allow offending behaviour to be addressed without the cost of formal court processing. In general, programmes that address offending behaviour instead of processing through the courts, and which are based in the community rather than in institutional settings, appear to have the most chances of success (Audit Commission, 1996, pp.46–7).

Despite such reported 'successes', community punishment in general came under most critical fire from the government itself. The period 1991–93 may well go down in the chronicles of youth justice as yet another watershed when the public, media and political gaze fixed on the perennial issue of juvenile crime and delivered a familiar series of knee-jerk and draconian responses. It was the image of the 'repeat' or 'persistent' young offender which provided the rationale for another U-turn in youth justice policy. The 1991 disturbances at Blackbird Leys (Oxford), Ely (Cardiff) and Meadowell (Tyneside) had already focused attention on young men in violent confrontations with the police (Newburn, 1996, p.69). The trial of two youngsters accused of killing James Bulger in 1993, although it involved the murder of a young child by two children barely at the age of criminal responsibility, also had a profound impact on the hardening of reaction to all young offending.

Fuelled by the Home Secretary's notion that 'prison works', plans were introduced in 1994 to build a network of secure training centres for 12 to 14 year-olds, and in 1996 US-style 'boot camps' were introduced in England. By 1997 a Crime (Sentences) Act had introduced mandatory minimum sentences for certain offences, extended electronic monitoring to the under 16s as part of a curfew order, and for the first time allowed convicted juveniles to be publicly named and shamed if the court was satisfied that this was in the interests of the public. One of the first priorities of the new Labour government in 1997 was a Crime and Disorder Act to ensure fast-track punishment for persistent young offenders and the adoption of 'zero tolerance' policies to prosecute even the most petty and minor of offences. It appeared that youth justice was once more to turn full circle, away from welfare, diversion or decarceration and back to an emphasis on punitive sentencing (see section 5).

4.3 Corporatism and managerialism

corporatism

With the expansion of stringent and punitive community corrections in the 1980s and 1990s, some commentators have come to argue that it makes little sense to talk of youth justice in terms of offering welfare and/or justice. Pratt (1989), for example, talks of a newly developing corporatist strategy which has removed itself from the wider philosophical arguments of welfare and punishment. Pratt and others describe the new strategies towards young offending as being characterized by administrative decision-making, greater sentencing diversity, the construction of sentencing 'packages', the centralization of authority and co-ordination of policy, the growing involvement of non-juridical agencies, and high levels of containment and control in some sentencing programmes (Pratt, 1989, p.245; Parker et al., 1987). The key players have become youth justice workers in multi-agency teams. The aim is neither necessarily to deliver 'welfare' or 'justice', but one of developing the most cost-effective and efficient way of *managing* the delinquent population. The issue of offending has come to be increasingly defined in scientific and technical terms, while political/moral debates about the causes of offending and the purpose of intervention are shifted to the sidelines (Pitts, 1992, p.142). In effect youth justice has been reconceptualized as a delinquency management service in which the hard core are still locked up, whilst an expanding range of statutory and voluntary community-based agencies devise non-custodial sentences which they hope will be stringent enough to persuade magistrates not to take the (more expensive) custodial option. The goal is not necessarily one of punishment, treatment or protection, but to retrain the offender and provide some reparation for victims. Within these new strategies, traditional problems and welfare-based interventions are excluded and replaced by the 'tougher' programmes of reparation, shaming, tagging and the admission of responsibility.

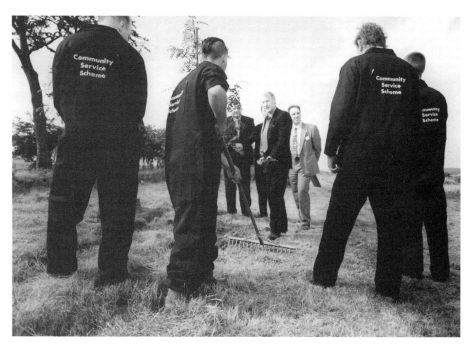

Designed to humiliate and shame? Community service in Scotland

This has led Rutherford (1993, p.160) to believe that an essential 'human face' of criminal justice will be lost and that its absence will produce 'apathy and ultimately violence' in all the probation and community service agencies involved. Whilst such corporatist and managerial strategies might be viewed as smokescreens to facilitate the depoliticization and dehumanization of the youth crime issue and to enhance more authoritarian means of control, it is also clear that, ironically, the concern for economy and pragmatism has the potential to temper the perennial 'clamour for custody' which routinely surrounds political decision-making. This certainly seemed to have been the case in the early 1990s (McLaughlin and Muncie, 1994).

An emphasis on the three Es of economy, effectiveness and efficiency was underlined when the Audit Commission published its report on the youth justice system in England and Wales in 1996. Noting that the public services (police, legal aid, courts, social services, probation, prison) spend around £1 billion a year processing and dealing with young offenders, it argued that much of this money was wasted through lengthy and ineffective court procedures. The report pointed to the need to shift resources from punitive to preventive measures. It was particularly critical of youth courts, where the process of prosecution takes on average four months, costs £2,500 for each young person processed, and half of the proceedings are ultimately discontinued, dismissed or discharged. The system has no agreed national strategies, and local authorities act more as an emergency service than as a preventive one. The report recommended the diversion of a fifth of young offenders away from the courts into programmes such as Northamptonshire's caution-plus, thus saving £40 million annually on costs. In short, the Audit Commission argued that:

> the current system for dealing with youth crime is inefficient and expensive, while little is being done to deal effectively with juvenile nuisance. The present arrangements are failing the young people – who are not being guided away from offending to constructive activities. They are also failing victims – those who suffer from some young people's inconsiderate behaviour, and from vandalism, arson and loss of property from thefts and burglaries. And they lead to waste in a variety of forms, including lost time, as public servants process the same young offenders through the courts time and again; lost rents, as people refuse to live in high crime areas; lost business, as people steer clear of troubled areas; and the waste of young people's potential.
>
> (Audit Commission, 1996, p.96)

The Commission's priority was clearly one of diversion, partly on the grounds of 'value for money' and partly because of the lack of effectiveness of formal procedures. Following a corporatist model, it advocated the development of multi-agency work, with parents, schools and health services acting in tandem with social services and the police. In line with managerialist objectives it argued that these goals could only be met by a clearer identification of objectives, more rigorous allocation of resources, and the setting of staff priorities. The aim was to build a pragmatic strategy to prevent offending rather than wed the system to any particular broad philosophy of justice or welfare. The issue of the causes of offending was side-stepped by the identification of 'risk conditions' (factors which correlate with known offending) such as inadequate parental supervision, truancy, the lack of a stable home, or the known use of drugs.

ACTIVITY 5.5

1   What do you now understand by the term 'diversion' in youth justice?

2   Why does it have a central role in corporatist and managerial strategies? In particular, think about whose 'needs' are met by diversion and community corrections: are they those of governments intent on cost-effectiveness or those of young offenders who are protected from the damaging consequences of custody?

3   Whose 'needs' are being overlooked in such developments?

In answering these questions you will find it useful to compare the key characteristics of diversionary strategies with those of 'welfare' and 'justice' (see Activities 5.2 and 5.3).

Diversion has had a recurring presence in youth justice for at least the past thirty years. However, it is a concept with multiple meanings. In the 1960s diversion largely meant developing community-based treatments as an alternative to custody. It was justified by the damaging and contaminating consequences for young people of incarceration. Whilst these early welfare-inspired efforts were overrun by a clear hardening of judicial attitudes towards young offending in the 1970s, by the mid 1980s dramatic reductions in youth custody were achieved. These were made possible through a complex of factors – not least a shift away from welfarism and the promotion of more punitive forms of community correction. These means, sponsored by government, were very often piecemeal and localized, but achieved some notable successes, particularly when young people were diverted from formal court processing through informal warnings, cautions and caution-plus schemes. By the mid 1990s multi-agency diversion schemes came to be lauded as not only effective but also more economical. Corporatist and managerial strategies emerged which were less interested in 'best interests' or 'protecting rights' and more concerned with achieving pragmatic and tangible outcomes. This entailed drawing educational, health and social services into the business of youth crime control. To this extent it may be noted that many aspects of social policy have become thoroughly 'criminalized'. In the 1980s many commentators warned that such an expansion of the control function of public services would necessarily draw more young people into the net of the youth justice system. However, detailed empirical research covering various diversionary projects revealed that this pessimism might in some respects be unfounded. Nevertheless, the goal of diversion always appears subject to political vulnerability. Progressive practice is forever prey to reactionary overhaul when 'get tough on crime' agendas achieve ascendancy. For example, in the mid 1990s the climate for practices such as diversion became decidedly chilly with the reassertion that 'prison works' and that specialized detention facilities (secure units, boot camps) should be expanded. By 1994 it was noticeable that the numbers in youth custody had once more started to rise.

■ ■ ■

5 The custodial imperative

Despite the emergence of welfare, justice and corporatist strategies, there is strong evidence to suggest that the custodial function of youth justice has always remained paramount. Even at moments of penal reductionism, the young offender institution, detention centre, youth custody centre, borstal, approved school, reformatory or youth prison have formed the cornerstone of youth justice against which all other interventions are measured and assessed. There has also persisted a strong law and order lobby which has forcibly argued that youth crime is caused by simple wickedness and that the only real punishment is incarceration. Consequently every decarcerative reform has been subject to either judicial or political backlash. Governments and policy-makers, it seems, are only prepared to sanction non-custodial options as long as custody is retained for particular groups of young offenders (Pratt, 1989, p.244). Moreover, the only elements of the prison system that have explicitly punitive aims always appear to be reserved for the young: namely detention centres and boot camps.

5.1   Detention centres and boot camps

Detention centres were introduced by the Criminal Justice Act 1948 and enabled the courts to sentence offenders aged 14 to 21 to short periods within an explicitly punitive regime. They were justified on the grounds that sending young offenders to adult prisons only helped to cement criminal careers, but there is strong evidence that their introduction was also a concession as corporal punishment was abolished (Muncie, 1990). Detention centres were established as an 'experiment', but lasted 40 years. Throughout they were dogged by a lack of any precise definition of purpose. Despite significant opposition, the only detention centre for girls was opened at Moor Court, near Stoke-on-Trent, in 1962. It was closed seven years later because military drill and physical education were not considered appropriate in the 'training' of young women. Whilst detention centres always promised the delivery of a 'short sharp shock', in the 1950s and 1960s their regime was not that far removed from that of borstals.

In the 1970s, in an effort to appease those who viewed the entire youth justice system as too soft, the Home Secretary announced the establishment of two 'experimental' regimes in which: 'life will be constructed at a brisk tempo. Much greater emphasis will be put on hard and constructive activities, and discipline and tidiness, on self-respect and respect for those in authority ... These will be no holiday camps' (Whitelaw, cited in Thornton *et al.*, 1984, para. 1). The regimes were subsequently evaluated by the Home Office's Young Offender Psychology Unit, which concluded that they had 'no discernible effect on the rate at which trainees were reconvicted' (Thornton *et al.*, 1984, para. 8.21). At one centre (Send, for 14–17 year-olds) reconviction rates remained at 57 per cent both before and after the experiment, whilst at the other (New Hall, for 17–21 year-olds) the rate rose from 46 to 48 per cent. Doubt was also expressed as to whether the new tougher regimes were actually experienced as more demanding. Indeed, some of the activities, such as drill and physical education, were fairly popular in comparison to the continuous chore of a humdrum work party which they replaced.

Despite such findings, the tougher regimes were not abandoned but rather extended to all detention centres. During the early 1980s the rhetoric and political expediency of 'short sharp shock' appeared to take precedence over research evaluation, logical argument or practical experience (Muncie, 1990, p.61). As Harris (1982, p.248) commented, 'punitive and liberal legislation are judged by different criteria, the latter being immediately at risk when it fails to reduce recidivism, but the former, however ineffective, appearing to a society in which to punish wrongdoing seems natural, to contain an intrinsic logic.' However, the new initiative was to misfire largely through the unintended consequences of the government's own legislation. Before the Criminal Justice Act 1982, magistrates had a vested interest in the detention centre network, since it was their main custodial resource. Following the Act, however, they could sentence directly to youth custody centres (previously borstals), so in the mid 1980s 6 per cent fewer 17–21 year-olds were sentenced to detention centres than in 1982, and youth custody receptions of 15 and 16 year-olds increased by 41 per cent. Occupancy levels at detention centres fell to about 60 per cent of total capacity, while youth custody centres were overflowing. Amidst a growing chorus of complaint from penal reform organizations and most significantly from the Magistrates Association about ineffectiveness, excessive cost, ill treatment, self-injury and inmate suicides, the experiments in 'short sharp shock' were formally abolished in 1988.

It took only another eight years for their revival. The introduction of US-style 'boot camps' in 1996–97 ignored all the lessons learnt in the previous fifty years. The origins of the boot camp lie in survival training for US military personnel during the Second World War. They were introduced for young offenders in the USA from 1983 in response to prison overcrowding and a belief that short periods of retributive punishment would change or deter offending behaviour: 'typically detainees might face pre-dawn starts, enforced shaved heads, no talking to each other, being constantly screamed at by guards, rushed meal times, no access to television and newspapers and a rigorous and abusive atmosphere for 16 hours a day' (Nathan, 1995, p.2). In the USA there has been evidence that such regimes have consistently failed to live up to expectations: the deterrent effect of military training has proved to be negligible; the authoritarian atmosphere has denied access to any effective treatment; there have been occasional lawsuits from inmates claiming that elements of the programme were dangerous and life-threatening; they have failed to reduce prison populations; and they distract attention from other policies that may work better (Parent, 1995).

Despite such warnings, the British government decided to go ahead. The first boot camp was opened in 1996 at Thorn Cross Young Offenders' Institution in Cheshire. Instead of a military-based regime, it employed a 'high intensity' mixture of education, discipline and training. A second camp was opened at the Military Corrective Training Centre in Colchester in 1997, and this promised a more spartan regime. However, its open prison conditions, aimed at 17–21 year-olds, excluded the most serious of offenders. Furthermore, the notion of handing over criminal cases to a military authority provoked an avalanche of complaints from virtually all sides of the criminal justice process.

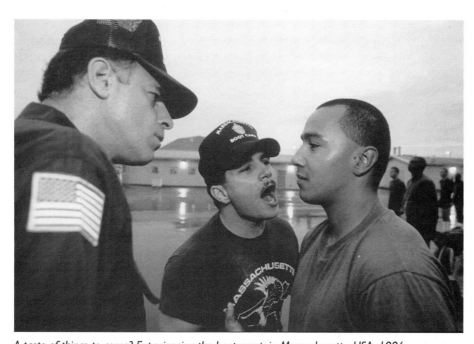

A taste of things to come? Experiencing the boot camp in Massachusetts, USA, 1996

5.2   Acting tough

Given the critiques of custody that were propounded not only in the 1980s but also in the 1960s, some have argued that it remains difficult to justify a custodial approach to youth crime (refer back to Extract 5.3). In the early 1990s the claim was made that crime was soaring out of control through the activities of small groups of 'hard core' persistent offenders.

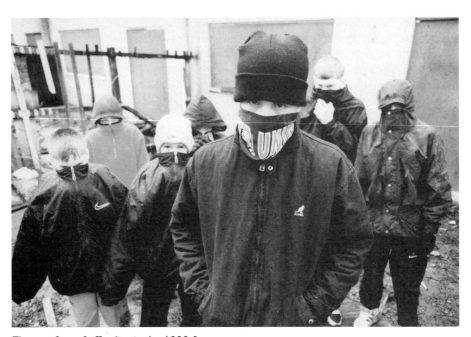

The new face of offending in the 1990s?

Although the notion of 'persistence' could not be substantiated by academic research (Hagell and Newburn, 1994), a clear hardening of political and judicial attitudes soon became evident. The percentage of convicted youths sent to young offender institutions started to grow in 1992, after reaching a low in 1990. By the mid 1990s it had yet to reach 1984 levels for males, but had already exceeded that for females (refer back to Table 5.1). In part this reflected recorded increases in levels of female violence, but, arguably, it also mirrored the historical tendency to deal with young women offenders more harshly because they contradict dominant images of women as nurturers and carers (see the article opposite from *The Independent*).

Such a recourse to custody is usually justified by increasing crime rates or by the effectiveness of punishment. However, as we saw in section 4.1, between 1983 and 1994 the recorded youth crime rate *declined* by 34 per cent. Moreover, the failure of custody to rehabilitate is repeatedly illustrated by reconviction rates of over 80 per cent. Although governments insist that custody at least ensures that offenders cannot re-offend whilst they are inside and thus is likely to reduce the crime rate, such assumptions have also been widely criticized. For example, Roger Tarling (1993), head of the Home Office Research Unit, re-examined crime and custody rates over forty years and concluded that a reduction in the crime rate of just 1 per cent would require an increase in the prison population of some 25 per cent.

One possible explanation for these anomalies lies in the way that progressive legislation, such as the 1969 and 1991 Acts, becomes perceived as being too liberal and 'soft'. A judicial and political backlash ensures that more authoritarian measures can be entertained in the future. Being seen to 'act tough' is widely assumed to be politically attractive.

Girls get angry, too

by Glenda Cooper

Home Office figures show the number of violent crimes committed by women has increased by 250 per cent since 1973. In 1987 women and girls accounted for just 10 per cent of violent crimes, but by 1995 the figure was 16 per cent. Psychologists agree that these figures mark a significant trend in female behaviour, particularly among younger women. If present trends continue, women's violent crimes will equal those of men by the year 2016.

Whereas 20 years ago girls accounted for only one in seven violent juvenile crimes, the ratio is now one in three. And there is no shortage of stories in the press about their aggression. Yesterday, 17 year old Sharon Carr was found guilty of the horrific murder of teenager Katie Rackliff, a crime committed when Carr was just 12. In May last year 13 year old Louise Allen was kicked to death near a fairground by a crowd of girls from a rival school. In Scotland a number of schoolgirls are alleged to have carried out a hate campaign against one of their teachers which allegedly involved paint and excrement being daubed on her door and petrol spread over her drive.

An increase in violent crime among female juveniles is clearly disturbing, but there may be a deeper problem still in the way these girls are treated when they enter the criminal justice system.

Last week two workers for the Women's Strategy Group, part of the Forum for Youth Justice, presented a paper at the National Association for the Care and Resettlement of Offenders conference warning that we need to rethink our treatment of girls if we are not [to] end up with a generation of alienated women. NACRO is presently pro-ducing a 10-point plan to deal with youth crime.

The theory has always been that girls get off lightly under the criminal justice system, whereas boys are hit hard. This is simply not true, say workers in the front-line, who are increasingly worried that girls are being penalised by a system that is unused to them and has no idea how to cope with them ...

'Do girls get it easy? Quite the opposite,' says Ros Price, one of the committee members of the Women's Strategy Group. 'They tend to get into the criminal justice system earlier. If there's a fight in a playground the young woman will end up in court; the young man won't.'

The establishment sees girls who use violence as less acceptable than boys who are expected to indulge in roughness. 'Generally the attitude of magistrates is to see young women as nurturers and carers,' says Cathy Phillips, another member.

At the moment, of 70 teenagers Phillips and Price are seeing under supervision orders, 12 are girls. But in the last two years they have seen a tremendous rise in girls going through the courts. And it is not for the traditional shoplifting. These girls steal cars, carry out burglaries and beat people up.

'One of the issues we are faced with is the frustration that young girls are feeling,' says Ms Price. 'They are repeatedly told that they have the same rights as young men but in reality they cannot see that they have the same status.

'Young men express their anger and frustration by smashing something. Young women are more likely to start off trying to express themselves through words. But when they realise that doesn't get as much attention as smashing a window they change their behaviour' ...

But what happens to girls when they get pushed into the criminal justice system? It is a system that is historically unused to them and is still struggling to cope with their influx.

Take attendance centres – where young people are deprived of their liberty for a set number of hours per week. They were set up originally for football hooligans and even though they are now mixed centres all they may be offering is PE and woodwork.

'We saw a young pregnant woman a year ago who had got into a scrap at school over her boyfriend,' says Ms Phillips. The girl was expected to fit in with what the boys were doing: 'Can you imagine the experience of being six, seven months pregnant with 15–20 young men around having to do PE in a T-shirt and shorts, doing 20 push ups? When we raised it with the police they just said "Well maybe you could get someone in to do knitting and embroidery". We managed to get her a conditional discharge in the end.

'Another young girl who had come out of a secure unit and was in a halfway house had been given a care plan that she didn't want anything to do with. She wanted it changed and we had a real struggle to get anyone to listen to her. Even when we took up her case we had difficulty enough and we are articulate adult women not 13 year olds' ...

'We must remember that they are children and we need to help them,' says Cathy Phillips. 'Otherwise we will be breeding another generation of offenders – and another generation of victims'.

(The Independent, 26 March 1997)

By the mid 1990s such an agenda appeared to cross party political boundaries. In 1994 the Home Secretary denounced 'do-gooders' who in his view simply rewarded offenders for their crimes (*The Independent on Sunday*, 21 August 1994), whilst in 1996 Labour's shadow Home Secretary blamed 'liberal elements' who used poverty and deprivation as an excuse for a do-nothing approach (*The Guardian*, 19 September 1996). For both, the faults of the present were laid firmly in the hands of inadequate parents, welfare professionals and penal reformers. In a series of initiatives and policy statements that preceded the 1997 General Election, both main political parties appeared to be pandering to a perceived public demand for retribution. Both pledged themselves to a policy of 'zero tolerance' towards young offenders, the Conservatives advocating a Parental Control Order and Labour a Parental Responsibility Order to make parents responsible in law for their children's behaviour, even at primary school age.

retribution

On coming to power in 1997, Labour committed itself to abolishing the *doli incapax* rule and to introducing legislation that would enforce parents to impose curfews on their children. The new government also retracted earlier plans and gave the go-ahead for the construction of the secure training centres for 12–14 year-olds that had been first proposed by the Conservatives in 1994 (*The Independent*, 5 July 1997; *The Guardian*, 22 September 1997). It was a climate in which the 'need' to 'act tough' seemed to take precedence over all others. It was clearly at odds with the simultaneous demands of corporate pragmatism to tighten budgets and to pursue policies that 'work' in delivering tangible and effective outcomes in reducing offending. The question remains whether this uneasy alliance of authoritarianism and pragmatism heralds the final demise of any legitimacy for welfare intervention in youth justice policy. If so, it will surely mark the end of almost two centuries of attempts to 'meet the needs' of young offenders.

6   Conclusion

A key question running through this chapter has been: whose 'needs' are met in the formulation and implementation of youth justice policy? We have considered the extent to which historical and contemporary youth justice has been and continues to be designed for, and capable of responding to, the individual needs of offenders. The chapter has provided a framework of welfare, justice, diversion and custodial strategies in order to disentangle some of the system's contradictory aims and outcomes.

As youth justice has developed in response to increases in the influence of those professionals working in the system and also to changes in the broader political climate, it is clear that it has evolved in a state of constant flux. No one of these approaches has achieved ascendancy. Instead, youth justice has expanded and oscillated to meet a variety of different demands and aspirations. The duty set out in the Children and Youth Persons Act 1933 and the Children Act 1989 to safeguard and promote the welfare of children in need sits uneasily against the competing objectives of punishment and protecting the public. Such an overriding goal may also be given little or no priority in those diversionary strategies of the 1990s which are simply geared to the delivery of efficient and cost-effective measures.

Youth justice, then, has evolved as a complex object incorporating elements of welfare, punitive justice and liberal justice. Furthermore, multi-agency work has drawn many aspects of public service into its remit. Wider goals of welfare or justice have become submerged in a more pragmatic and managerial assessment of 'what works'.

Above all, notions of welfare and punishment, treatment and control, 'moral danger' and wilful criminality continue to circulate around, and inform, the various contradictory policies and practices of contemporary youth justice. Having 'invented' the juvenile delinquent in the early nineteenth century, an 'army' of social workers, probation officers, youth workers, child-care workers, police, magistrates and the prison service have come to do battle over their respective place in the control and supervision of the young. However, youth justice reform is not simply driven by an increase in crime or by rational assessments of 'what works'. It also appears to reflect sudden and volatile shifts in political mood in which short-term political gain and the need for the state to assert itself can override all other concerns. Indeed, in the final analysis the study of youth justice tells us more about the political 'need' for order than it does about the nature of young offending itself.

Further reading

There are numerous reviews of post-war developments in juvenile and youth justice. Harris and Webb (1987), Gelsthorpe and Morris (1994) and Pitts (1988) are all well worth consulting. Hudson (1987) provides a radical critique of both welfare and justice strategies. The Audit Commission (1996) is the clearest example of how diversionary strategies are embedded in a corporatist and managerial approach. NACRO regularly produces briefing papers which would help you to keep up to date on contemporary issues in youth crime and youth justice.

References

Alcock, P. and Harris P. (1982) *Welfare, Law and Order*, London, Macmillan.

Allen, R. (1991) 'Out of jail: the reduction in the use of penal custody for male juveniles 1981–88', *Howard Journal*, vol.30, no.1, pp.30–52.

Anderson, D. (ed.) (1992) *The Loss of Virtue: Moral Confusion and Social Disorder in Britain and America*, London, Social Affairs Unit.

Asquith, S. (1983) 'Justice, retribution and children', in Morris, A. and Giller, M. (eds) *Providing Criminal Justice for Children*, London, Edward Arnold.

Association of County Councils, Association of Metropolitan Authorites, Association of Directors of Social Services, National Association for the Care and Resettlement of Offenders and Association of Chief Officers of Probation (1996) *National Protocol for Youth Justice Services*, London, AMA.

Audit Commission (1996) *Misspent Youth*, London, Audit Commission.

Black Committee (1979) *Report of the Children and Young Persons Review Group*, Belfast, HMSO.

Bottoms, A. (1974) 'On the decriminalization of the juvenile court', in Hood (ed.) (1974).

Bottoms, A. (1995) *Intensive Community Supervision for Young Offenders*, Cambridge, Institute of Criminology.

Burney, E. (1985) *Sentencing Young People*, Aldershot, Gower.

Carpenter, M. (1853) *Juvenile Delinquents, Their Condition and Treatment*, London, Cash.

Casburn, M. (1979) *Girls Will Be Girls*, London, Women's Research and Resources Centre.

Children's Society (1989) *Penal Custody for Juveniles – The Line of Least Resistance*, London, Church of England Children's Society.

Clarke, J. (1975) *The Three R's – Repression, Rescue and Rehabilitation*, Birmingham, Centre for Contemporary Cultural Studies, University of Birmingham.

Clarke, J. (1985) 'Whose justice? The politics of juvenile control', *International Journal of the Sociology of Law*, vol.13, no.4, pp.405–21.

Clarke, R.V.G. and Sinclair, I. (1974) 'Toward more effective treatment evaluation', *Collected Studies in Criminological Research*, vol.xii, pp.55–82, Strasbourg, Council of Europe.

Cohen, S. (1985) *Visions of Social Control*, Cambridge, Polity.

Cullen, F. and Gilbert, K. (1982) *Reaffirming Rehabilitation*, Cincinnati, Anderson.

Davies, B. (1982) 'Juvenile justice in confusion', *Youth and Policy*, vol.1, no.2, pp.33–6.

Department of Health and Social Security (1981) *Offending by Young People: A Survey of Recent Trends*, London, DHSS.

Dickie, D. (1979) 'The social work role in Scottish juvenile justice', in Parker, M. (ed.) *Social Work and the Courts*, London, Edward Arnold.

Fitzgerald, M. (1993) *Ethnic Minorities and the Criminal Justice System*, Royal Commission on Criminal Justice, Research Study no.20, London, HMSO.

Gelsthorpe, L. (1984) 'Girls and juvenile justice', *Youth and Policy*, no.11, pp.1–5.

Gelsthorpe, L. and Morris, A. (1994) 'Juvenile justice 1945–1992', in Maguire, M., Morgan, R. and Reiner, R. (eds) *The Oxford Handbook of Criminology*, Oxford, Clarendon.

Gill, K. (1985) 'The Scottish hearing system', *Ajjust*, no. 5, pp.18–21.

Hagell, A. and Newburn, T. (1994) *Persistent Young Offenders*, London, Policy Studies Institute.

Harris, R. (1982) 'Institutionalised ambivalence: social work and the Children and Young Persons Act 1969', *British Journal of Social Work*, vol.12, no.3, pp.247–63.

Harris, R. and Webb, P. (1987) *Welfare, Power and Juvenile Justice*, London, Tavistock.

Home Office (1927) *Report of the Departmental Committee on the Treatment of the Young Offender* (The Molony Committee), Cmnd 283, London, HMSO.

Home Office (1968) *Children in Trouble*, Cmnd 3601, London, HMSO.

Home Office (1990) *Crime, Justice and Protecting the Public*, Cm 965, London, HMSO.

Home Office (1996) *Criminal Statistics for England and Wales 1995*, London, HMSO.

Home Office (1997a) *Preventing Children Offending*, Cm 3566, London, HMSO.

Home Office (1997b) *Tackling Youth Crime*, London, HMSO.

Hood, R. (ed.) (1974) *Crime, Criminology and Public Policy*, London, Heinemann.

Hudson, A. (1988) 'Boys will be boys: masculinism and the juvenile justice system', *Critical Social Policy*, no.21, pp.30–48.

Hudson, B. (1987) *Justice Through Punishment*, London, Macmillan.

Hudson, J., Morris, A., Maxwell, G. and Galaway, B. (1996) *Family Group Conferences*, Annandale, Australia, Federation Press.

Hughes, G., Leisten, R. and Pilkington, A. (1998) 'Diversion in a culture of severity', *The Howard Journal*, vol.37, no.1, pp.16–33.

Kettle, M. (1982) 'The racial numbers game in our prisons', *New Society*, September.

Landau, S. and Nathan, G. (1983) 'Selecting delinquents for cautioning in the London Metropolitan area', *British Journal of Criminology*, vol.23, no.2, pp.128–49.

Lipsey, M. (1995) 'What do we learn from 400 research studies?', in McGuire (ed.) (1995).

Lloyd, C., Mair, G. and Hough, M. (1994) 'Explaining reconviction rates: a critical analysis', *Research Findings*, no.12, London, HMSO.

McGhee, J., Waterhouse, L. and Whyte, B. (1996) 'Children's hearings and children in trouble', in Asquith, S. (ed.) *Children and Young People in Conflict with the Law*, London, Jessica Kingsley.

McGuire, J. (ed.) (1995) *What Works: Reducing Reoffending*, London, Wiley.

McLaughlin, E. (1998) 'Social work or social control? Remaking probation work', in Hughes, G. and Lewis, G. (eds) *Unsettling Welfare: The Reconstruction of Social Policy*, London, Routledge in association with The Open University.

McLaughlin, E. and Muncie, J. (1993) 'Juvenile delinquency', in Dallos, R. and McLaughlin, E. (eds) *Social Problems and the Family*, London, Sage.

McLaughlin, E. and Muncie, J. (1994) 'Managing the criminal justice system', in Clarke, J., Cochrane, A. and McLaughlin, E. (eds) *Managing Social Policy*, London, Sage.

Martinson, R. (1974) 'What works? – questions and answers about prison reform', *The Public Interest*, no.35, pp.22–54.

May, D. (1977) 'Delinquent girls before the courts', *Medical Science Law*, vol.17, no.2, pp.203–10.

May, M. (1973) 'Innocence and experience: the evolution of the concept of juvenile delinquency in the mid-nineteenth century', *Victorian Studies*, vol.17, no.1, pp.7–29.

Mooney, G. (1998) '"Remoralizing" the poor?: gender, class and philanthropy in Victorian Britain', in Lewis, G. (ed.) (1998) *Forming Nation, Framing Welfare*, London, Routledge in association with The Open University.

Morgan, P. (1978) *Delinquent Fantasies*, Aldershot, Temple Smith.

Morris, A. (1974) 'Scottish juvenile justice: a critique', in Hood (ed.) (1974).

Morris, A. and McIsaac, M. (1978) *Juvenile Justice?*, London, Heinemann.

Morris, A., Giller, H., Geach, H. and Szwed, E. (1980) *Justice for Children*, London, Macmillan.

Muncie, J. (1990) 'Failure never matters: detention centres and the politics of deterrence', *Critical Social Policy*, no.28, pp.53–66.

Muncie, J. (1997) 'Shifting sands: care, community and custody in youth justice discourse', in Roche, J. and Tucker, S. (eds) *Youth in Society*, London, Sage.

NACRO (1993) *Community Provision for Young People in the Youth Justice System*, London, National Association for the Care and Resettlement of Offenders.

NACRO (1995) 'Family group conferencing', *NACRO Briefing Paper*, September, London, National Association for the Care and Resettlement of Offenders.

Nathan, S. (1995) *Boot Camps: Return of the Short Sharp Shock*, London, Prison Reform Trust.

Newburn, T. (1996) 'Back to the future? Youth crime, youth justice and the rediscovery of "authoritarian populism"', in Pilcher, J. and Wagg, S. (eds) *Thatcher's Children*, London, Falmer.

Parent, D.G. (1995) 'Boot camps failing to achieve goals', in Tonry, M. and Hamilton, K. (eds) *Intermediate Sanctions in Over-Crowded Times*, Boston, North Eastern University Press.

Parker, H., Jarvis, G. and Sumner, M. (1987) 'Under new orders: the redefinition of social work with young offenders', *British Journal of Social Work*, vol.17, no.1, pp.21–43.

Pitts, J. (1988) *The Politics of Juvenile Crime*, London, Sage.

Pitts, J. (1992) 'The end of an era', *The Howard Journal*, vol.31, no.2, pp.133–49.

Pratt, J. (1989) 'Corporatism: the third model of juvenile justice', *British Journal of Criminology*, vol.29, no.3, pp.236–54.

Radzinowicz, L. and Hood, A. (1990) *The Emergence of Penal Policy*, Oxford, Clarendon.

Riddell, P. (1989) *The Thatcher Effect*, Oxford, Blackwell.

Rutherford, A. (1989) 'The mood and temper of penal policy', *Youth and Policy*, no.27, pp.27–31.

Rutherford, A. (1993) *Criminal Justice and the Pursuit of Decency*, Oxford, Oxford University Press.

Shacklady Smith, L. (1978) 'Sexist assumptions and female delinquency', in Smart, C. and Smart, B. (eds) *Women, Sexuality and Social Control*, London, Routledge.

Springhall, J. (1986) *Coming of Age: Adolescence in Britain 1860–1960*, London, Gill and McMillan.

Tarling, R. (1993) *Analysing Offending: Data, Models and Interpretations*, London, HMSO.

Taylor, L., Lacey, R. and Bracken, D. (1979) *In Whose Best Interests?*, London, Cobden Trust/Mind.

Thornton, D., Curran, C., Grayson, D. and Holloway, V. (1984) *Tougher Regimes in Detention Centres*, London, HMSO.

Thorpe, D.H., Smith, D., Green, C.J. and Paley, J.H. (1980) *Out of Care: The Community Support of Juvenile Offenders*, London, Allen and Unwin.

Von Hirsch, A. (1976) *Doing Justice: The Choice of Punishments*, New York, Hill and Wang.

Weiner, M.J. (1990) *Reconstructing the Criminal: Culture, Law and Policy in England, 1830–1914*, Cambridge, Cambridge University Press.

CHAPTER 6

Legitimate Membership of the Welfare Community

by Lydia Morris

Contents

1   Introduction

Welfare provision is about catering for certain basic needs, and minimally ensuring survival, and so raises questions about acceptable minimum standards of living. However, it is also about identifying those groups whose needs should be met and it is this question of 'inclusion' or 'membership' which will be the main concern of this chapter. We will be asking you to consider the position of certain key groups in our society in terms of the claim they can make on public funds, and also to address political debates about the moral foundation for their claims. Can the long-term unemployed, single mothers and migrant groups reasonably expect the welfare state to meet their most basic needs or are they to be excluded from the collective community of mutual responsibility?

These issues have been apparent throughout the 1980s and 1990s in both political and academic debate about the concept of the 'underclass', and a central aim of this chapter is to examine this term and some of the criticism it has attracted. It has been used by people of different political persuasions to refer to a group in some way outside 'mainstream' society, either in terms of material standards of living, or in relation to their core values and attitudes. The meaning of this will become clearer as we move through the chapter. We will also be examining the way in which national boundaries of membership are drawn, and the implications of this for migrant groups.

Before exploring these ideas we take a brief look backwards to consider the repeated appearance of the 'social outsider' in history, and the light this can throw on contemporary thinking. The chapter divides into five main sections:

- Section 2 looks at some forerunners of the recent 'underclass' debate, and the challenge that 'outsider' groups have always posed for welfare policy. We pay particular attention to the early promise of the post-war welfare state to eradicate need and guarantee 'social inclusion' for all citizens in the common standards of society. However, we also find that the idea of an 'excluded' group is a persistent presence in social commentaries from the 1800s to the 1990s.

- Section 3 looks in more detail at a recent debate in the UK, and its roots in US literature on the 'underclass' which is fraught with disagreement. We consider the competing positions in this literature, and the way in which they have been adopted and applied to UK society. Are members of the 'underclass' the innocent victims of social forces, or must they individually take responsibility for their own position in society? Have social rights been superseded by social obligations?

- Section 4 takes up a very specific issue which runs through the underclass debate – its gender subtext. Here we consider the gendered assumptions which permeate much of the thinking on the 'underclass', and focus on the particular dilemma confronting single mothers. Does their obligation to their children conflict with the principle of self-reliance? And which of these duties earns them the public recognition of their needs? Are they inevitably to be dependent on either a partner or the state?

- Section 5 takes some of the ideas we have considered and applies them in a slightly different context. Here we ask what the position is of the strangers in our society. Those who cross national boundaries to establish themselves in a 'foreign' country can become particular objects of suspicion in relation to national resources. Do they have a legitimate claim on the welfare state, or are there reasonable grounds for their exclusion from the welfare community?

- Section 6 looks at these questions through the logic informing EU migration policy. Is there a move afoot to create a 'Fortress Europe', protection against the dangerous demands of the less affluent populations beyond the borders of the EU? In this context, we look at some specific examples from UK welfare policy which seem designed to limit the claims of 'outsiders' on the welfare system.

To express these sorts of questions in more abstract terms we can say that the modern welfare state represents a community of interests which is at once financial and moral. It is faced with both the (financial) administration of national resources, and the (moral) identification of a legitimate claim. Correspondingly, there is a population of people with a responsibility to contribute to the funding of welfare, and there are criteria of membership which confer the legitimate expectation of support in times of crisis. These two categories of contributor and recipient overlap substantially, but not completely, and thus considerable significance attaches to the definition of both genuine need and a legitimate claim. In Freeman's (1986 p.52) words: 'The welfare state requires boundaries because it establishes a principle of distributive justice that departs from the distributive principles of the free market.' While the free market operates through the interaction of supply and demand, distributive justice requires judgements about material need and moral desert.

2 Forerunners of the 'underclass'

2.1 Social outsiders in history

In this chapter we are largely concerned with those moral judgements, which have throughout history been reflected in a struggle to identify the truly deserving. We see this most overtly in the classic distinction between the worthy and unworthy poor which runs throughout the history of British social assistance. The construction of a category of outsiders, who were morally blameworthy and in some way set apart from the bulk of the population, has been recurrent in the history of the UK since the industrial revolution. Examination of a range of writing throughout the nineteenth century reveals a vocabulary of contagion, and the idea that certain sections of the population can contaminate society's more respectable members. The behaviour of the 'polluting' group is also usually thought to be underpinned by some moral incapacity, manifest in criminality, sexual license, work avoidance, and dependence on charity or the state. The 'underclass' is only the most recent version of these ideas.

unworthy poor
outsider

For Malthus (1806) it was the redundant population who reproduced irresponsibly, without the means of survival; for Marx and Engels (1853) the lumpenproletariat, stood apart from the real working class, and they describe them in pejorative terms as the scum of the earth, the depraved element of all classes; for Mayhew (1861) it was the 'social outcasts' – a race apart, a wandering tribe, with a 'repugnance towards civilization' and a 'psychological incapacity for steady work'. This idea of a race apart was also echoed in the eugenics movement and its attack on the degenerate hordes who threatened social stability (see Jones, 1980). Even Booth's (1902) path-breaking work, which revealed poverty in sections of the working population, still claimed to identify a group incapable of improvement who 'degrade whatever they touch'.

ACTIVITY 6.1

You do not need a detailed knowledge of these works but you may be interested to look at some of the descriptions of the 'outsider groups' and particularly the graphic imagery which is used. Pick out some of the more powerful words and consider their implications.

> Educated in workhouses where every vice is propagated, or bred up at home in filth and rags, and with an utter ignorance of every moral obligation.
>
> [On provision for the poor:] We shall raise the worthless above the worthy; we shall encourage indolence and check industry.
>
> *(Thomas Malthus, 1806)*

> Often hardly human in appearance, they had neither tastes nor sympathies, not even human sensations, for they revelled in the filth which is grateful to dogs.
>
> *(Edwin Chadwick, 1842)*

> The dangerous class, the social scum, that passively rotting mass thrown off by the lowest layers of the old society.
>
> *(Karl Marx, 1848)*

> As the streets grow blue with the coming light ... they come sauntering forth, the unwashed poor, some with greasy wallets on their back, to haunt over each dirt heap, and eke out life by seeking refuse, bones or stray rags and pieces of old iron.
>
> [Of street people:] ... imbibing the habits and the morals of the gutters along with their mother's milk ... the child without training goes back to its parent stock the vagabond savage ... a foul disgrace ... the utter depths of barbarism ... beasts of the field ... instinctless animals.
>
> *(Henry Mayhew, 1861)*

> [On emigration:] While the flower of the population emigrate, the residuum stays, corrupting and being corrupted, like the sewage of the metropolis which remained floating at the mouth of the Thames last summer.
>
> *(Samuel Smith, 1885)*

COMMENT

Much of the descriptive vocabulary calls up pictures of dirt, waste, contagion, immorality and passivity. See, for example, references to sewage, filth, rags, refuse and so on. This imagery was used, by association, to support the argument that there existed a worthless, decadent section of the population, who should not be encouraged in their idleness and vice through provisions for the poor.

■ ■ ■

*Beggars leaving town
for their workhouse*

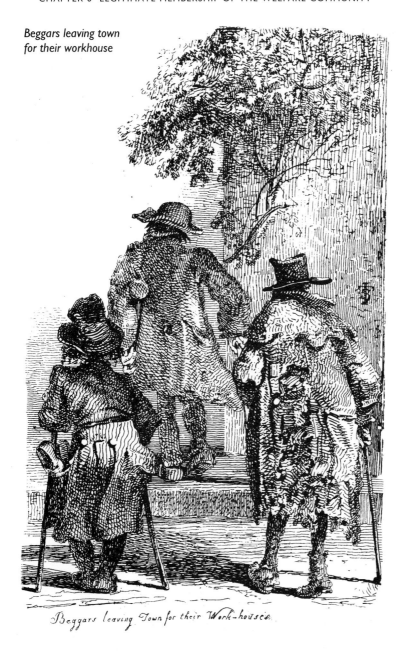

Beggars leaving Town for their Work-houses.

2.2 Sturdy beggars

Protection against poverty caused by the loss or absence of employment has posed a problem ever since the industrial revolution transformed a semi-subsistence society into a society of workers dependent for a livelihood upon selling their labour in the open market. It was this transition which created the very concept of unemployment and fuelled related problems concerning both the funding of social assistance and the potential conflict between meeting the needs of the unemployed and maintaining the incentive to work. A source of **work incentive** much political concern was the fear that any provision for poverty would undermine the work ethic.

These difficulties were apparent as early as 1350, when legislation defined the 'sturdy beggar' as those able to labour and without other means of support, evoking hostility against any 'who do refuse to labour, giving themselves only to idleness and vice ... so that they may be through want, compelled to labour for their necessary living' (quoted in Fulbrook, 1978, p.83). In subsequent legislation the distinction between the 'impotent' (unable to work) and the 'able-bodied' became increasingly important. In fact, this classification of the poor was the key to the seventeenth-century Elizabethan Poor Law:

> Essentially the Elizabethan Poor Law identified three main groups to be dealt with. The impotent poor (the aged, the chronic sick, the blind, the lunatic), who really needed institutional relief, were to be accommodated in 'poor houses' or 'almshouses'. The able-bodied were to be set to work ... and for this a 'house of correction' ... was to be established ... Finally, the able-bodied who absconded ... or the persistent idler who refused to work were to be punished in this 'house of correction'.
>
> (Fraser, 1986, p.33)

The nature of these provisions reveals anxiety about the inculcation of a work ethic also apparent in later legislation, notably the Poor Law of 1834, which embraced the principle of 'less eligibility': 'The first and most essential of all conditions is that the situation of the individual relieved should not be made really or apparently so eligible as the situation of the independent labourer of the lowest class' (see Brown, 1988, p.1). In other words, relief for the poor must never even appear to be preferable to reliance on earned income. It should therefore be set at a level below the wages of the poorest paid. Relative (and probably absolute) poverty was therefore inevitable, and the 'able-bodied' in receipt of assistance would necessarily be viewed with suspicion. The principle of less eligibility has, in fact, been an enduring feature of social security provision, while related concern about the maintenance of the work ethic implicitly questions the legitimacy of claims for support by the long-term unemployed.

2.3   Social citizenship

The long history of concern to identify the undeserving was briefly challenged by post-war thinking which was focused on securing the material position of all members of the population. When William Beveridge was appointed to review the provision of social insurance in the UK (Beveridge Report, 1942), in the aftermath of the Second World War, it was felt for a brief period that a turning-point had been reached. There was optimism at the same time about what Marshall (1950) terms the guarantee of 'social inclusion' through 'social citizenship'. This was defined as 'full membership of the community', and was lodged in the belief that welfare provisions should offer material security to all, ensuring full participation in society. In this sense the idea of social inclusion stands as a counterpart to the notion of the underclass or the unworthy poor – terms designating social, material and moral exclusion, and referring to a condition it was thought the UK welfare state under the Beveridge plan would eradicate (see Chapter 1).

There have been attempts to appropriate the term 'underclass' (for example, Field, 1989), to argue that the welfare state has failed in its aims, that the commitment to full employment was never strong enough, social provision for

social
inclusion
social
citizenship

the unemployed was never adequate, and the administration of the system was always punitive. The dominant rhetoric, however, comes from the right, where we see the underclass debate imbued with a moral panic. Thus we find a condemnation of the alleged 'culture of dependency', which argues that the welfare state has gone too far, and turns state dependence into a badge of exclusion rather than a guarantee of inclusion. The right to social inclusion has increasingly been called into question, and we find the growth of arguments stressing social obligations above social rights (for example, Mead, 1986), the major obligation being to work for a living. This *reverses* the original promise of social citizenship, and is based on the view that those dependent on the state must be compelled to give something back to society. This shift in thinking is the foundation of the Conservative position, as expressed by Michael Howard at the 1993 Conservative Party Conference: 'Social Security benefits all too often appear as an entitlement rather than something which should be earned.' We will come back to these ideas later in the chapter.

ACTIVITY 6.2

1 What do you think is meant by 'social citizenship'?

2 Should it be guaranteed by social security for all who need it?

3 Should there be clearly stated obligations attached to benefits?

4 If so, what would those obligations be?

COMMENT

You may find these questions difficult to answer, but keep them in mind as you work through the chapter. They involve complex and competing issues concerning the financial viability of systems of welfare, the need to establish clear boundaries of eligibility, anxiety about maintaining a work ethic, and ideas about moral desert. There are no easy answers to these questions.

■ ■ ■

2.4 Cycles of deprivation?

Even before the notion of an underclass took hold, there were periodic panics about 'problem' groups in society, most notably the 'cycles of deprivation' hypothesis, framed by Sir Keith Joseph in 1972 when Secretary of State for Education. His concern was why it is that, 'in spite of long periods of full employment and relative prosperity and the improvement in community services since the Second World War, deprivation and problems of maladjustment so conspicuously persist' (Rutter and Madge, 1976, p.3). A series of projects was set up to explore the possibility that disadvantage was reproduced in a particular form within families, and passed on from one generation to the next.

cycles of deprivation

The general orientation of the research centred on a set of interests very close to investigations into a 'culture of poverty' as, for example, in Extract 6.1. This idea was developed by Oscar Lewis (1968) in research suggesting that the poor develop ways of coping through a set of attitudes and behaviour which then reinforces their position.

Extract 6.1 Lewis: 'The culture of poverty'

As an anthropologist I have tried to understand poverty and its associated traits as a culture or, more accurately, as a subculture with its own structure and rationale, as a way of life that is passed down from generation to generation along family lines. This view directs attention to the fact that the culture of poverty in modern nations is not only a matter of economic deprivation, of disorganization, or of the absence of something. It is also something positive and provides some rewards without which the poor could hardly carry on.

…

The culture of poverty is both an adaptation and a reaction of the poor to their marginal position in a class-stratified, highly individuated, capitalistic society. It represents an effort to cope with feelings of hopelessness and despair that develop from the realization of the improbability of achieving success in terms of the values and goals of the larger society. Indeed, many of the traits of the culture of poverty can be viewed as attempts at local solutions for problems not met by existing institutions and agencies because the people are not eligible for them, cannot afford them, or are ignorant or suspicious of them. For example, unable to obtain credit from banks, they are thrown upon their own resources and organize informal credit devices without interest.

The culture of poverty, however, is not only an adaptation to a set of objective conditions of the larger society. Once it comes into existence, it tends to perpetuate itself from generation to generation because of its effect on the children. By the time slum children are age six or seven they have usually absorbed the basic values and attitudes of their subculture and are not psychologically geared to take full advantage of the changing conditions or increased opportunities that may occur in their lifetime.

(Lewis, 1968, pp.4,5–6)

underclass

The contemporary equivalent of this argument is the idea of an underclass which recreates itself though poor socialization and the absence of appropriate role models. In other words, children are taught the wrong attitudes and behaviour at home and so reproduce their own disadvantage. Findings from the 'cycles of deprivation' projects seem to cast doubt on such a view (see Rutter and Madge, 1976). Broadly speaking, there is some evidence of family continuity, but over half of all forms of disadvantage are found to arise anew in every generation. Even where continuity is strongest, many individuals break out of the cycle, while others become disadvantaged without having been brought up by disadvantaged parents. Certainly when it comes to explaining unemployment, the impact of economic change on particular workers and regions seems to carry much more weight than explanations rooted in family background.

2.5 Scroungerphobia

One perennial concern in British policy-making which also precedes the interest in the 1990s in the notion of the underclass is 'scroungerphobia' – the conviction that welfare has undermined the will to work. However, alongside this view of the unemployed as habitually dependent lurks the suspicion that they are in fact working. Both views have been expressed by the Department of Employment:

There is evidence that a significant minority of benefit claimants are not actively looking for work. Some are claiming benefit while working at least part-time in the black economy. Others seem to have grown accustomed to living on benefit and have largely given up looking for work, despite the high level of job vacancies which are increasingly available throughout the country.

(Department of Employment, 1988, p.55)

Thus, charges that over-generous welfare has created a dependency culture in the UK, sit alongside charges that many of the unemployed have been working all along. These arguments must be set against ample evidence of extreme poverty experienced by many of the benefit-dependent population. A study by Morris and Ritchie (Morris, 1996), for example, found that a large proportion of income support recipients were unable to meet basic needs for food and clothing.

ACTIVITY 6.3

There are periodic revivals of these ideas, often in the form of campaigns against 'benefits cheats':

Everyone who is a dole cheat is taking money away from the unemployed and training councils. We cannot allow that to happen ... Everyone wants to see law and order restored, and the weeding out of people who do not respect it.

(David Hunt, Employment Secretary, Conservative Party Conference, 1993)

In August 1996 billboard posters appeared in towns across the UK bearing the advertisement reproduced here. What do you think would be the likely effect of these campaigns on social cohesion?

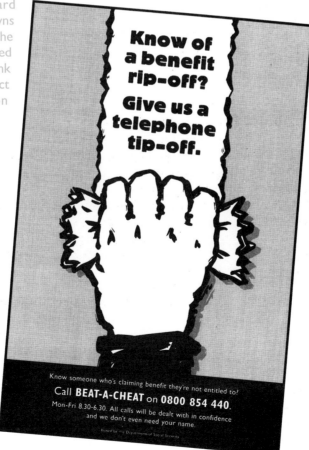

'Beat-a-cheat'

Optimistic approaches to social provision (such as Marshall, 1950) argued that social cohesion would be achieved by guaranteed standards for all. Concern about the escalating costs of welfare and anti-fraud campaigns challenge such a view and encourage suspicion and stigmatization. *The Independent* (29 January 1996) reported that officials expected 2,000 calls a week in response to 'Beat-a-Cheat', but in fact received 8,000. David Donnison (a distinguished academic who chaired the Supplementary Benefits Commission from 1975–80) is quoted as stating, 'The Benefit Fraudline could be used to stoke up hostility towards the poorest people in society'.

■ ■ ■

Small-scale studies of unemployment do reveal that some unemployed claimants take occasional opportunities for paid work, though even official estimates of the numbers involved are no more than 10 per cent. Jordan *et al.* (1992) emphasize the enduring significance of work as a basis for identity and self-respect, noting: 'The men described themselves as actively needing to work to fulfil their personal needs as well as their roles as providers'. However, all writers stress the limited nature of the work available: 'Earnings tend to be occasional lump sums rather than regular weekly incomes and as a result, although individuals have earned more than the legal amount in one particular week, over a longer period their earnings have often averaged out at less than this amount' (McLaughlin *et al.*, 1989, p.82).

Evidence of this kind points to an enduring need for the self-respect attached to work, and also the contradictions of a benefit system which wishes to preserve independence but stifles initiative in a climate in which regular employment for a certain section of the population is no longer embraced as a feasible aim.

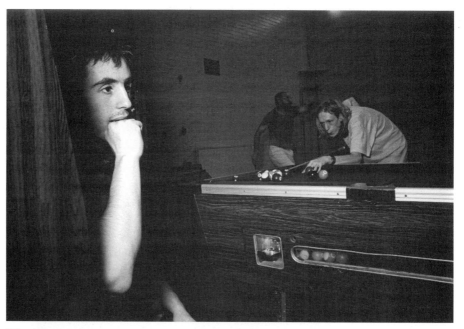

Life without work

2.6 The incentive to work

A 'softer' version of the 'work-shy' position is that workers are pricing themselves out of jobs and have an unrealistically high 'reservation wage', i.e. the lowest wage at which they would accept employment. But does the obligation to accept available work – which is a condition of social citizenship – extend to any work, whatever the terms and conditions? Or is one of the rights of citizenship the right to command a reasonable wage, i.e. one sufficient to secure a reasonable standard of living, and in that sense to facilitate inclusion in the social and cultural expectations of the community of membership? The argument is anyway too narrow, being based only on financial motivation. A number of studies demonstrate the significance of employment for a sense of personal worth, and suggest that the wage is only one of many reasons for working.

One approach to the issue of reservation wages and low pay is the view that if benefits fall low enough, then the unemployed will start to accept jobs they would not previously have considered, and it will become financially viable for employers to create work which at higher wage levels would not have been possible. However, despite falls in the value of benefit in the 1980s (Micklewright, 1986), unemployment continued to rise, and meanwhile the unemployed became more impoverished in relation to the majority of the population. Field (1989) adopted the notion of the underclass to make this point. For him the underclass was not principally to be defined in terms of a problem of social order or dependency, but rather as those who have been excluded from the increased affluence of the majority population:

> They increasingly live under what is a subtle form of political, social and economic apartheid. Indeed the emergence of an underclass marks a watershed in Britain's class politics. Today the very poorest are separated, not only from other groups on low income, but more importantly, from the working class.
>
> (Field, 1989, p.4)

ACTIVITY 6.4

The gap between rich and poor grew more quickly in Britain during the 1980s than in any other industrialized country.   *(The Guardian, 1 February 1994)*

Here are some of the findings of the Joseph Rowntree Foundation report, *Income and Wealth* (Hills, 1995) which suggest a process of **'social polarization'**. Read through them and then consider the three questions which follow.

social
polarization

- Income inequality in the UK grew rapidly between 1977 and 1990, reaching a higher level than recorded since the war.

- Between 1979 and 1992 the poorest 20–30 per cent failed to benefit from economic growth, in contrast to the rest of the post-war period.

- The income gap widened between those dependent on benefits and those with earnings.

- Since the early 1980s, benefit levels have generally been linked to prices so that the incomes of those dependent on benefits have fallen behind those of the working population.

- After 1978 the hourly wages of the lowest paid men hardly changed in real terms, and by 1992 were lower than in 1975; median wages grew by 35 per cent, but high wages grew by 50 per cent.

- In many areas of the UK the living standards and life opportunities of the poor are simply unacceptably low in a society as rich as ours.

- Regardless of any moral arguments or feelings of altruism, everyone shares an interest in the cohesiveness of society. As the gaps between rich and poor grow, the problem of the marginalized groups which are being left behind rebound on the more comfortable majority.

1 Is evidence of poverty sufficient to support the idea of an underclass?

2 Is collective responsibility for the poor a matter of morality or of self-interest for the majority?

3 Is the 'moral' position to help the poor or to encourage self-reliance?

Frank Field's more recent views, outlined in an article from the *Independent on Sunday* reprinted here as Extract 6.2, suggest a policy response which raises problems of its own.

Extract 6.2 Field: 'The poison in the welfare state'

The underclass, a category of people that vanished in the post-war era of full employment and welfare reform, has reappeared in Britain.

There are families now that have totally abandoned the idea that paid work has any relevance for them at all, such is the impossibility of finding a job. There are schoolchildren who, because no member of the family is in work, have not the slightest idea of what it means to earn one's living. I have become hardened to the brave men with laughing mouths but wintry eyes who tell me that it doesn't matter that they may never work again …

…

… Many young women are moving away from their parents and starting their own families, often with a succession of boyfriends. Their male counterparts have three main options: they can leave home and become drifters, often ending up begging; they can try their hand at the drugs trade or they may be forced back on to their parents and into a state of permanent adolescence.

…

A deadly lesson is being taught: the only way to survive is to cheat. Because means-tested help is reduced as income rises, people on low or no wages have no incentive to improve their lot. Suppose that a married wage earner with two children earns £60 a week. With means-tested benefits, the net family income will be £125 a week (after housing costs), which is not much more than he would get without a job. Just to add £10 per week to the family income, he would need to increase his gross wages by around £140 a week and earn a total of £200 a week.

The alternative – unless he decides to sit tight and do nothing – is to take work but not declare additional income. This is fraud. And fraud is a criminal offence. Welfare is therefore having the opposite effect from that for which it was devised. The welfare state was constructed as a means of extending full citizenship to the entire population, many of whom might otherwise remain outside civil society. Welfare fraud now acts as an expelling agent, encouraging people into criminal activity.

Means tests poison the welfare state. They paralyse self-help, discourage self-improvement and tax honesty. They reward claimants for being either inactive or deceitful. They penalise all those values which make strong, vibrant communities
…

...

We should, therefore, phase out means tests. Instead, a National Insurance Corporation, comprising representatives of employers, employees and government, should run a new national insurance scheme. Those paying into it should be known as 'stakeholders'. They would receive protection against unemployment, illness and disability. But levels of benefits should be clearly linked to levels of contributions. In other words, stakeholders should be clear that the money they pay into the scheme will not be used to redistribute their income to other people.

What about those who cannot pay adequate contributions – because their wages are too low, because they cannot get jobs, because they are sick or disabled or because they are caring for elderly relatives? The Exchequer would pay contributions into the scheme on their behalf. In this way, redistribution would be clear and above-board. It would come, and would be seen to come, from generation taxation and not from some sleight of hand within the national insurance scheme.

...

Income support should continue but should be transformed into an opportunities agency developing career plans. It should act as a life-raft taking people back into work rather than, as at present, as a sink into which they are dumped.

In addition social security fraud should be recognised as the very big business it is. Imaginative counter-action needs to be driven by a core of SAS-style anti-fraud officers. Benefit savings from successful anti-fraud campaigns should be ring-fenced and used for tax cuts and increases in child benefit.

The growth of individualism is not going to be arrested by talk about rebuilding the community. Welfare has to be shaped so individual wishes can simultaneously promote new senses of community.

(*Independent on Sunday*, 14 May 1995, p.27)

COMMENT

The UK post-war welfare state was based on the ideal of shared risk and collective responsibility through insurance. Contributions paid while in employment were to cover the periods without work – through sickness, retirement or unemployment, and necessarily involved some redistribution to the more vulnerable. The system, however, could only sustain fairly limited demand and became overly reliant on non-contributory, means-tested supplements. Field's position represents a shift away from collective responsibility, arguing that the existing benefit system encourages fraud, that what people pay in should be tied to their own individual benefit, and that those unable to pay should be placed in a different category. This solution does not confront the unequal distribution of risk and need in society, and arguably opens up new social divisions rather than offering a new basis for community.

■ ■ ■

3 Understanding the underclass debate

3.1 Back to basics?

*Raising the welfare
drawbridge*

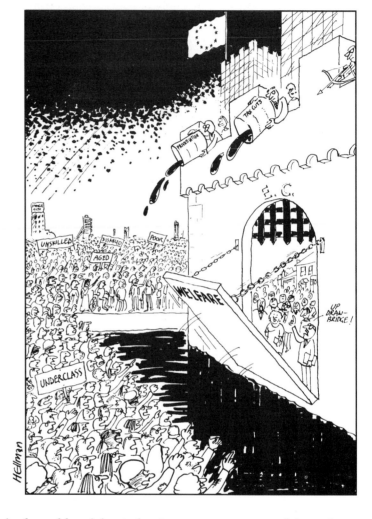

So intractable is the fear of fraud that it dominates contemporary debate about
the existence of an underclass through the view that welfare provisions have
been over-generous and are abused by many. The underlying assumption is
that state provision has created a culture of dependency which has both
undermined the work ethic and been damaging to family stability, and this taps
into more general feelings of uncertainty. Thus, the anxiety evoked by the image
of an underclass in 1990s' Britain, and its political purchase, is rooted in the
growing instability of two traditional building-blocks of social life – secure full-
time employment for men, and the nuclear family household. We will later
introduce a third source of concern, and further challenge for welfare – the
increasing fragility of the boundaries of the nation-state.

Both UK and US societies are based on assumptions about a division of
labour which has produced a particular combination of work, family and welfare.
Over the last three decades the fit between them – whilst never perfect – has

gradually become dislocated and much of the underclass debate revolves around where explanation (or blame) for this dislocation lies. In particular, attention has focused on growing male unemployment and rising single parenthood, both argued to be linked to aspects of welfare provision, and there has been some suggestion that the two phenomena are interrelated. Certainly doubts have been raised about the stability of two key social institutions.

In some ways the notion of the underclass, and the public attention it has attracted, can be seen as an exercise in *conceptual containment*. Rather than revise our understanding of social organization to accommodate a number of rather complex changes, some explanation is sought which leaves the social world as we understand it more or less intact. The policy of 'Back to Basics', embraced by nineties' Conservatism, was a symptom of the same unease and search for containment, and was based on an over-idealized belief in 'traditional' values. A dominant view in the underclass literature defines a group which rejects the norms and values of mainstream society, and the evidence cited for this argument is state dependency, denial of the work ethic, the failure of morality, and the rejection of family norms, often also argued to be linked with criminality (see, for example, Auletta, 1982). Popular usage of the term thus groups these disparate features together into a residual category, located 'outside' of a society which remains otherwise cohesive and free from internal challenge.

underclass

3.2 The US influence

Political and academic interest in the notion of the underclass was imported into the UK from the USA, though the situation there differs in important respects. Most notably, the history and structure of welfare provision in the two countries has been sharply divergent (at least until recently), and crucially the US system offers no 'as of right' provision for unemployed men without eligibility for the *contributory* insurance benefit. Whilst both countries operate such a system of unemployment benefit, there are growing numbers of workers who do not qualify, a result of rising unemployment and increasing job insecurity. In the UK the means-tested income support fills this breach, but there is no direct US equivalent.

The major means-tested benefit in the US has been directed through *Aid to Families with Dependent Children (AFDC)*, and this has usually meant single mothers. Although since 1989 AFDC has been available in all states to homes with dependent children in which there is an unemployed father present, there are tight conditions attached. The main recipients have overwhelmingly been single mothers, and certainly not young unmarried or childless men, who have no automatic right to benefit on their own behalf. This is still not the case in the UK, though single people aged under eighteen now only receive support as part of a programme of training, and the rate of benefit for those aged under 25 has been reduced.

The functioning of AFDC has been at the heart of a US literature arguing that welfare provision has undermined the institution of the family and the work ethic. State dependency is seen as one defining feature of an underclass made up of single mothers, associated with young men living on the criminal fringe but assumed to have oblique access through these women to welfare for which they are not themselves eligible. This is perceived to be a predominantly black way of life.

The central character in this debate is Charles Murray (1984) who argues on the basis of 'rational choice theory' that young women are in fact better off living independently on their welfare cheques than throwing in their lot with the father of their children, hence the argument that welfare has undermined the institution of the nuclear family. These single mothers, it is argued, then foster a culture of the underclass which reproduces the pattern in the next generation. Furthermore, this culture is thought to take its hold because of the absence of a viable male role model offering an alternative way of living. It is this alleged *cultural* reproduction of the underclass which is offered as evidence of a rejection of the mainstream norms and values of society.

The counter-position is taken up by William Julius Wilson (1987) who argues that the high proportion of single mothers – particularly in the black population – is to be explained by the *structural* factors which have produced high levels of male unemployment, together with the high mortality and incarceration rates among young black men. The pool of marriageable men is thus argued to be far too low for the nuclear family household to be a viable option, having been undermined by the disadvantaged position of poor black men in the labour market. Murray and Wilson appear to agree, however, in seeing single parenthood as anomalous, and at least by implication holding up the nuclear family household as the ideal. For Murray, the central issue is ultimately an ethical one, concerning correct upbringing and maintenance of the work ethic; for Wilson, it is economic, with structural change in the economy undermining the viability of traditional gender arrangements.

ACTIVITY 6.5

Compare and contrast the approaches to the underclass by Murray and Wilson outlined in the following quotes.

[Phyllis has become pregnant by her boyfriend, Harold, and now faces a dilemma.] To keep the baby or give it up? To get married or not? What are the pros and cons? ... If Phyllis and Harold marry and he is employed, she will lose her AFDC benefits. His minimum wage job at the laundry will produce no more income than she can make, and, not insignificantly, he, not she, will have control of the [pay cheque]. In exchange for giving up this degree of independence, she gains no real security. Harold's job is not nearly as stable as the welfare system ... [H]er child provides her with the economic insurance that a husband used to represent.

(Murray, 1984, p.160)

... historical discrimination and a migration to large metropolises that kept the urban minority population relatively young created a problem of weak labor-force attachment among urban blacks and, especially since 1970, made them particularly vulnerable to the industrial and geographic changes in the economy. The shift from goods-producing to service-producing industries, the increasing polarization of the labour market into low-wage and high-wage sectors, innovations in technology, the relocation of manufacturing industries out of central cities, and periodic recessions have forced up the rate of black joblessness ... The rise in joblessness has in turn helped trigger an increase in the concentrations of poor people, a growing number of poor single-parent families, and an increase in welfare dependency.

(Wilson, 1993, p.12)

While Murray emphasizes the active decisions made by individuals, based on conscious calculation, Wilson is concerned to explain the forces which place certain groups at a disadvantage, and which operate outside of their control. Both Murray and Wilson have similar *definitions* of the underclass, but they emphasize different issues in their *explanations*. Murray's approach to explanation can be termed 'behavioural', and is based on incentives and penalties which might influence individual behaviour. In general, he argues, the expansion of the welfare state in the 1960s meant that 'pride in independence was compromised' (p.185), though he seems to concede that poor job prospects for men play a part. In contrast Wilson emphasizes not individual behaviour, but economic structure.

■ ■ ■

Murray more recently collaborated with Herrnstein to produce their book, *The Bell Curve*. They analyse data which appear to demonstrate that 'for that minority of men who are either out of the labour force or unemployed the primary risk factor seems to be neither socio-economic background nor education but low cognitive ability' (Herrnstein and Murray, 1994, p.155). The book goes on to argue that there are also patterns of association between divorce and illegitimacy and low IQ. Herrnstein and Murray interpret this as meaning that women of low intelligence fail to appreciate the severe problems posed by a life on welfare and are more likely to produce illegitimate children. These women are also argued to figure in the 'culture of poverty' syndrome, transmitting welfare dependency from one generation to the next. In addition, there are data (for example, pp.279, 452) purporting to show that blacks score lower than whites on IQ tests.

The book has been heavily criticized, not least because such data are taken at face value when, as Liam Hudson (1994) argues, 'there are good and obvious reasons ... why whole segments of society should become disaffected with the educational process; and why many individuals should fail to do themselves justice on mental tests'. The book is also argued by Hudson to be irresponsible in raising policy questions which are not fully explored. The article from the *Daily Mail*, by Richard Lynn, Professor Emeritus, University of Ulster, reproduced as Extract 6.3, illustrates one of the more extreme policy responses to the kind of argument offered by Herrnstein and Murray.

Read through Extract 6.3. What is the author's explanation of the growth of the underclass and what policies could arise out of this analysis?

Extract 6.3 Lynn: 'Why, as we grow richer, does our underclass get bigger every year?'

There is no more serious problem facing Britain and other economically developed countries than the growth of the underclass.

The underclass consists of those who choose not to work and would rather live on social security benefits, topped up by the proceeds of crime. Its size has roughly doubled in Britain and other Western countries over the past 30 years.

The number of able-bodied men who are long-term unemployed, who could work but have opted not to, has increased from about half a million to around one million. Many of them are criminals and this is the main reason why crime rates have also risen approximately six-fold since the 1960s. Most people have had personal experience of this shocking increase by being burgled or mugged.

As well as this unwillingness to work, members of the underclass are often handicapped by low intelligence, a poor educational record and weak moral character. They tend to lack the sense that everyone in society should pull their weight by working or that it is wrong to steal.

They are less likely to marry or form stable partnerships, the women instead having illegitimate children by men who enter their lives for a while and then move on. The underclass has become the dominant culture in many housing estates.

One of the reasons for the growth of the underclass is that they have more children than the law-abiding majority – half as many again, in fact. Their lifestyle is transmitted from parents to children, and inevitably, with the tendency to have more children, the size of the underclass goes on increasing.

...

The transmission of the underclass culture from parents to children takes place in two ways. First, children generally copy the lifestyle of their parents by the process known to psychologists as modelling: typically, the children of professional parents go to university and themselves become professionals.

...

Second, there are genetic factors in the transmission of lifestyles from parents to children.

...

The conclusion that low intelligence and weak moral character are transmitted genetically in underclass families is established beyond dispute.

...

In an ideal world, the professional and middle classes would have the largest numbers of children, because they would give them the best heredity and the best upbringing, while the underclass would have the fewest.

For the past century or so it has been the other way around. We have come to live in a topsy-turvy world.

(*Daily Mail*, 23 December 1996, p.8)

COMMENT

This article comes close to recommending the enforced management of reproduction. It encourages an explanation of disadvantage based on individual (genetic) defects rather than inherited cultural and material advantage. 'Intelligence' is itself a disputed concept, while the argument that 'moral character' is genetically transmitted is inherently implausible. Morality is a social product embedded in a particular culture; it is necessarily learnt.

■ ■ ■

3.3 'Race' and the underclass

There has been a strong 'racial' dimension to much of the underclass debate in the USA. In his book *Losing Ground*, Murray is at pains to point out that, just as there are affluent black Americans, there are also poor whites:

> But we are speaking of proportions. The comparison between black (or 'black and others') and white is an imprecise but nevertheless useful comparison over time between 'disadvantaged' Americans in general (blacks) and 'advantaged' Americans in general (whites), blurred by the members of both groups who fail to fit their category.
>
> (Murray, 1984, p.55)

Later in the book, however, a central point turns on the 'destruction of status rewards'. His argument is that expanded welfare provision in the 1970s removed the stigma from dependence and so destroyed the status attached to self-reliance. The recipients were principally black people, and according to Murray (1984, pp.178, 187) they were persuaded by white guilt into the view that they were irresponsible victims. In other words, their receipt of assistance was legitimized by their own sub-cultural values. This view is, of course, contested – not least by Fainstein's argument (1987, p.438) that 'black males almost never receive welfare benefits, and they must be supported clandestinely on the meagre allotments handed to females with dependent children'.

'Race' also has a central position in Wilson's writing, but in a different way. In an earlier work, *The Declining Significance of Race*, he makes reference to 'a vast underclass of black proletarians – that massive population at the very bottom of the social class ladder plagued by poor education and low-paying, unstable jobs' (Wilson, 1978, p.1). They were disproportionately affected by inner-city job loss, but not real contenders for new opportunities in the suburbs. More highly skilled sections of the black community did benefit from these opportunities, he argues, thus polarizing the black population. For him, then, the 'underclass' phenomenon is driven primarily by class disadvantage rather than racial discrimination. Again there is disagreement, with Fainstein (1987, p.416) arguing that even middle-class blacks are disadvantaged in relation to their white counterparts and that racial discrimination permeates the whole US class structure.

While there have been periodic scares in the UK about allegedly high rates of black street crime, *explicit* concern about a specifically black underclass is less central to British debate. One early study which is unusual in this respect was conducted in the 1960s by Rex and Moore (1967). They examined the position of black and Asian workers in Sparkbrook, Birmingham, and the way in which discrimination in access to housing led to their concentration in particular areas and types of accommodation. Rex and Tomlinson (1979, p.33) later developed these ideas to argue that 'there is some tendency for the black community to operate as a separate class or underclass in British society'. The emphasis in the Sparkbrook study was on the struggle over scarce resources, in this case housing. In fact, much of the more recent political debate about migration, documented in sections 5 and 6 of this chapter, is quite explicitly about defending 'national resources' more generally. However, as we will see, limiting the rights of 'foreigners' creates a new source of inequality and a new basis for 'stratification' in our society.

Murray's concern is with the emergence of a distinctively black value frame; Wilson's lies with the class disadvantage affecting inner-city blacks. Rex and Moore offer a perspective in which access to state resources itself generates a form of racial inequality.

3.4   The British picture

It is Charles Murray, however, who has played the central role in placing the concept of the underclass on the agenda of contemporary debate in the UK. His contention is that, 'The difference between the United States and Britain is that the United States reached the future first' (Murray, 1990, p.2). With metaphors of 'plague' and 'disease' he argues that an underclass defined by illegitimacy, violent crime and drop-out from the labour force is growing, and will continue to do so because there is a generation of children being brought up to live in this manner. This, of course, is in direct contradiction to the findings from the cycles of disadvantage research, but is an argument which reiterates Murray's depiction of a US underclass.

The first issue Murray addresses is that of illegitimacy, which he argues to be strongly associated with social class. Areas with a high concentration of class V (unskilled manual) workers showed high rates of illegitimacy (about 40 per cent), in contrast with areas with a high concentration of class I household 'heads' (about 9 per cent) – but see Figure 6.1 below. Unlike the situation in the US, these births are not predominantly to black women, although black women do have a somewhat higher 'illegitimacy' rate than white women. Like the US, however, he argues that the UK shows a higher proportion of never-married women (as opposed to divorced women) becoming benefit-dependent. Benefit dependence, especially when combined with the absence of a father, is argued to provide poor socialization into work identities. The interpretation of the statistics in terms of the availability of a father is not clear, however, in that 69 per cent of 'illegitimate' births are registered by both parents.

The benefit system in the UK has, since its inception, been more generous than the US system in that the unemployed, with or without children, can claim benefit as of right. Although under-18s are required to undergo training in order to qualify for benefit, it is not possible to make the direct connection between single parenthood and male unemployment that has been made in the US. Young adults do not have to produce children to get access to welfare, although their benefit rights have been somewhat eroded in recent years. Nevertheless, the availability of support for single mothers, and their rising numbers, led to the argument that British welfare has been undermining the nuclear family. This was part of the rationale for cuts in 1996.

Joan Brown (1990) is generally critical of Murray's view of the UK situation. Whilst agreeing with much of his data she points out that never-married mothers still constitute a minority of single mothers (38 per cent in 1997), and that long-term benefit dependence is greater for divorced mothers than never-married mothers. She argues that increased numbers of long-term claimants among never-married mothers throughout the 1980s may be linked to male unemployment, but to date never-married mothers do not spend long years on benefit because they usually marry (Ermisch, 1986).

Furthermore, particular concentrations of single mothers in certain areas are argued by Brown to be a result of housing policy rather than any 'contaminating' cultural influence of the kind Murray suggests. High priority cases for public housing tend to be offered the accommodation which is in least demand – in hard-to-let blocks or estates. This low popularity housing occurs in areas of generally poor appeal, and hence the concentration of class V workers alongside high levels of single parenthood. A correlation – i.e. the association of two different characteristics – does not always imply a direct explanatory link, as Figure 6.1 explains. Thus, two factors may coincide without being directly related; both may be explained by something else, in this case the dynamics of the housing market.

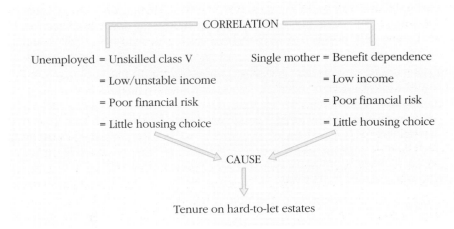

Figure 6.1

Finally, as others have argued for the USA, Brown suggests that marital, residential and child-rearing patterns are undergoing a revolution, which may pose a particular problem at the lower end of the income scale, but which is nevertheless a feature of society as a whole, reflected in high and rising rates of divorce. The stability of the nuclear family cannot be taken for granted as a cornerstone of social organization.

Criticisms such as those offered by Joan Brown and others (see Lister, ed., 1996) have encouraged a rejection of the *concept* of the underclass, as being tainted by its use as a tool of political rhetoric. This view is expressed by Ruth Lister in Extract 6.4, taken from her own introduction to the debate, which engages with the opposition between structure and agency apparent in our earlier extracts from Murray and Wilson.

Extract 6.4 Lister: 'Blaming the "underclass"? Reconciling structure and agency'

[The] explicit moralising agenda underlying Murray's [1990, 1994] account of the 'underclass' has prompted accusations, such as Alan Walker's in this volume, of 'blaming the victim'. Explanations of poverty which focus on the behaviour and values of those deemed to be members of the 'underclass' divert attention from wider social, economic and political causes. This ... has led many to prefer the less pejorative term of social exclusion. This is a more dynamic language which encourages a focus on the processes and institutions which create and maintain disadvantage rather than what can become a voyeuristic preoccupation with individual poor people and their behaviour. Social scientists are thereby encouraged no longer to gaze only in the direction of the poor and powerless, but also at the rest of society and in particular, the powerful. 'An "overclass", Mr Murray?' asks Walker. And indeed, [others have] identified just such an overclass or élite who have excluded themselves from society and from the responsibilities of citizenship associated with membership of a society. The concept of social polarisation, which would capture what is happening at the top as well as the bottom of society, has thus been advanced to complement that of social exclusion.

This is how the battle lines have been drawn up between those who subscribe to structuralist and behaviouralist approaches in explaining poverty, ... the 'classic polarity' between structure and agency. [... O]ther commentators ... suggest that the notion of an 'underclass' might offer a way of breaking down this polarity in recognition of the possible interplay between structural and cultural or behavioural factors.

Certainly, we can observe in the literature about poverty a shift away from what could be interpreted as a structural determinism in which the poor are presented as simply powerless victims. An emphasis on the structural constraints which limit the opportunities of disadvantaged groups needs to be balanced with a recognition that members of these groups are also agents or actors in their own lives. As actors there is ample evidence of the ways in which, both individually and collectively, people in poverty (and especially women) struggle to gain greater control over their own lives and to improve their situation and that of the communities in which they live. However, as actors they will make mistakes and 'wrong' decisions, like the rest of us, and there is a fine line between acknowledging the agency of people in poverty and blaming them for that poverty.

It is partly because the notion of an 'underclass' now carries such strong connotations of blame that I do not believe that it offers the means of reconciling structure and agency in helping us to understand poverty and thereby do something about it. Moreover, as I have argued, its imprecision renders it an unhelpful concept for shaping sociological research. The danger is that in searching for the 'underclass', social scientists, politicians and the media will fail to see on the one hand the structural forces which are pushing more and more people into poverty and on the other the resourcefulness and resilience with which many of these 'victims' respond.

References

Murray, C. (1990) *The Emerging British Underclass*, London, IEA.

Murray, C. (1994) *Underclass: The Crisis Deepens*, London, IEA/Sunday Times.

Walker, A. (1996) 'Blaming the victims' in Lister, R. (ed.).

(Lister, 1996, pp.11–12)

4 Gender and the underclass

At this point I would like to examine the gender subtext of the underclass debate, for although gender differentiation permeates the substance of discussion of the underclass, it is rarely made explicit in analysis. Murray sees the absence of a male role model in the family unit as central to explanation of the alleged growth of the 'underclass', and seems implicitly to suggest that the underclass is made up of men but reproduced by women. The task of socialization is thus firmly located in the family unit, and the generation of a subculture of the underclass is argued to emerge because the single mother is unable to perform that duty. There have been varied responses to this situation, as Activity 6.7 will demonstrate.

ACTIVITY 6.7

These arguments again derive originally from a US literature with each position citing different empirical evidence:

Argument A: Whereas 25 per cent of the poor were living in female-headed families in 1960, by 1980 about 35 per cent were, and by 1987 perhaps 40 per cent (Peterson, 1991, p.7). Their poverty is for the most part attributable to the low incomes provided by AFDC.

Similarly, for Britain we find 57 per cent of single mothers on incomes below £100 a week, and only 4 per cent of married couples. Conversely, 62 per cent of married couples have incomes of £350 or more per week, and only 9 per cent of single mothers (Office of National Statistics, 1996).

Argument B: In 1959, 32 per cent of the heads of poor families worked full-time, and only 31 per cent did not work at all. By 1984 these figures were 17 per cent working full-time, and 51 not working at all. Mead (1993, pp.174–9) explains this by 'rising welfare dependency by single mothers, and less regular work by single men, many of them the fathers of welfare children' … He sees the major policy task as the restoration of 'conventional work norms', especially for single parents.

In Britain it is in fact the case that single (never-married) mothers are less likely to be employed than divorced mothers – though when they are employed are more likely to work full-time (Office of National Statistics, 1996). A possible reason for their lower levels of employment is that the age of the youngest child is likely to be lower, and therefore child care will be more of a problem.

COMMENT

Argument A is the feminization of poverty argument (see, for example, Bane, 1988) which maintains that women are being forced to carry the burden of society's poverty, and that better provision should be made for them.

feminization of poverty

Argument B presents the other, more dominant, view that some work requirement is necessary for single mothers, both as a deterrent to welfare dependency and presumably to foster the work ethic in their children (see, for example, Mead, 1986).

Which position do you find more convincing, and why?

■ ■ ■

The second of the positions sketched out above shows a social control dimension to welfare, which seeks to influence behaviour by imposing conditions on welfare support, the most extreme example of which was the workhouse system. Oddly enough, this contemporary manifestation of control seems not to address the real concern expressed in the debate which centres on the alleged withdrawal of young men from the labour force. It offers a solution which, at least in traditional terms, brings women's work role and family obligations into conflict, but does not confront the problem of male unemployment.

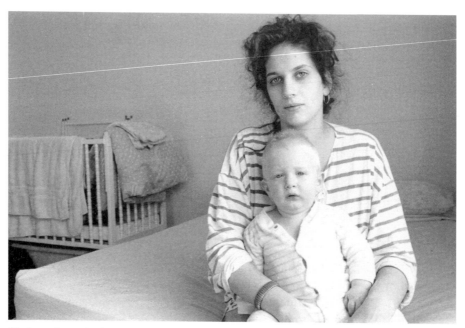

Single mother in bed and breakfast accommodation

4.1 Gendered citizenship

There is, in fact, a more fundamental problem here. To understand it we must return to the issue of social citizenship or social inclusion. Citizenship embodies a set of rights which are held by the individual in relation to the state. One of the obligations required in exchange for these rights has traditionally been the readiness of the able-bodied to work for a living. UK and US welfare provision were both originally designed to exempt married women from these obligations. Thus, AFDC was intended:

> ... to release from the wage earning role the person whose natural function is to give her children the physical and affectionate guardianship necessary ... to rear them into citizens capable of contributing to society.
>
> (Congressional Budget Office, 1987, p.7)

Similarly, for Beveridge: 'The ideal social unit is the household of man, wife and children maintained by the earnings of the first alone ...' (quoted in Land, 1980).

In other words, in both the UK and the USA one aim of the welfare system was to protect mothers from the need for employment, and so the basis for social citizenship was gendered. This is expressed most clearly in the role of work in demonstrating men's personal and social worth, while the traditional obligations of women revolved around home and family. These prescriptions do not entirely hold good for either men or women, but nor has a viable alternative been fully established in terms of work, family and welfare arrangements. The whole set of relationships is in the process of being renegotiated.

ACTIVITY 6.8

Consider the merits of these different arguments:

1   Society is pushing responsibility for its poverty onto a vulnerable population of single mothers.

2   Society in its affluence has encouraged irresponsible behaviour among women. Single mothers should have to work for their benefit.

3   Women are being forced to carry the family burden of high levels of male unemployment.

4   Welfare encourages irresponsible behaviour among men, who can avoid the responsibilities of fatherhood and employment.

5   Single mothers fail in their task of socialization and reproduce their own problems in the next generation.

Do you agree or disagree with each of these statements – and why?

COMMENT

These assertions rest on different assumptions concerning the degree of choice single mothers have about both their personal and employment circumstances. It could be that their situation is due to *male* unemployment, or to *male* irresponsibility, or a result of inadequate child care provision and poorly paid employment for *women*.

■ ■ ■

4.2   The sexual division of labour

In relation to the underclass, single mothers and social inclusion, perhaps there is an argument to say traditional gender roles have been undermined; that, at the end of the twentieth century, a majority of women are in paid employment and single mothers should be no exception to this trend. It still remains to consider the employment options which are generally available to low-skilled women in the UK and the US, and which account for the rise in recent years of married women in the labour force. Wages available to most women are not adequate for family maintenance (see Jencks, 1992, on the US, and Brown, 1989, on the UK), especially where employment opportunities are concentrated in part-time work constructed on the assumption of women's domestic role – increasingly the case in the UK. The corollary of this is that many married women are working for a secondary wage, viable only because there is another wage in the household. They are working not only for a secondary wage, but in secondary employment: low-paid, insecure and designed for cheapness and disposability. For many women, paid employment, together with mothering obligations, still requires some kind of dependency – whether it be on the state or on a husband/partner.

Thus the gender-related issues which arise from the debate about the underclass partly stem from unresolved questions about the sexual division of labour in society. Women's position in the household, and particularly the situation of single mothers, raises a number of problems for conceptions of social inclusion. As welfare dependants, they become stigmatized members of the underclass, failing in their role of socialization. Their weak position in the labour market, which is partly a result of gender segregation, means they are for the most part unable to earn sufficient to be self-supporting, and full-time employment would anyway conflict with their mothering role. It is hard to see what full social inclusion would look like for these women and, without some reassessment of the sexual division of labour in society, this will continue to be the case.

Women's full social inclusion would involve the breakdown of gender divisions in the private sphere, the removal of much private labour into the public sphere, or a more public appreciation of that private labour, as well as fundamental labour market reform. The underclass debate evades these issues by marginalizing the status of single mothers; thus single motherhood is presented as a moral issue, and as a departure from the norms and values of mainstream society. Yet the break-up of the nuclear family household is happening at the centre of society; changes to household structures and the decreasing viability of marriage as a lifetime condition are more far-reaching, and more centrally placed in society than the underclass debate has ever suggested. So, too, is a dependent status for women.

Developments in the conceptualization of social citizenship in the 1980s and 1990s have placed at least as much emphasis on obligations as on rights, the prime obligation being work as a means to self-reliance, but not care of the next generation of citizens (cf. Pateman, 1989). This places women in an ambiguous position: either they earn their 'public' citizenship rights by their own paid employment, or they perform their 'private' family obligations and remain dependent. The situation obtaining in the 1990s, however, left individual women in something of a dilemma, especially if the fathers of their children were unwilling or unable to perform *their* traditional role. These women became the new 'undeserving poor'.

Thus, the underclass debate stigmatizes women's dependency in the context of a tradition which has constructed women as dependent. This tradition has been challenged but not overcome, and is still maintained by beliefs about appropriate gender roles, beliefs about the significance of motherhood, and also by the disadvantaged position of most women in the labour market. For single mothers the dilemma is particularly clear. It is argued that the children in such households suffer from the absence of a breadwinning role model, and yet the weak position of the majority of sole mothers in the labour market prevents them from easily assuming this role themselves. Even were they to do so, this would raise the problem of child care, and more generally of whether they were meeting their traditional obligations as mothers. One response to this complex of problems has been to reaffirm strongly the logic of traditional arrangements, but any more radical solution to the impasse over women's rights to social inclusion can only be achieved by a fundamental and far-reaching review of many taken-for-granted aspects of social life.

ACTIVITY 6.9

The 'traditional' view is illustrated by the following quotes:

> I've got a little list ... (of) young ladies who get pregnant just to jump the housing list.
> *(Peter Lilley, Secretary of Sate for Social Security, Conservative Party Conference, 1992)*

> It must be right, before granting state aid, to pursue the father and see whether it is possible for him to make a financial contribution.
> *(John Redwood, Secretary of Sate for Wales, July 1993)*

> Putting girls into council flats and providing taxpayer funded childcare is a policy from hell.
> *(Stephen Green, Chairman, Conservative Family Campaign, 1993)*

1   What view of single mothers do these comments suggest?

2   Do you agree?

3   Is there an alternative view?

COMMENT

Again, you need to think here about the constraints under which single parents are living. What are their realistic possibilities of being self-reliant, and why should they attract condemnation when marriage and the nuclear family seem increasingly unstable throughout society?

■ ■ ■

What we are witnessing in the 1990s is a breakdown in the family/work/welfare nexus on a number of fronts: employment for men is in decline, the nuclear family is under challenge, and the use of welfare to fill the breach is increasingly being questioned. Yet women with children have no easy route to independence, because of their principal role in child care and their limited labour market opportunities. The public anxieties surrounding these issues have been captured by the rhetoric of the underclass, which by isolating and stigmatizing single mothers seems to offer at least a containment of the problem. That problem, however, pervades the whole of society, which is undergoing some renegotiation of the organization of work, family and welfare. The nature of that change cannot be understood through a focus on a residual group, argued to be inadequately socialized, and without whom it is believed the problems will go away.

It is interesting that concern in the UK about single mothers has not focused on their high concentrations in the black population. In part this is because *numerically* these black families are a tiny proportion of the total of single mother families. However, Phoenix (1996) makes a further comment on the UK Conservative campaign against single mothers: 'It is insiders, whose belonging to the nation cannot be easily challenged, who are the targets in such campaigns. The omission of lone black mothers in this instance still renders them pathological since it indicates they are not genuinely British.' This leaves open the possibility of an attack on other grounds, as section 5 will show.

We have so far reviewed a political debate which revolves in part around moral questions concerning acceptable behaviour, particularly as applied to men's and women's traditional work and family roles. The debate is also rooted in a growing anxiety about what the nation can afford, and the increasing size of social security spending. We are now going to shift our focus to a very different area of social concern, but one in which a similar set of issues has emerged – the challenge of international migration.

5 Migration and the national community

5.1 Strangers and citizens

The discussion so far has focused on the decreasing viability of two traditional social institutions – the nuclear family household, and the male principal earner. It was suggested earlier in this chapter that a third institution is under challenge – that of the nation-state. In addition to the male unemployed and single parents there is a third group with a precarious claim to social inclusion: members of the diverse migrant population, and particularly undocumented (or 'illegal') migrants. The distrust awakened by the 'stranger' is apparent in popular responses to migrant labour in eighteenth-century England, with settlement regulations designed to protect parishes against the costs of the 'wandering poor'. The idea was that parishes should only be called upon to support their own members. Where movements occur across national boundaries these issues are all the more salient, and necessarily involve questions of citizenship and the social rights which follow from citizenship.

An obvious example concerns the circumstances and conditions of labour migration across socio-political boundaries, the place of the new arrival in the social and economic structures of the receiving 'community', and the rights of this individual to the resources and protections the 'community' conventionally offered to its citizens. As we shall see, the acceptance of migrant labour has often been designed to be partial; to take the labour without conferring the rights of membership. We see below how Carens (1988) has considered the philosophical roots of such issues in the context of Mexican migration into the United States. In the next section we examine the negotiation and renegotiation of these matters in relation to migration into the European Union.

Note that the terms 'migration' and 'immigration' tend to be used interchangeably. While *migration* perhaps implies temporary flows, and *immigration* more permanent settlement, this distinction is by no means clear in usage or in practice.

undocumented migrants
'stranger'

5.2 The morality of membership

The conventional moral view is that a country is justified in restricting immigration whenever it serves the national interests to do so.

(Carens, 1988, p.207)

In contemporary society concern about accelerating demands upon the welfare state is an issue that commonly arises in relation to immigration. The usual fear is that large-scale migration will undermine the will and the capacity to support the institutions of welfare. Conversely, we also find the popular argument that immigrants are taking employment from the indigenous population. However:

Almost all of the illegal immigrants and many of the legal immigrants are unskilled people eager to find jobs of any kind and prepared to accept difficult, unpleasant work at rates of pay that are low by American standards because these jobs are much better than whatever work (if any) they can find in their native land.

(Carens, 1988, p.210)

Jobs of the kind conventionally filled by migrant labour in the US offer terms and conditions which fail to live up to the promise of full participation in the accepted standards of life for US citizens. They do not rival even the precarious existence available outside of employment, and can be filled only by workers with origins outside that 'community' of reference – usually the nation-state. Temporary migrants are not normally granted access to welfare supports, and undocumented migrants are particularly vulnerable in this respect, afraid to declare their presence to any 'official' organization. Carens goes on to argue that: 'The existence of such a vulnerable, exploited *underclass* is incompatible with the goal of creating a society in which all members are regarded as having "equal social worth" and equal social, legal and political rights.'

If this group's passage across national borders was against the laws and conditions of entry, what could be the legitimate basis of their claim to such rights? Yet if they are recruited to perform the least rewarding and most poorly paid tasks by another society, then arguably their exclusion from full membership in the community of rights is on dubious grounds. Access to 'membership', and the rights it carries, thus raises a number of difficult questions, both moral and financial.

community of rights

Are you able to distinguish between those who belong in our society and those who do not? Should people arriving in this country from abroad have a right to claim social support from our health and social security system?

These questions are compounded if the migrant can be deemed to be in some sense inherently 'foreign', i.e. to be of different 'racial' or ethnic or cultural origin. The receiving 'communities' may then object to their presence in defence of a claimed common identity and distinctive way of life.

ACTIVITY 6.10

The link between nationalist sentiments of this kind and 'racism' are discussed in Extract 6.5 from Balibar's (1991) work. As you will see on reading this piece, the precise role of 'race' in relation to migration, citizenship and national identity poses complex questions.

Extract 6.5 Balibar: 'Racism and nationalism'

Racist organizations most often refuse to be designated as such, laying claim instead to the title of *nationalist* and claiming that the two notions cannot be equated. Is this merely a tactical ploy or the symptom of a fear of words inherent in the racist attitude? In fact the discourses of race and nation are never very far apart, if only in the form of disavowal: thus the presence of 'immigrants' on French soil is referred to as the cause of an 'anti-French racism'. The oscillation of the vocabulary itself suggests to us then that, at least in already constituted national states, the organization of nationalism into individual political movements inevitably has racism underlying it.

At least one section of historians has used this to argue that racism – as theoretical discourse and as mass phenomenon – develops 'within the field of nationalism', which is ubiquitous in the modern era. In this view, nationalism would be, if not the sole cause of racism, then at least the determining condition of its production. Or, it is also argued, the 'economic' explanations (in terms of the effects of crises) or 'psychological' explanations (in terms of the ambivalence of the sense of personal identity and collective belonging) are pertinent in that they cast light upon presuppositions or subsidiary effects of nationalism.

Such a thesis confirms, without doubt, that racism has nothing to do with the existence of objective biological 'races'. It shows that racism is a historical – or cultural – product, while avoiding the equivocal position of 'culturalist' explanations which, from another angle, also tend to make racism into a sort of invariant of human nature. It has the advantage of breaking the circle which traces the psychology of racism back to explanations which are themselves purely psychological. Lastly, it performs a critical function in relation to the euphemistic strategies of other historians who are very careful to place racism *outside* the field of nationalism as such, as if it were possible to define the latter without including the racist movements in it, and therefore without going back to the social relations which give rise to such movements and are indissociable from contemporary nationalism (in particular, imperialism). However, this accumulation of good reasons does not necessarily imply that racism is an inevitable consequence of nationalism, nor, *a fortiori*, that without the existence of an overt or latent racism, nationalism would itself be historically impossible. These categories and the connections between them continue to be rather hazy. We should not be afraid to investigate at some length why no form of conceptual 'purism' will work here.

(Balibar, 1991, pp.37–8)

COMMENT

The question being posed here is whether assertions of national distinctiveness are by their nature racist, and even whether an opposing racism is activated against the host society by the presence of migrant groups. Certainly the exclusive claims to membership on which nationalism is founded seem, at the least, to provide a good breeding-ground for racist sentiment. This drawing of boundaries of inclusion and exclusion is not, however, on grounds of *biological* difference. Rather, it is grounded in the emotions attaching to 'nationhood', prompted either by resource protectionism, or identity formation. While nationalism may not be inherently racist, it is conducive to racism and may serve to legitimize it.

■ ■ ■

5.3 The boundaries of membership

We have already considered some aspects of social exclusion in relation to the concept of the 'underclass'. We have also looked at its counterpart, social citizenship, defined by T.H. Marshall as 'full membership of a community', for purposes of civil, political and social rights and duties. However, Marshall's treatment of citizenship has been argued by various writers (Yuval-Davis, 1990; Held, 1989) to be deficient in a number of ways, notably through its emphasis on social class as the main social differentiator, and through an implicit confinement to the nation-state. Yuval-Davis (1990, p.3), in arguing this point, problematizes the notion of 'community': 'It assumes a given collectivity ... (not) an ideological and material construction, whose boundaries, structures and norms are a result of constant processes of struggles and negotiations, or more general social developments. Any dynamic notion of citizenship must start from the processes which construct the collectivity.'

The determinants of community membership need therefore to be brought to the fore, an issue which Marshall fails to address. Traditionally we have assumed that the boundaries of society coincide with the territory of the nation-state, but increasingly there are both economic and political dynamics which challenge this assumption. Writers are beginning to identify a tension between citizenship, national sovereignty and international law (see, for example, Held, 1989). The construction of a labour supply with a particular, disadvantaged relation to the nation-state and therefore with limited claims to membership of the 'community' which that state represents, is one particular aspect of this tension. It poses a knot of problems for the relationship between the construction of an 'underclass' of foreign workers, the status of outsider, and claims to social rights.

Access to welfare is one of the central issues in the denial of full membership for foreign workers and there has been a number of different ways of restricting these rights. The presence of such a population, however, offers support for the view that there are jobs available for those willing to work, and that welfare dependants thus constitute an 'underclass' in the sense of optional withdrawal from the labour market. These concerns have long been identified in the United States (for example, Mead, 1986), but in the 1990s emerged in the very particular context of the European Union.

5.4 The case of post-war Europe

In the post-war period the industrialized countries of Western Europe faced a labour crisis: there was insufficient indigenous labour to fill the less desirable jobs in their growing economies. The problem was principally solved in two different ways: countries with access to a colonial labour force (such as the UK, France and the Netherlands) could encourage inward migration, while others relied on recruitment through a 'guestworker' system (for example, Germany, Belgium and Switzerland), though both categories of worker were expected to be temporary:

> Jobs filled by these workers were ones which were less acceptable to the indigenous workforce. They were disproportionately employed in jobs which required arduous physical effort, had poor working conditions, had little security and in some instances their employment was subject to seasonal variation and redundancy. These features of the work experience were common to ex-colonial labour and guestworkers alike.
> (Nanton, 1991, p.92)

guestworker

Thus the common pattern was confinement to a narrow range of low status, insecure jobs, which would otherwise be difficult to fill, and which is often subject to fluctuations in demand. Like Mexican labour in the USA, foreign workers were employed where they were willing to work on terms unacceptable to indigenous labour and were intended to be expendable. The rights and status of foreign workers show some variation between countries. While colonial labour more often carried access to formal citizenship, true guestworkers were more precariously placed, granted only legal residence and often with conditions attached.

By the early 1970s the demand for labour had fallen in all receiving countries, who by then wished to limit entry. They began to seek ways of restricting or dismissing their foreign workers, some of which were inherent in the original terms permitting entry. The guestworker systems in Germany and Switzerland were arguably most severe in these terms, and these countries had more success than others in immediately reducing (though not eliminating) their foreign workforce. In the UK, however, there were legislative changes over a longer period which removed the right of people from black Commonwealth countries to full UK citizenship. In all cases the 'temporary' workers proved more difficult to remove than had been anticipated, many having settled and produced second and third generations.

5.5   A changing pattern of entry

reserve army of labour

While the nation-states of Europe were implicated in the structuring of a reserve army of labour, whether from their colonies or as 'guestworkers', the neat coincidence between economic demand and political supply was short-lived. As temporary migrants started to look permanent, political concern became more narrowly focused on securing the resources of the welfare state and the closure of national boundaries. There was also concern about 'racial' tension. However, despite explicit attempts to limit entry by all EU countries, they have only succeeded in changing its form. The workers brought in as labour for the post-war expansion have, in many cases, settled permanently and acquired a wide range of associated rights, including welfare rights. Although state initiatives to recruit labour no longer existed in the 1990s, a continuing flow of clandestine migrants was still welcomed by a number of employers – typically, but not exclusively, in agriculture and construction.

transnational human rights

However, 'legal' migration also continued to grow, despite explicit policies to the contrary. Against the logic of national and regional exclusion came another distinctive post-war development: the emergence of rights located outside of national belonging, in the form of transnational human rights. These rights are by nature universal, and are given their form by international conventions. Their growing importance has been at the heart of speculation about an emergent 'post-national' citizenship (Soysal, 1994) or a 'global society' (Giddens, 1992), and potentially cuts across any specifically national set of concerns. It is in fact through the assertion of rights to asylum and to family reunification that migration has continued to grow in the face of explicit attempts since the 1970s to bring it to an end.

asylum-seeker

By 1990 there were 13 million legally settled non-Europeans (i.e. non-citizens of any EU country) in the twelve countries of the EU, and an unknown number of undocumented migrants. The figures in Table 6.1 show inflows of foreign population for selected years to the UK, France and Germany, followed by the inflow of asylum-seekers, that is, those arrivals seeking protection against persecution under the 1951 Geneva Convention. While these *inflow* figures are reasonably reliable, statistics on *settled* populations present more problems.

ACTIVITY 6.11

Migration statistics are notoriously misleading, partly because they include only officially recognised residents, thus omitting the 'illegal' or 'undocumented' migrants. They also tend to be records of nationality, and many of the early colonial immigrants either arrived with or subsequently acquired the nationality of their 'host' country. In this respect there is considerable variation between countries and across time.

Table 6.1 Immigrants and asylum-seekers to United Kingdom, France and Germany (thousands)

	Inflow of (total) foreign population				
	1985	*1990*	*1992*	*1993*	*1994*
United Kingdom	55.4	52.4	52.6	55.5	–
France	43.4	102.4	116.6	99.2	–
Germany*	398.2	842.4	1207.6	986.9	–

	Inflow of asylum-seekers				
	1985	*1990*	*1992*	*1993*	*1994*
United Kingdom	6.2	38.2	32.3	28.5	41.0
France	28.8	54.8	28.9	27.6	26.0
Germany	73.8	193.1	438.2	322.6	127.2

Note: *West Germany upto 1990; the re-unified Germany from 1991 on.

Source: SOPEMI, 1995, Tables A.2 and A.3, p.195

In the UK, for example, there was automatic citizenship for Commonwealth immigrants until a series of restrictions were introduced, beginning in 1962. Similarly, many immigrants from the French colonies have French citizenship, while German citizenship is extremely difficult to acquire, in part because of the refusal to allow dual citizenship – immigrants therefore have to give up their original citizenship to acquire German citizenship. Figures based on 'nationality' do, however, serve to reveal the size of the officially recognized population who nevertheless lack full citizenship rights. The 1993 figures of 'foreign' residents (i.e. non-citizens) for selected EU countries, as a percentage of total population, are as follows: Britain 3.5 per cent; France 6.3 per cent; Germany 8.5 per cent; Belgium 9.1 per cent; Italy 1.7 per cent (SOPEMI, 1995, p.194).

1 What are the problems attaching to comparisons of this kind?

2 Why are statistics based on citizenship misleading?

3 Why would data on 'illegal' migrants be difficult to gather?

COMMENT

The most disadvantaged members of the migrant population, and those about whom least is known, are the undocumented or 'illegal' migrants. They are not represented in official statistics by virtue of their necessarily hidden presence, and fear of all contacts with 'authority'. Conversely, other migrants who arrived with citizenship of the 'host' society, or subsequently acquired it, still experience many disadvantages but are recorded as nationals in official statistics on migration. These statistics thus give only a partial and possibly misleading picture of the make-up of the total population and the social position of different migrant groups.

6   A European single market

6.1   Fortress Europe

The circumstances described so far combine to pose a challenge to the idea of European citizenship and European integration. The principal objective of the European Union has been the realization of a common market, envisaged in the Treaty of Rome 1957 and given urgency by the Single European Act 1986. This Act contained a commitment to establishing, by 1992, a frontier-free area for the movement of goods, persons, services and capital. It immediately raises two questions which have proved contentious: what categories of person are to be granted free movement; and, in the absence of frontiers between member-states, where will ultimate authority over entry lie?

By the late 1990s the decision had been to extend free movement only to citizens of the member-states of the EU, and not to the many non-EU citizens legally resident: 'Member countries do not want them to demand work in their countries because up until now they did not have any say in the way the entrance policies of the other member countries have worked' (House of Lords, 1992, p.9). In fact, even for nationals of member-states, the 'right' to residence is largely conditional upon not being a charge on the state, i.e. having no recourse to public funds. For non-economically active groups, residence in another member-state requires sufficient resources for maintenance, while those seeking employment must be established as workers before full benefit rights are granted.

At least one source of resistance to extending free movement to non-EU citizens is the defence of national resources. As we have seen, Freeman (1986, p.51) has argued that the welfare state is necessarily bounded, indeed that 'national welfare states cannot co-exist with the free movement of labour'. Its financial logic depends on the designation of a limited community of people

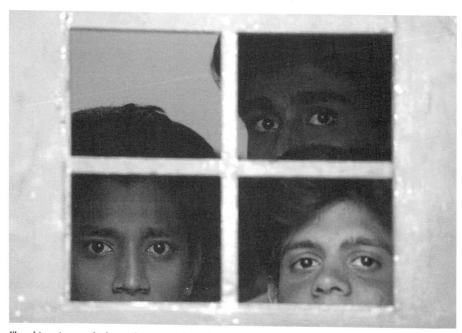

Illegal immigrants look out from a prison cell window in Greece

who can make a claim. Developing hand in hand with the nation-state, it has traditionally required the exclusion of less affluent peoples, and for Freeman, this is the central concern in control over entry to the national territory. Thus, in Baubock's (1991, p.3) terms: 'The more substance the internal rights of citizenship acquire, the more important it seems to police the frontiers of the state.'

Attempts to establish a frontier-free Europe, together with the contested status of non-EU citizens, immediately sets up a series of tensions. If free movement were granted to these populations from outside Europe, then the immigration decisions of one country would have an ultimate impact on those of another. The member-states differ both in terms of the nature and structure of their economies, and also the nature of their policies and degree of practical control over migration. The countries of southern Europe – Spain, Greece, Italy – have fewer 'official' entries but higher levels of undocumented migration, which have in part been dealt with by offers of 'regularization', i.e. the legalization of their status in periods of amnesty.

An extension of free movement to these non-EU residents would mean that the greater accessibility of Europe's southern countries to clandestine migrants from the third world would ultimately affect the populations and resources of the more developed countries of the north (the UK, France, Germany). One of the fears which underlies resistance to extending free movement to all is that it opens up the possibility of 'social dumping' – complete freedom of movement in an integrated labour market could mean that countries with high unemployment or low social welfare provision would effectively export their unemployment to countries with jobs to offer or better welfare systems – unless there was a shift to a European-wide system of social protection. So far, the emphasis has been rather on attempts to harmonize the conditions and control of entry across Europe, to restrict free movement to EU citizens, and to limit eligibility for social support. These decisions rebound disproportionately on non-white populations from impoverished third world countries, and also on non-EU countries of the old Soviet bloc.

6.2 The British response

In so far as nationals of other member-states have welfare rights in the UK, they are narrowly defined, and derive from their status as workers. Contributory benefits are transferable across Europe, but means-tested social assistance is not. This distinction became an issue in the UK in October 1993, when the Secretary of State for Social Security, Peter Lilley, speaking on the right to free movement declared: 'Community rules have opened up a new abuse: "benefit tourism". People travelling round pretending to look for work, but really looking for the best benefits. Not so much a Cook's tour as a Crook's tour' (Conservative Party Press Release, 6 October 1993).

The vast majority of arrivals in the UK are admitted on the condition of no 'recourse to public funds'. EU citizens (who automatically have the right to work and reside) were, however, permitted six months on income support while seeking employment. It was this entitlement which came to be the focus of a 'habitual residence' test, denying means-tested benefit to those who had not already established residence. This is not necessarily out of line with the practice in other EU countries, which is quite varied. It does, however, move the UK from the more generous to the less generous end of the scale, and serves as an example of the link between welfare protectionism and the restriction of migrants' rights.

A further effect of the rule is to deny benefit to UK citizens who have, for various reasons, spent time abroad, possibly exercising their right of free movement in Europe. As with controls on entry, this disproportionately affects black and ethnic minority residents – often UK citizens, with ties outside the UK. In a discussion of the UK citizens affected by the test, the Parliamentary Under Secretary of State for Social Security told the House of Lords: 'These people were strangers to this country and were certainly strangers to the Pay-As-You-Earn system, the tax system or the national insurance system' (*Lords Hansard*, 20 October 1995, col. 394).

Separate proposals also undertake to deny non-contributory benefits for those whose entry was 'sponsored' by other residents who undertook to provide for them; even before this, their sponsors could be faced with a demand for financial compensation for a claim for non-contributory benefit.

Can you see any parallels between debates about the 'underclass' and the treatment of 'strangers' discussed above?

6.3   Asylum-seekers and benefits

Another change in social security legislation in the 1990s, also designed to limit access to benefits, has been aimed at asylum-seekers. There has been a rapid growth in their numbers across Europe since the mid 1980s, and many believe that a majority of asylum-seekers are 'bogus', that is they are not genuinely fleeing persecution but are in fact 'economic migrants'. Without solid evidence to this effect, but as part of an attempt to discourage their arrival in the UK and, it is argued, to defend national resources, a change was made in the benefit rules.

In the UK, until February 1996, those seeking asylum were eligible for benefits until a judgement on their case had been made. New regulations were introduced such that while those seeking asylum at their point of entry to the country would continue to qualify, those whose entry is on other grounds, but who later make an asylum claim, would not. The regulation was over-ruled by the appeal court which concluded it was 'uncompromisingly draconian' and produced 'a life so destitute that … no civilized nation can tolerate it' (*The Guardian*, 22 June 1996). It was, however, re-established in the Asylum and Immigration Bill 1996.

Seventy per cent of asylum claims are made by people who enter the country as tourists, students, business people, or 'illegally', and subsequently make an asylum claim. It is argued that the experience of persecution, and the general personal confusion associated with their flight, make many asylum-seekers wary of authority. They are therefore inclined to gain entry to a country and seek advice and support before officially declaring themselves. The new legislation means that, in doing so, they will forfeit their claim to benefit. A more recent ruling, however, upheld the responsibility of local authorities to make provision for the destitute – setting the scene for a struggle between central and local government. These decisions are traced in two articles from the *The Guardian* reproduced here. While the Labour government elected in May 1997 undertook to study the position of asylum-seekers, six months after their election there had been no commitment to reinstate benefit rights for all.

Lilley evades asylum ruling

Alan Travis
Home Affairs Editor

THE Government is to overturn last week's Appeal Court judgement on withdrawing welfare benefits from most asylum seekers by rushing emergency asylum legislation through Parliament.

Social Security Secretary Peter Lilley insisted the measures were essential if Britain was to remain a safe haven for genuine refugees and not a 'soft touch' for false claimants. 'We are determined that this judgment will not provide a blank cheque for bogus asylum seekers,' he said.

But his Commons statement caused an outcry. Labour said the plan to rush though a series of amendments to the Asylum and Immigration Bill was an 'abuse of process', while immigrants' rights groups called it a 'moral outrage'.

...

Mr Lilley said the new legislation would write into statute the power to exclude benefits from asylum seekers who failed to claim refugee status when they first arrived, or whose claim had been rejected but were appealing.

He offered one small concession by saying that those whose asylum claims were eventually granted in full would receive a welfare benefit payment backdated to the day they lodged a claim for refugee status.

...

Refugee Council director, Nick Hardwick, was disturbed about the details of the package: 'The new proposals won't work because it takes an average of 18 months to have asylum claims finally determined – how is a person supposed to survive in the meantime?'

Labour's Social Security spokesman, Chris Smith, said the decision to 'judgeproof' the legislation only highlighted the Government's incompetence.

He told Mr Lilley: 'In a supposedly civilised country, you are leaving people to starve. You have acted with both inhumanity and injustice. Will you now think again and abandon your foolish intention to legislate your way around the problem?'

In their ruling last Friday, the senior judges described Mr Lilley's policy of withdrawing welfare benefits as 'uncompromisingly draconian' and ruled it illegal. They said Mr Lilley and Michael Howard, the Home Secretary, had been less generous towards 'poor foreigners' than the government had been in Napoleonic times and were effectively denying asylum seekers appeal rights.

More than 8,000 people seeking asylum in Britain have been left without official means of support since their entitlement to claim benefits was withdrawn on February 5.

...

(The Guardian, 25 June 1996, p.1)

In what way do these developments serve as an example of the tension between the assertion of human rights, the defence of national sovereignty and the protection of 'national resources'?

The overall result of differing forms of migration has been a proliferation of statuses in relation to social citizenship. This constitutes what might be termed a form of civic stratification, an emerging form of inequality in which groups of people are differentiated by the legitimate claims they can make on the state (Morris, 1997). The weakest position is occupied by those who entered the country clandestinely. While they may be paying into the welfare state by virtue of their employment, their illegal status and fear of discovery makes any claim on public provisions impossible. In fact, public services and employers are increasingly being used as a means of policing immigration.

Slightly better placed than 'illegal' migrants are the asylum-seekers described above, whose entry into the country was on other terms and who, as a result, must sacrifice the right to benefits. There are other legally resident groups who have no legitimate claim on state support, notably the non-economically active groups exercising their rights to free movement in Europe. In so far as citizens of other member-states have a legitimate claim to benefit, it is narrowly tied to their status as workers. Only contributory unemployment benefit is transferable

Ministers acted illegally in leaving 10,000 destitute

Judge's swipe at new asylum law

Alan Travis
Home Affairs Editor

A HIGH Court judge yesterday told the Government it was illegal for ministers to leave 10,000 asylum seekers destitute on the streets of Britain, facing the risk of serious illness or death.

Mr Justice Collins, giving judgment in four test cases, said local authorities had a duty dating back to welfare state legislation passed by the 1945 Labour government to provide 'the basics for survival' for those in need.

The judgment strikes at Home Secretary Michael Howard's policy of trying to deter asylum applicants coming to Britain, enshrined in the Asylum and Immigration Act which reached the statute book only three months ago.

While refugee groups were jubilant at the ruling the Home Office expressed its disappointment. Local authorities, now facing a bill which would run into millions, started preparations to set up a temporary tent city on Wormwood Scrubs, west London, to house some of the refugees.

Mr Howard's Asylum and Immigration Act reached the statute book only three months ago and was supposed to have removed the access of would-be refugees to welfare benefits and public housing.

The case yesterday was brought by the Refugee Council on behalf of four asylum seekers, a Chinese, an Iraqi Kurd, a Romanian and an Algerian, against Westminster, Hammersmith and Fulham, and Lambeth councils.

David Pannick, QC, argued that the three councils had breached their duties under the 1948 National Assistance Act to provide housing for destitute applicants who could not look after themselves.

Mr Justice Collins not only agreed but challenged ministers in his ruling. He said he found it impossible to believe that Parliament intended that asylum seekers 'should be left destitute, starving and at risk of grave illness and even death'. None is allowed to work during the first six months while the asylum application is considered.

In his judgment Mr Justice Collins said: 'No doubt it was hoped that the bogus would thereby be deterred from coming or forced to return whence they came, but if an entrant faced the dilemma and decided he had to stay because to return would be to court persecution, I am sure Parliament would not have intended he be left to starve.'

The Home Office said it was disappointed by the decision. 'It cannot be right that people who enter the UK on the basis that they can maintain and accommodate themselves without resort to public funds should become eligible simply by claiming asylum,' said a Home Office spokeswoman.

A similar High Court ruling in June that the Social Security Secretary Peter Lilley had acted unlawfully in withdrawing benefit from refugees who failed to claim asylum on arrival in Britain, was reversed by the introduction of emergency legislation.

(The Guardian, 9 October 1996, p.10)

across member-states, and a job-seeker is anyway limited to three months in receipt of such benefit. The habitual residence test denies means-tested benefit to those who have not first established themselves in the labour market, and in doing so rebounds on UK citizens who spend time abroad. Most of the indigenous unemployed are better placed, though even their right to benefit has gradually been eroded over the years, with ever-tightening conditions of job search.

7   Conclusion

In this chapter you have been asked to think about how the 'welfare community' is constructed. Given finite resources there will always be limits to provision, and we have been concerned here with debates on the position of three key groupings – the long-term unemployed, single parents and migrants. We began by noting the persistence throughout history of 'outsider' groups, whose claims for support have been viewed with suspicion. The basis of such suspicion has often been grounded in doubts about moral desert, and we briefly considered some of the forms this has taken.

These moral judgements strike an odd note when set against the ideals of the UK welfare system established under the Beveridge plan. The intention of securing reasonable standards for all, what T.H. Marshall (1950) termed social citizenship, seems inconsistent with judgements about worth and desert. Such questions have nevertheless been an element of contemporary debate about the 'underclass', generally understood to refer to those either materially or behaviourally 'outside' mainstream society. The all-important *explanation* for their position, however, is contested, and with it the validity of their claim to public funds. Broadly speaking we identified a *structural* approach which emphasized changing economic conditions, and a *behavioural* or *cultural* approach which emphasized individual motivation. The former position tends to be associated with collective responsibility for disadvantage, and the latter with individual responsibility.

The two principal target groups in this debate are the long-term unemployed and single mothers. Those seeking to limit claims on the public purse call into question the individual motivations of both groups by postulating the creation of a 'dependency culture'. Linked to this position we find a growing emphasis not simply on social rights but also social obligations. The foremost of these is self-reliance, and with it the readiness to work for a living. Hence the scrutiny of the unemployed, and the 'actively seeking work' conditions attached to their receipt of benefit.

If readiness to work is to be the basis of social inclusion then single parents are placed in something of a dilemma. To explore this dilemma we asked what the basis for women's social citizenship could be, given a tradition of child care and domesticity which constructs women as dependent. Most markedly for single mothers, but also for many other women, the work role and the family role are in conflict. Often commanding only poor employment and inadequate income, mothers of young children must depend either on the state or on a partner. The debate about the underclass thus serves to open up a series of wider questions about gender roles in society, and the viability of traditional models of behaviour.

In the last two sections we moved to consider an apparently different issue, that of the position of migrant groups in society. In fact, we found parallel questions about legitimate membership of the welfare community. The position of migrant workers and asylum-seekers highlighted a set of problems relating to the right to social inclusion. If a society appropriates labour, must it also confer rights, and is the narrow defence of national resources overridden by the assertion of universal human rights? As with the long-term unemployed and single mothers, questions are being raised about the foundations for a legitimate claim to social support. Just as the mesh between work, family and welfare is being unravelled, so too is that between nation, citizenship and rights – but not without resistance from the nation-state. What is difficult to assess, at the end of the 1990s, is how far the developments documented here are the product of eighteen years of Conservative government, and how far they represent broader features inherent in late capitalism.

Further reading

The two books central to the US debate about the underclass are Charles Murray's (1984) *Losing Ground* and William Julius Wilson's (1987) *The Truly Disadvantaged*. Murray's book focuses on the US welfare system and its escalating costs over the period 1950–80. His argument is that, by encouraging dependence, welfare actually exacerbates the problems it is supposed to address. Wilson's book reviews the US underclass debate and various policy responses. His argument emphasizes the social effects of changes in the economic structure which leave a section of the working-class black population suffering the impact of decline of heavy industry, and marooned in inner-city areas which offer no alternative employment opportunities. He is critical of welfare-based explanations of inner-city problems. Jencks (1992) re-opens many of these issues in his *Rethinking Social Policy*.

The British debate on the underclass, however, has been more immediately influenced by Murray, who visited the UK to announce that we were following the same path as the USA. *The Emerging British Underclass* (Murray, 1990) features his comments on the UK, together with a number of responses from British writers. This debate has been updated in a collection of further contemporary comment from British writers and a substantial introduction by Ruth Lister (Lister, ed., 1996). She argues against the term 'underclass' and its inevitable simplifications. A more specialized book by Kirk Mann (1992), *The Making of an English 'Underclass'?*, gives a historical class-based account of the construction of social divisions in relation to the the UK welfare system.

For a historical classic, see Stedman Jones' (1971) *Outcast London* on the class relations of Victorian London; this provides considerable detail of the stigmatization of the poor in the nineteenth century. Morris (1994) reviews the development of the UK and US debates on the underclass, but also includes a chapter on its historical precursors, and extends the debate to consider gender divisions and migrant groups in Europe.

The issue of the rights of migrants in Europe is addressed by Soysal (1994), who argues that we are moving towards a post-national society in which national citizenship is no longer the exclusive basis for social rights. For a critique of this argument, see Morris (1997).

References

Auletta, K. (1982) *The Underclass*, New York, Random House.

Balibar, E. (1991) 'Racism and nationalism' in Balibar, E. and Wallerstein, I., *Race, Nation, Class: Ambiguous Identities*, London, Verso.

Bane, M.J. (1988) 'Politics and policies of the feminization of poverty' in Weir, M., Orloff, A. S. and Skocpol, T. (eds) *The Politics of Social Policy in the United States*, Princeton, NJ, Princeton University Press.

Baubock, W. (1991) *Immigration and the Boundaries of Citizenship*, Warwick, Centre for Research in Ethnic Relations.

Beveridge Report (1942) *Social Insurance and Allied Services*, Cmnd 6404, London, HMSO.

Booth, C. (1902) *Life and Labour of the People of London*, London, Macmillan.

Brown J. (1988) *Victims or Villains?*, Studies of the Social Security System No. 16, London, Policy Studies Institute.

Brown, J. (1989) *Why Don't They Go to Work?*, London, HMSO.

Brown, J. (1990) 'The focus on single mothers' in Murray, C. (1990).

Carens, J.H. (1988) 'Immigration and the welfare state' in Gutman, A. (ed.) *Democracy and the Welfare State*, Princeton, NJ, Princeton University Press, pp.201–30.

Chadwick, E. (1842) *Report on the Sanitary Conditions of the Labouring Population of Great Britain*, Parliamentary Paper XXVI.

Congressional Budget Office (1987) *Work-related Programs for Welfare Recipients*, Washington, DC, CBO.

Department of Employment (1988) *Employment for the 1990s*, Cm. 540, London, HMSO.

Ermisch, J. (1986) *The Economics of the Family: Applications to Divorce and Remarriage*, Discussion Paper 40, London, Centre for Economic Policy Research.

Fainstein, N. (1987) 'The underclass mismatch hypothesis as an explanation for black economic deprivation', *Politics and Society*, vol.15, pp.403–51.

Field, F. (1989) *Losing Out*, Oxford, Basil Blackwell.

Fraser, D. (1986) *The Evolution of the British Welfare State*, London, Macmillan.

Freeman, G. (1986) 'Migration and the political economy of the welfare state', *Annals of the American Academy of the Political and Social Sciences*, vol.526, pp.51–63.

Fulbrook, J. (1978) *Administrative Justice and the Unemployed*, London, Mansell.

Giddens, A. (1992) *The Consequences of Modernity*, Cambridge, Polity Press.

Held, D. (1989) 'Citizenship and autonomy' in Held, D. and Thompson, J.B. (eds) *Social Theory and Modern Societies*, Cambridge, Cambridge University Press, pp. 162–84.

Herrnstein, R.J. and Murray, C. (1994) *The Bell Curve*, New York, Free Press.

Hills, J. (1995) *Income and Wealth: Report of the JRF Enquiry Group*, York, Joseph Rowntree Foundation.

House of Lords (1992) *Community Policy on Migration*, HL Paper 35, London, HMSO.

Hudson, L. (1994) 'The wretched connection', *Times Literary Supplement*, 2 December.

Jencks, C. (1992) *Rethinking Social Policy*, Cambridge, MA, Harvard University Press.

Jones, G. (1980) *Social Darwinism and English Thought*, Brighton, Harvester Press.

Jordan, B., James, S., Kay, H. and Redley, M. (1992) *Trapped in Poverty*, London, Routledge.

Land, H. (1980) 'The family wage', *Feminist Review*, vol.6, pp.55–77.

Lewis, O. (1968) *A Study of Slum Culture*, New York, Random House.

Lister, R. (ed.) (1996) *Charles Murray and the Underclass: The Developing Debate*, London, Institute of Economic Affairs.

McLaughlin, E., Millar, J. and Cooke, K. (1989) *Work and Welfare Benefits*, Aldershot, Avebury.

Malthus, T.R. (1806/1989) *An Essay on the Principle of Population*, vol.2, James, P. (ed.), Cambridge, Cambridge University Press.

Mann, K. (1992) *The Making of an English 'Underclass'? The Social Divisions of Welfare and Labour*, Buckingham, Open University Press.

Marshall, T.H. (1950) *Citizenship and Social Class*, Cambridge, Cambridge University Press.

Marx, K. and Engels, F. (1848/1853/1951) *Karl Marx and Frederick Engels, Selected Works*, vol.1, London, Lawrence and Wishart.

Mayhew, H. (1861) *London Labour and the London Poor: The Condition and Earnings of Those that Will Work, Cannot Work and Will Not Work*, vol.1, London, Griffin, Bohn and Co.

Mead, L.M. (1986) *Beyond Entitlement*, New York, Free Press.

Mead, L.M. (1993) 'The logic of workfare' in Wilson, W.J. (ed.).

Micklewright, J. (1986) *Unemployment and Incentives to Work: Policy Evidence in the 1980s*, Discussion Paper 92, ESRC Programme on Taxation Incentives and the Distribution of Income, London, London School of Economics.

Morris, L. (1994) *Dangerous Classes: The Underclass and Social Citizenship*, London, Routledge.

Morris, L. (1996) 'Researching living standards', *Journal of Social Policy*, vol.25, pp.459–83.

Morris, L. (1997) 'A cluster of contradictions: the politics of migration in the EU', *Sociology*, vol.31, pp.241–59.

Murray, C. (1984) *Losing Ground*, New York, Basic Books.

Murray, C. (with commentaries by others) (1990) *The Emerging British Underclass*, Choice in Welfare Series No. 2, London, Institute of Economic Affairs.

Nanton, P. (1991) 'National frameworks and the implementation of local policies', *Policy and Politics*, vol.19, pp. 191–7.

Office of National Statistics (1996) *Living in Britain*, London, HMSO.

Pateman, C. (1989) *The Disorder of Women*, Cambridge, Polity Press.

Peterson, P.E. (1991) 'The urban underclass and the poverty paradox' in Jencks, C. and Peterson, P.E. (eds) *The Urban Underclass*, Washington, DC, Brookings Institute.

Phoenix, A. (1996) 'Social constructions of lone motherhood' in Bortolaia Silva, E. (ed.) *Good Enough Mothering? Feminist Perspectives on Lone Motherhood*, London, Routledge, pp.175–90.

Rex, J. and Moore, R. (1967) *Race, Community and Conflict*, London, Oxford University Press.

Rex, J. and Tomlinson, S. (1979) *Colonial Immigrants in a British City*, London, Routledge and Kegan Paul.

Rutter, M. and Madge, N. (1976) *Cycles of Disadvantage*, London, Heinemann.

Smith, S. (1885) 'The industrial training of destitute children', *Contemporary Review*, vol.XLVII.

SOPEMI (1995) *Trends in International Migration, Annual Report 1994*, Paris, OECD.

Soysal, Y.N. (1994) *Limits of Citizenship*, Chicago, IL, Chicago University Press.

Stedman Jones, G. (1971) *Outcast London*, London, Oxford University Press.

Wilson, W.J. (1978) *The Declining Significance of Race: Blacks and Changing American Institutions*, Chicago, IL, Chicago University Press.

Wilson, W.J. (1987) *The Truly Disadvantaged: The Inner City, The Underclass and Public Policy*, Chicago, IL, Chicago University Press.

Wilson, W.J. (ed.) (1993) *The Ghetto Underclass: Social Science Perspectives* (updated edn), London, Sage.

Yuval-Davis, N. (1990) *Women, the State and Ethnic Processes*, paper presented at the Racism and Migration Conference, Hamburg.

CHAPTER 7

Review

by John Clarke and Mary Langan

Contents

1   Introduction

This book has explored the central role that the idea of need plays in the provision of social welfare. In the process, we have seen that this role is not the obvious one that is usually assumed in descriptions of welfare services. The conventional model of welfare provision is one that treats needs as a set of conditions, states or properties that people – or specific groups of people – have. The main issue then becomes how best to meet these needs – both in the sense of what types of intervention or service are most appropriate or most likely to be effective, and in the sense of how to organize the most efficient provision of these services. So, to take one example, we might see that young people have a need to learn things as their minds develop. We might also think that the best way of making this happen is to put them together in large groups in large buildings to be directed by people who are specialists at getting others to learn things. However, as will be obvious from your reading so far, this view of providing services to meet needs begs a few difficult questions.

ACTIVITY 7.1

Based on what you know from reading the other chapters of this book, what difficult questions are missed by the brief description of educational 'needs' and ways of meeting them that we gave above?

COMMENT

We can think of several clusters of questions that should be asked, all of which deal with issues about the ways in which 'needs' are being socially constructed:

- What do we mean when we say 'young people'? Do all young people have the same needs? Are they a homogeneous group – or are there significant differences within this age band (of class, gender or ethnicity, say)? How do we know what sort of needs they have? Who says they have these needs? Why is the emphasis on 'learning things' rather than on, say, 'doing things'?

- There are also questions about the 'things' young people need to learn. What sorts of things are involved – and why these things rather than other things? Who gets to decide which things young people get to learn? Who gets to decide how they should learn them?

- Why do we think these needs are best met by putting young children in groups in specialized buildings? What sorts of groups should they be in? Why do we have specialists in learning? What sort of power do they have to direct young people?

■ ■ ■

Our aim here is not to write another chapter for this book about education, but to remind you of the pivotal role that the word 'need' plays in the way we think about and organize social welfare. One reason for the significance of the idea of need is that it links common-sense understandings of the social world with the language and ways of thinking (discourses) of social policy and technical expertise. We all think of ourselves – and other people – as having needs. It is a description that we can readily recognize. Even as you are reading this chapter, you may be thinking of yourself as a person who has needs. For example, you may be saying to yourself: 'I need a break', 'I need a drink' or, possibly, 'I need this to stop'. Similarly, we think of others as having needs – needs for a job, money, a home, affection, being looked after. At times, we also think that people need other people to 'do something' – make them better, make them happier, make them safer, make them behave.

There are points of connection and overlap between our everyday usage of the idea of need and the more formal discourses of social policy. These discourses define specific forms of need (for health or social care) and how they are to be addressed by welfare-providing organizations. In some respects these overlaps or connections make it harder to disentangle the processes of social construction that are at stake in the identification, attribution and meeting of need. But these processes are fundamental ones in the organization of social welfare.

Though the condition of being in need may be regarded as self-evident, the question of how the needs of different individuals, or groups of individuals, are met in our society is not so straightforward. There is a general expectation that some needs will be met by individuals themselves: most adults work to provide an income that enables them to fulfil most – if not all – of their needs. Some needs, including those associated with children, people with minor illnesses and disabilities, and those of old people, are met within the family. In the course of the twentieth century the state in all industrial societies has undertaken to provide for an expanding range of social needs, though there have been significant moves towards retrenchment since the 1970s.

It is immediately apparent that there is considerable scope for conflict over the ways in which society defines and meets the needs of particular individuals or sections of society. What happens if somebody is unable to secure a basic income from work, as a result of sickness, disability or age, or simply because of the lack of availability of jobs? What if a family is unable or unwilling to meet the needs of its members who are too young or too old, or otherwise incapable of providing for their own needs? What happens when the state insists that it cannot continue to meet the apparently inexorably expanding needs of a growing population?

We can summarize our discussion of the social construction of need by focusing on three aspects of the conflicts that arise around the issues of the definition of need and the provision of welfare services.

1   Entitlement: who gets what? The definition of 'need' forms the crucial point of connection between welfare services and those who receive them.

2   Provision: how are needs met? The ways in which 'need' is defined imply sets of relationships between welfare services and those who receive them.

3   Contestation: who decides? Conflicts around need involve issues of power – both the power to define needs effectively and the power in relationships that are enmeshed in 'meeting needs'.

The following three sections deal with each of these issues in turn, even though they are clearly interconnected.

2   Entitlement: who gets what?

When it comes to gaining access to welfare services, the question of how need is defined is crucial. The distinction we have already noted between the familiar usage of the term 'need' in everyday conversation and the formal definition of need as a precondition of welfare provision now becomes clearer. Thus, we may experience many needs – for a holiday, a swimming pool or a sexual partner – that we would not seek to define in terms of an application to a welfare agency (or if we did make the attempt the inevitable disappointment would certainly deter any further application). We may also be disappointed if we express a need for a service – like council housing or IVF fertility treatment – that is less and less available in the public sector.

Another area of tension arises in relation to needs that may not be recognized by individuals themselves, but are defined by society in relation to a particular welfare service. Thus we may say that all young people need education and training, and that some also need the services of the criminal justice system, though neither of these needs is likely to be articulated by young people themselves. We may take the view that all people with psychiatric illness need treatment, but that some need it more than others – to the extent that if they do not receive it they may be a risk to themselves or others and should therefore, if necessary, be detained against their will (under the provisions of the Mental Health Act) to receive it. Again, these needs are unlikely to be perceived in this way by the individual concerned, and a degree of conflict is inevitable.

Yet another focus of conflict surrounds needs articulated by particular individuals or communities which are not recognized – or are contested – in society. For example, demands for advocacy services from people with learning difficulties or from migrant groups have received only a limited and often token response. The long-running controversy over abortion centres on the morality of terminating pregnancy at different stages, but also involves the question of whether this is a service that should be provided through the health service, or at the expense of the individual (or individuals) concerned in the private sector. A person with disabilities affecting mobility may assert a need for an electric wheelchair; the care manager responsible for drawing up the community care package may decide that the budget only stretches to a manually operated chair. The question of who gets what is partly a matter of the rights of citizenship, partly a matter of professional risk assessment, and partly also a matter of resource rationing. Let's look further at the different levels at which need is defined and the provision of welfare services are sanctioned.

2.1   Citizenship rights: membership of the nation state

The simplest answer to the question of who is entitled to have their needs met by welfare services in Britain is: all British citizens. This seems straightforward enough, yet it is worth noting that it marks a significant retreat. In the past mere residence was sufficient to gain access to most welfare services in Britain. It was only with the immigration and nationality legislation of the 1980s that services were formally restricted to British citizens, thus excluding many long-term residents, migrants and visitors from welfare. In Chapter 6, Lydia Morris drew attention to the issues involved in defining 'legitimate membership' of the community that may benefit from welfare provision. The conflicts over who is included and excluded at this level determine whose needs will be met by publicly funded or provided services. For example, those categorized as 'illegal aliens' will be unable to have needs for housing, health or income support met by public services. Indeed, as Morris indicated, such services might indeed act as 'internal' border guards, testing the legitimacy of 'membership' claims made by individuals.

Non-citizens may have needs but not the capacity to turn these into a legitimate claim on the nation's resources or services. The concern to limit membership, protect national boundaries and distinguish legitimate members from 'aliens', 'fraudulent' claimants and 'scroungers' means that public resources are expended on testing 'legitimacy' or 'genuineness' in a range of ways. So, even before we get to the social construction of particular needs, we need to remember that only some groups of people are allowed to have needs in the context of specific national welfare systems.

Furthermore, citizenship does not carry an absolute right to welfare services. The most familiar device for restricting claims on public welfare is the means test: only those citizens who can satisfy the authorities that they lack the means to meet their own needs are deemed entitled to state benefits. The 'workfare' proposals of the new Labour government in 1997 marked a further significant restriction on the rights of citizenship: jobless young people would continue to receive benefit only if they attended job creation or training schemes.

2.2 'Priority needs': the politics of rationing

Although, as we have seen, every citizen is entitled to welfare services, it is also the case that some are more entitled than others. It was Aneurin Bevan, the Labour Minister of Health and founder of the National Health Service, who famously declared that 'the language of priorities is the language of socialism', thus giving legitimacy to the rationing of resources through the imposition of charges in the early years of the service. One of the simplest methods of allocating resources is through the principle of 'first come, first served', formalized in the time-honoured British institution of the queue. Crude though it may be, this device, in the modified form of the waiting list, has retained a key role in deciding on priority for hospital admission for elective (non-urgent) surgery from the dawn of the NHS up to today. It also continues to play a role in the allocation of housing and community care services.

The queue and the waiting list work well when the level of need is uniform. For example, the waiting list provides a fair enough system for organizing admissions of fit people for minor surgical procedures, such as varicose veins and hernias, which are not too distressing (though as the months drag into years, some undoubtedly find the delay more onerous than others). However, it is apparent that most of the need for health care is not uniformly distributed in the population: some have greater needs than others. When the distinction is between a life-threatening case requiring urgent treatment and a condition causing minor discomfort that can be dealt with as a routine case, there is unlikely to be much disagreement. But what if the problem is, like most health problems, somewhere in between, not life-threatening perhaps, but causing pain and incapacity, as well as fear and anxiety? No doubt such a problem will be differently perceived by the patient and by the doctor, and the scope for conflict is considerable, particularly if the patient fears that the doctor's judgement may be influenced by considerations of resource allocation as well as clinical need.

In Chapter 2, Mary Langan discussed conflicts over needs and resources in the context of health care. These arguments take place on top of an assumption that 'health needs' are naturally existing phenomena – they are distributed in the population, they can be counted, and the costs of meeting them can be determined (more or less accurately). We may have to stop and think about this proposition for a moment. If we think about health needs we are forced to deal with a diversity of conditions that range from the biologically clear-cut (some illnesses and injuries) through a variety of conditions about which there is considerable uncertainty or dispute (psychiatric disorders, experiences of chronic fatigue with indeterminate causes, or even simply 'not feeling well') but where 'needs' may be constructed in the process of consulting with a medical professional ('I'm going to give you some of this'), to self-diagnosis and need determination.

For example, think about deciding for yourself whether you have a headache or a migraine, whether your upset stomach is serious enough to see a doctor, and so on. Indeed, as Chapter 2 indicated, one of the aims of 'health promotion' is to curtail the demand for health services, by cultivating a sense of individual responsibility both for becoming ill (by failing to adopt a healthy lifestyle) and for getting better (by taking the path of righteous living). If people could be converted to the causes of disease prevention and early detection (through screening tests) then they would make fewer demands on the health services.

At an aggregate level, national debates about health needs and service priorities proceed as if these ambiguities and processes of constructing and defining needs did not take place. The public debate about rationing and priority-setting treat these needs as objective fact. In this setting, the arguments concern two issues about need – what needs are more or less important, and how to determine what needs are more or less important. In the case of the latter, as Chapter 2 showed, there are disagreements about who should determine priorities and through what means. Should it be politicians, the public, medical professionals or even economists (providing cost-benefit analysis of different types of treatment)? But these are only routes to determining the 'big question' – which needs should be met and for whom? It is clear from Chapter 2 that these needs are not discussed in isolation from the social groups that 'possess' them.

Chapter 2 revealed not just that needs are socially constructed, but that debate about priorities involves 'moral evaluations' of different groups and their needs. Thus, a variety of features may make my 'health needs' less of a priority for the nation: my age (older people may be 'worth less' in terms of what they can contribute); my occupation (am I somebody that it is worth keeping in service?); my 'race' (do I look like a legitimate member of the welfare community?) and especially my own 'health management' (have I looked after myself 'properly'; am I a 'good investment'?).

Chapter 2, then, identified public debate about health needs (and who possesses them) as a central point of connection between services and the potential recipients of them, but this is not the only way in which 'need' acts as the pivot between people and services.

2.3   'What you need is …': attributed need

Whereas in section 2.2 we suggested that the identity attributed to social groups might make their needs be seen as more or less worthy, here we want to concentrate on how needs are attributed to particular social groups. Can you think of any examples from earlier chapters? The chapters that spring to mind are those which dealt with children and young people (Chapters 4 and 5). In both of these we saw how the 'needs' that were attributed to young people – in political, professional and legal discourses – shaped how they were dealt with by public agencies such as the courts, the police, social services departments, and so on. Theories of how children develop, of what their place in family relationships and dynamics should be, and of how 'things go wrong', all speak of the 'needs' of young people and imply particular forms of intervention. Both chapters also made clear that the 'needs' of young people are a highly contested subject. For example, in Chapter 5 John Muncie explored the differences and tensions between the 'welfare' and 'justice' models of dealing with young offenders. Each rests on a different view of young people, their needs and capacities, and their relationship to the adult world. Similarly, in Chapter 4, Esther Saraga shows that arguments about how a child's needs can best be met have been at the centre of shifting relationships between the state and the family in the last century.

Other examples from the book would be the arguments, discussed by Marian Barnes in Chapter 3, over who has the power to define the needs of disabled people. We will be looking at this issue in more detail later, so here we just want to note two things. The first is the way in which the determination or construction of these needs has historically been the province of policy-makers and welfare professionals. So, just like children and young people, disabled people have been 'spoken for' by others and have been told what they need.

The second point is that disabled people tend to be defined by their 'special needs'; these needs dominate how they are perceived, spoken of and represented, so that other social distinctions are flattened or even obliterated. The attributed need becomes the attributed identity. Medicalized models of need, like the dominant models of disability, often involve this totalizing quality, such that people become defined in terms of their 'condition'. This reflects relationships of power, since it is the definition of the condition or the need that determines the person's relationship to the service provider (as a patient, client, or whatever). These relationships and definitions are carried – at this level – in political, policy and professional discourses that shape the systems of welfare services and the forms of provision and intervention that they offer. 'Needs', however, are also constructed and negotiated within these systems.

2.4   'What I want is …': assessing need

Chapter 3 also pointed to processes of assessment as the pivot on which relationships between service users and service providers turn, and it is here that the social construction of need is visible at the level of individualized interactions. The wider political formulations of 'legitimate' needs and the policy and professional discourses of 'attributed' needs are *enacted* in these processes of assessment. Although Chapter 3 deals primarily with social care, processes of assessment or evaluation take place at the points where people meet welfare systems. In these processes, decisions are taken about the legitimacy of the claim, the type of needs, the worth of the applicant, the priority attached to this type of need, and how the need may be met.

Welfare discourses about needs work through these millions of individualized interactions – whether at the Benefits Agency, the GP's surgery or the social work interview. The processing of people is conducted through the categories of need. It is also the process in which 'lay' perceptions of need (the perceptions of the would-be service user) meet 'professional' constructions of need – sometimes matching, sometimes conflicting, but always a process that requires negotiation of some kind. This may be a matter of persuading the 'user' about 'what they need' and then providing it, but it may also be a matter of explaining that they don't 'really need' what they thought they needed. It may also be a matter of persuading them to 'do it themselves' – to 'take responsibility' for meeting their own needs, rather than being 'dependent' on public services.

What we can see, then, is that the social construction of need operates as the point of connection between the public and welfare services at a number of different levels and through different discourses. In the social construction of need we can trace a range of contested decisions that involve determining:

- Whose needs are legitimate (discourses about membership of the welfare 'nation').
- Which needs are most important to meet (discourses of priority setting, evaluation and worth).
- Who has what needs (discourses about the attribution of needs and how they are to be met).
- Which individuals have which needs and how they are to be met (discourses and practices of assessment, testing or diagnosis).

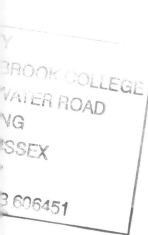

3   Provision: how needs are met

In this section we want to look at the way in which the definition of need implies particular sets of social relationships. Think, for example, of how we might say that 'children need a mother'. What patterns of relationship are evoked by this statement? The way we think about children's needs carries implications about how those needs might be met and by whom. In this section we want to consider these issues in a little more detail by exploring two different dimensions that have been visible in the earlier chapters of this book. The first concerns a set of distinctions between family, market and state as settings or sectors through which needs might be met. The second concerns the character of the social relationships that are involved in addressing particular conceptions of need.

Turning to the first of these, the distinction between family, state and market is, of course, an extremely crude abstraction, but it is nonetheless helpful for thinking about how different types of need are met and about arguments over how needs should be met. Many public and political disputes over needs in different areas of welfare involve claims about who – that is, what agency – should be responsible for addressing these needs. In the course of the twentieth century the boundary between the state and the market has shifted backwards and forwards in the course of hard-fought political struggles. The role of the family in the social division of welfare has also been a recurrent focus of controversy.

As Mary Langan indicated in Chapter 1, the post-war welfare state was constructed around an assumption that publicly recognized ('legitimate') needs would be met by the efforts of public agencies. In the terms used by some social policy analysts (such as Esping-Anderson, 1990), the process of turning such needs (for protection from unemployment, old age and sickness, for example) into the business of public services could be described as *de-commodification*. Such needs were taken out of the realm of the market-place, where previously insurance, pensions or health care had been traded – bought and sold as commodities – and moved into the realm of the state, where they became provided on the basis of 'entitlements' rather than being purchased. In the 1980s and 1990s, however, political arguments and reforms led to many public services and provisions being returned to the market-place (in the form of private pensions, education, health insurance, and so on), and so becoming commodities once again. Not surprisingly, the debate over the relative importance of the market and the state as mechanisms of provision or servicing needs has remained at the centre of discussions of social policy.

One way of reflecting back on the earlier chapters is to think about where the 'needs' that they described were to be met in terms of this distinction between 'commodified' and 'de-commodified' settings. One can also trace changes, as certain sorts of needs move from one setting to another – and possibly even back again. Nevertheless, this is clearly an inadequate framework for examining how welfare needs are met. Even in the heyday of welfare states, public provision still rested on assumptions that many needs would be provided for within the 'private' realm, beyond the state or the market. The family (or household or networks of social relationships) has been a third setting in which needs are addressed – ranging from primary or informal care to the young, sick or old to transfers of money and other resources to enable family members to meet their needs (intra-family loans, parental contributions to schooling and other education, and so on).

However, it is difficult to describe the patterns of relationships in the family and the processes through which it meets the diverse needs of its members in terms comparable with those we apply to the state and the market. Despite the fact that some family relationships may involve contracts (marriage, for example), we think of household or family arrangements as something other than market-like interactions. We expect them to be based on something other than the buying and selling of commodities or services, and we use terms like love, care, affection, obligation or duty to describe the motive forces that drive these relationships.

On the other hand, family relationships are also quite different from the self-consciously de-commodified encounters between service users and public welfare agencies. They do not operate through legal or bureaucratic definitions of rights, entitlements and conditions. They are not anonymous and universal. They have not been intentionally removed from their marketed or commodified form as a deliberate act of policy-making. These private processes are simultaneously more deep-rooted (lodged in hard-to-articulate conceptions of obligation and the duty of care owed to one's 'nearest and dearest') and more intangible: they are not written out in public statutes as a series of entitlements that can be claimed formally. It has always been difficult to conceptualize the role of family relationships in the provision of welfare. This is partly because of the emotionally charged character of family relations, and partly because of the problem of separating the rhetoric from the practical reality of meeting needs in such a private setting. As a result, rather awkward terms like 'non-commodified' or even 'pre-commodified' have been used to indicate the different relationships that underpin the family/household/private realm of servicing welfare needs. However, this provides us with a triangular model for describing how responsibilities for meeting welfare needs are distributed:

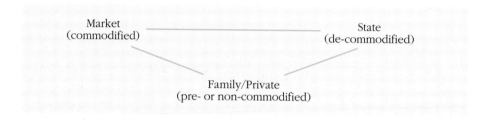

Market
(commodified)

State
(de-commodified)

Family/Private
(pre- or non-commodified)

Taking the distinction between family, market and state, think about particular sorts of needs that have been discussed in chapters in this book. Where does the main responsibility for meeting those needs fall in this model? Have there been any distinctive changes in where particular sorts of needs are supposed to be met?

COMMENT

There are many issues highlighted in the book. For example, in the areas of health and social care discussed in Chapters 2 and 3, there have been important shifts of emphasis in recent years. In both areas the family is an important provider. In the immediate post-war years the state assumed a significant responsibility in practice, but also in the political imagination. In the 1980s the emphasis was moved to the market as an appropriate area for providing services. For 'dangerous families', the underclass and young offenders – discussed in Chapters 4, 5 and 6 – the state has continued to exert the role of authority, at the same time exerting pressure on the family to reform or contain its recalcitrant members.

These are not the only relationships in which the social construction of need is enmeshed. The chapters of this book have highlighted ways in which the construction of needs brings with it a particular pattern or quality of relationship. The meeting of needs sounds like a benevolent process, but the practices described in the other chapters should give us reason to stop and think about this imagined benevolence. We can conceive of social welfare as a process in which a self-identified need is met in full, unconditionally and ungrudgingly, but this does not capture the complexities of conflict and negotiation that we have seen in the production of social welfare. So, in Chapter 6, we saw the struggle of 'excluded' social groups to establish their legitimate claims to have their welfare needs recognized – whether as migrants or as morally excluded members of an 'underclass'. However, in Chapters 4 and 5 we saw that being the recipients of welfare interventions may not be a desired or sought-after goal. Thus, the attribution of 'needs' to young people may lead to them receiving forms of 'treatment'. On the other hand, disabled people may find their needs being 'spoken for' by professionals or experts who 'know best'. As a result, the social construction and attribution of needs implicates people in a variety of relationships. For example, think about the attribution of needs to children (a process in which most adults play a role: as parents, other relatives, child psychologists, teachers or even politicians, most of us are willing to express a view about what children need). But different sorts of attributed need imply very different sorts of relationships.

What relationships do you think are associated with the following childhood 'needs': love; attention; watching; discipline; role models; clear boundaries; father figures; protection?

There is a reason for focusing this discussion on childhood. This stage of life makes explicit what is often implicit in the relationships associated with meeting need – that those who have their needs met are in a position of dependency. We treat dependency as a 'natural' corollary of childhood, assuming that it is both necessary and right and proper that children will be dependent on the adults who are responsible for them (despite the potential for abuse that goes with such adult power). Think back to Chapter 4, which discussed this issue at length. The relationship between adults and young people or the state and young people discussed in Chapter 5 also highlights the issues of power, dependency and responsibility in welfare relationships and the youth justice system. But other need-meeting relationships are constructed around axes of power and dependency. By analogy with the place of childhood within the authority of the family, we might say that these other relationships could be described as 'paternalist'.

ACTIVITY 7.3

Think back over the earlier chapters and note down examples of where you think positions of dependency were constructed in the process of meeting need.

COMMENT

Here are some of our examples:

- Being dependent on the state for your income exposes you to 'morality tests' of proving yourself worthy.

- Being dependent on health care services exposes you to decisions about whether you are 'worth' medical investment.

- Being defined as in 'need of care and control' as a young person makes you vulnerable to others' decisions about punishment and/or treatment.

- Being dependent on public services for assistance or social care makes you vulnerable to the choices and decisions of health and social care agencies.

These (and other) examples remind us that power is implicated in the social construction of need. The processes through which definitions of need are constructed and attributed to particular groups or classes of people also position those 'in need' in relationships which are both dependent and subservient. Part of the struggle over need is to construct ways of receiving care or assistance that do not mean that being dependent is also being subservient. Thus, in Chapter 3 on social care, Marian Barnes discussed the efforts of disabled people's movements in demanding 'rights' and 'entitlements' as a way of underpinning new forms of relationships. The idea of 'rights' rather than 'needs' challenges the paternalist patterns of relationship between service user and service provider.

■ ■ ■

4   Contestation: who decides?

What is the significance of the insistence throughout this book that 'need' is a contested concept? It seems to us that there are a number of conclusions that we might draw from this argument. The first is that needs are not essential properties of particular groups of people, given in their biological or psychological make-up. The variations in the types of 'need' that are attributed to groups of people – or which they define themselves as having – are too substantial to allow us to fall back on assuming an essentialist view of need. The historical and cultural shifts in what groups 'need' are enormous and cannot be seen simply as progress towards a better understanding of what needs 'really' are. So, a view of needs as socially constructed begins by taking us away from this conception of needs as the fixed or static attributes of a particular group of people (whether these be children, adolescents, disabled people, or even economic migrants).

The second conclusion that we might draw from studying need as a contested concept is that historical and cultural variations in what is seen as 'need' are interesting because they are the result of contested processes of social construction. They are not of interest just because they show 'differences' – this book has not assembled a museum or a zoo of exotically 'different conceptions of needs'. These differences are important because they are the visible points – the outcomes – of processes of contestation, conflict and negotiation around what counts as 'need' and who is allowed, or required, to have needs. Some of the chapters here have revealed these processes – the large and small conflicts around the meaning of need and the consequences of whose definitions come to command the public resourcing of providing for needs.

This leads to our third conclusion: that need as a contested concept leads us to issues of power. Central to this argument is that the power to define 'need' and the processes, practices and relationships associated with needs has been and continues to be central to the organization and provision of social welfare. Forms of economic, social, political and organizational power are involved – in different ways and at different levels – in constructing definitions of legitimate need.

In the course of this book, we have seen issues about the exercise of economic and political power in struggles over who is allowed 'membership' of the nation-as-welfare-community. We have seen issues about the relationship between parental and patriarchal power within families and the political and professional powers of the state in relation to children. We have seen political and professional power exercised in relation to 'managing' the rationing of resources in health care, and using a mixture of social, professional and political judgements to determine what and who count as priorities. But we have also seen that each of these is the subject of challenges, resistances and refusals – the expressions of other views about needs and who is entitled to have them met. We have also seen that, for some groups, 'need' itself is not how they wish to define their relationship to public services. Thus, one form of conflict around 'need' is the struggle to replace it with forms of access built around ideas of 'rights' and 'entitlements'.

In this sense, need as a contested concept is used – or mobilized – in different ways. 'Need' can be a focus for the campaigning efforts of particular groups, as a means of making demands upon the welfare system. But it can also be the term around which group or 'community' identities are built – the process of articulating or defining 'our needs' can be the process of defining who 'we' are as a recognizable social grouping. In contrast, though, 'needs' can be things to be resisted. For example, many of the campaigns to close institutions 'treating' people defined as mentally ill or handicapped challenged the way the 'needs' of those groups were defined (and the implication that 'secure' facilities were the best setting). And, as we have seen, the word 'need' itself (rather than particular definitions of what counts as need) may be resisted in defence of less paternalistic patterns of relationship expressed in terms of needs or rights.

This leads to a final conclusion about need as a contested concept. It is contested not just because there are arguments about who has or can have certain sorts of needs. As we have seen, this is certainly one central element in the conflicts and negotiations around need, but it is not the only one. How needs are constructed also implies social positions and relationships. Need is the focus of conflict because of where it places those who have needs (and those who do not). Some of this contestation is about social and political recognition – to be defined as an individual or group who/which has needs is to be admitted to a place within the 'welfare community'. Having (legitimate) needs means social inclusion rather than exclusion.

There are, however, other issues about places and relationships within the 'welfare community'. Some of these are about 'whose needs' have priority (as we saw in the chapters on health and social care). Some of them, however, are about being the forced beneficiary of others' definition of your needs. Finally, these issues also hinge around whether 'having needs' necessarily means being in a position of subservient dependency in relation to paternalist service provisions. We started this chapter by arguing that 'needs' act as a point of connection between people and welfare provision. In this role they also allow us to see the conflicts, tensions and ambiguities that are embedded in social welfare.

Reference

Esping-Andersen, G. (1990) *The Three Worlds of Welfare Capitalism*, Cambridge, Polity Press.

Acknowledgements

Grateful acknowledgement is made to the following sources for permission to reproduce material in this book:

Text

Chapter 1: Dennis, N. (1997) *The Invention of Permanent Poverty*, © The IEA Health and Welfare Unit 1997; ***Chapter 2:*** Smith, R. (1995) 'Rationing: the debate we have to have', *British Medical Journal*, vol.310, no.6981, BMJ Publishing Group; Brindle, D. (1996) 'Hospital in cash crisis bars many elderly', *The Guardian,* 14 October 1996, © Guardian Newspapers Ltd; Mihill, C. (1996) 'Authority rules out vasectomy ops on NHS', *The Guardian*, 27 November 1996, © Guardian Newspapers Ltd; Klein, R., Day, P. and Redmayne, S. (1996) *Managing Scarcity: Priority Setting and Rationing in the National Health Service*, Open University Press; Kitzhaber, J.A. (1993) 'Prioritising health services in an era of limits: the Oregon experience', in Smith, R. (ed.) *Rationing in Action*, BMJ Publishing Group; Hart, J.T. (1994) *Feasible Socialism: The National Health Service, Past, Present and Future*, Socialist Health Association; ***Chapter 3:*** Valios, N. (1997) 'Law lords give green light to slash services', *Community Care*, 27 March–2 April 1997. Published by permisson of the editor of *Community Care*; ***Chapter 4:*** Coles, B. (1995) *Youth and Social Policy: Youth Citizenship and Young Careers*, UCL Press Ltd; Carvel, J. (1997) 'Parents told to sign reading pledge', *The Guardian*, 29 July 1997, © Guardian Newspapers Ltd; Rickford, F. (1997) 'Right or duty?', *Community Care*, 9–15 January, 1997. Published by permisson of the editor of *Community Care*; ***Chapter 5:*** Black Committe (1979) *Report of The Children and Young Persons Review Group*, December 1979, © Crown Copyright is reproduced with the permission of the Controller of Her Majesty's Stationery Office; *Penal Custody for Juveniles – The Line of Least Resistance* (1989) The Children's Society; Cooper, G. (1997) 'Girls get angry, too', *The Independent*, 26 March 1997; ***Chapter 6:*** Field, F. (1995) 'The poison in the welfare state', *Independent on Sunday*, 14 May 1995. Extracted from *Making Welfare Work* (1995), published by the Institute of Community Studies; Lynn, R. (1996) 'Why, as we grow richer, does our underclass get bigger every year?' *Daily Mail*, 23 December 1996; Lister, R. (1996) *Charles Murray and the Underclass: The Developing Debate*, IEA Health and Welfare Unit; Travis, A. (1996) 'Lilley evades asylum ruling', *The Guardian*, 25 June 1996, © Guardian Newspapers Ltd; Travis, A. (1996) 'Judge's swipe at new asylum law', *The Guardian*, 9 October 1996, © Guardian Newspapers Ltd.

Photographs/Illustrations

pp.9 & 11: Reproduced with permission of Punch Ltd; *p.18:* Martin Rowson/ *The Observer*. Photo courtesy of the Centre for the Study of Cartoons and Caricatures at the University of Kent; *p.22:* Emmwood, *Daily Mail*, SOLO Syndication. Photo courtesy of the Centre for the Study of Cartoons and Caricatures at the University of Kent; *p.25:* Chris Priestley/*The Economist*, 13 August 1994; *p.29:* David Simonds/*The Guardian*, 7 April 1997. Photo courtesy of the Centre for the Study of Cartoons and Caricatures at the University of Kent; *p.37:* John Stillwell/PA News; *p.44:* SOLO Syndication Ltd on behalf of Associated Newspapers; *p.45:* Getty Images; *p.49:* SOLO Syndication Ltd; *pp.51, 53:* Brenda Prince/Format; *p.55:* Geoff Tompkinson/Science Photo Library;

Figures

Tables

Index

The Open University Course Team

The Open University

Sally Baker	*Liaison Librarian/Picture Researcher*
Melanie Bayley	*Editor*
David Calderwood	*Project Controller*
Hilary Canneaux	*Course Manager*
John Clarke	*Author/Course Team Chair*
Allan Cochrane	*Author*
Lene Connolly	*Print Buying Controller*
Troy Cooper	*Author*
Nigel Draper	*Editor*
Ross Fergusson	*Author*
Sharon Gewirtz	*Reading Member*
Fiona Harris	*Editor*
Rich Hoyle	*Graphic Designer*
Gordon Hughes	*Author and Editor, Books 4 and 5*
Jonathan Hunt	*Co-publishing Co-ordinator*
Maggie Hutchinson	*Reading Member*
Sue Lacey	*Secretary*
Mary Langan	*Author and Editor, Book 3*
Patti Langton	*Producer, BBC/OUPC*
Helen Lentell	*Author*
Gail Lewis	*Author and Editor, Books 2 and 4*
Vic Lockwood	*Producer, BBC/OUPC*
Lilian McCoy	*Author*
Eugene McLaughlin	*Author*
Tara Marshall	*Print Buying Co-ordinator*
John Muncie	*Author/Co-Course Team Chair*
Pam Owen	*Graphic Artist*
Doreen Pendlebury	*Secretary*
Sharon Pinkney	*Author*
Michael Pryke	*Author*
Esther Saraga	*Author and Editor, Book 1*
Paul Smith	*Liaison Librarian/Picture Researcher*
Pauline Turner	*Course and Discipline Secretary*

External Contributors

Marian Barnes	*Author, Department of Social Policy and Social Work, University of Birmingham*
Janet English	*Tutor Panel, Region 11, The Open University*
Ian Gazeley	*Author, School of Social Sciences, University of Sussex*
Catherine Hall	*Author, Department of Sociology, University of Essex*
Mary J. Hickman	*Author, Irish Studies Centre, University of North London*
Eluned Jeffries	*Tutor Panel, Region 02, The Open University*
Chris Jones	*External Assessor, Professor of Social Work, University of Liverpool*
Gerry Mooney	*Author, Department of Applied Social Studies, University of Paisley*
Lydia Morris	*Author, Department of Sociology, University of Essex*
Janet Newman	*Author, School of Public Policy, University of Birmingham*
Lynne Poole	*Tutor Panel, Region 11, The Open University*
Pat Thane	*Author, School of Social Sciences, University of Sussex*